Frailty Models in Survival Analysis

Chapman & Hall/CRC Biostatistics Series

Editor-in-Chief

Shein-Chung Chow, Ph.D.
Professor
Department of Biostatistics and Bioinformatics
Duke University School of Medicine
Durham, North Carolina, U.S.A.

Series Editors

Byron Jones
Senior Director
Statistical Research and Consulting Centre
(IPC 193)
Pfizer Global Research and Development
Sandwich, Kent, U. K.

Jen-pei Liu
Professor
Division of Biometry
Department of Agronomy
National Taiwan University
Taipei, Taiwan

Karl E. Peace
Georgia Cancer Coalition
Distinguished Cancer Scholar
Senior Research Scientist and
Professor of Biostatistics
Jiann-Ping Hsu College of Public Health
Georgia Southern University
Statesboro, Georgia

Bruce W. Turnbull
Professor
School of Operations Research
and Industrial Engineering
Cornell University
Ithaca, New York

Chapman & Hall/CRC Biostatistics Series

Published Titles

1. *Design and Analysis of Animal Studies in Pharmaceutical Development,* Shein-Chung Chow and Jen-pei Liu
2. *Basic Statistics and Pharmaceutical Statistical Applications,* James E. De Muth
3. *Design and Analysis of Bioavailability and Bioequivalence Studies, Second Edition, Revised and Expanded,* Shein-Chung Chow and Jen-pei Liu
4. *Meta-Analysis in Medicine and Health Policy,* Dalene K. Stangl and Donald A. Berry
5. *Generalized Linear Models: A Bayesian Perspective,* Dipak K. Dey, Sujit K. Ghosh, and Bani K. Mallick
6. *Difference Equations with Public Health Applications,* Lemuel A. Moyé and Asha Seth Kapadia
7. *Medical Biostatistics,* Abhaya Indrayan and Sanjeev B. Sarmukaddam
8. *Statistical Methods for Clinical Trials,* Mark X. Norleans
9. *Causal Analysis in Biomedicine and Epidemiology: Based on Minimal Sufficient Causation,* Mikel Aickin
10. *Statistics in Drug Research: Methodologies and Recent Developments,* Shein-Chung Chow and Jun Shao
11. *Sample Size Calculations in Clinical Research,* Shein-Chung Chow, Jun Shao, and Hansheng Wang
12. *Applied Statistical Design for the Researcher,* Daryl S. Paulson
13. *Advances in Clinical Trial Biostatistics,* Nancy L. Geller
14. *Statistics in the Pharmaceutical Industry, Third Edition,* Ralph Buncher and Jia-Yeong Tsay
15. *DNA Microarrays and Related Genomics Techniques: Design, Analysis, and Interpretation of Experiments,* David B. Allsion, Grier P. Page, T. Mark Beasley, and Jode W. Edwards
16. *Basic Statistics and Pharmaceutical Statistical Applications, Second Edition,* James E. De Muth
17. *Adaptive Design Methods in Clinical Trials,* Shein-Chung Chow and Mark Chang
18. *Handbook of Regression and Modeling: Applications for the Clinical and Pharmaceutical Industries,* Daryl S. Paulson
19. *Statistical Design and Analysis of Stability Studies,* Shein-Chung Chow
20. *Sample Size Calculations in Clinical Research, Second Edition,* Shein-Chung Chow, Jun Shao, and Hansheng Wang
21. *Elementary Bayesian Biostatistics,* Lemuel A. Moyé
22. *Adaptive Design Theory and Implementation Using SAS and R,* Mark Chang
23. *Computational Pharmacokinetics,* Anders Källén
24. *Computational Methods in Biomedical Research,* Ravindra Khattree and Dayanand N. Naik
25. *Medical Biostatistics, Second Edition,* A. Indrayan
26. *DNA Methylation Microarrays: Experimental Design and Statistical Analysis,* Sun-Chong Wang and Arturas Petronis
27. *Design and Analysis of Bioavailability and Bioequivalence Studies, Third Edition,* Shein-Chung Chow and Jen-pei Liu
28. *Translational Medicine: Strategies and Statistical Methods,* Dennis Cosmatos and Shein-Chung Chow
29. *Bayesian Methods for Measures of Agreement,* Lyle D. Broemeling
30. *Data and Safety Monitoring Committees in Clinical Trials,* Jay Herson
31. *Design and Analysis of Clinical Trials with Time-to-Event Endpoints,* Karl E. Peace
32. *Bayesian Missing Data Problems: EM, Data Augmentation and Noniterative Computation,* Ming T. Tan, Guo-Liang Tian, and Kai Wang Ng
33. *Multiple Testing Problems in Pharmaceutical Statistics,* Alex Dmitrienko, Ajit C. Tamhane, and Frank Bretz
34. *Bayesian Modeling in Bioinformatics,* Dipak K. Dey, Samiran Ghosh, and Bani K. Mallick
35. *Clinical Trial Methodology,* Karl E. Peace and Ding-Geng (Din) Chen
36. *Monte Carlo Simulation for the Pharmaceutical Industry: Concepts, Algorithms, and Case Studies,* Mark Chang
37. *Frailty Models in Survival Analysis,* Andreas Wienke

Chapman & Hall/CRC Biostatistics Series

Frailty Models in Survival Analysis

Andreas Wienke

Institute of Medical Epidemiology, Biostatistics, and Informatics
Martin-Luther-University Halle-Wittenberg, Germany

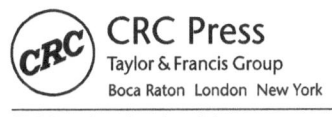

CRC Press
Taylor & Francis Group
Boca Raton London New York

CRC Press is an imprint of the
Taylor & Francis Group, an **informa** business
A CHAPMAN & HALL BOOK

First published in paperback 2024

First published 2011
by Chapman & Hall/CRC Press
2385 NW Executive Center Drive, Suite 320, Boca Raton FL 33431

and by Chapman & Hall/CRC Press
4 Park Square, Milton Park, Abingdon, Oxon, OX14 4RN

CRC Press is an imprint of Taylor & Francis Group, LLC

© 2011, 2024 by Taylor and Francis Group, LLC

Library of Congress Cataloging-in-Publication Data

Wienke, Andreas.
   Frailty models in survival analysis / author, Andreas Wienke.
     p. cm. -- (Chapman & Hall/CRC biostatistics series)
   "A CRC title."
   Includes bibliographical references and index.
   ISBN 978-1-4200-7388-1 (hardcover : alk. paper)
   1. Failure time data analysis--Mathematics. 2. Survival analysis (Biometry)--Mathematics. 3. Mortality--Mathematical models. 4. Demography--Mathematics. I. Title. II. Series.

QA280.W54 2011
519.5'46--dc22   2010021869

ISBN: 978-1-4200-7388-1 (hbk)
ISBN: 978-1-03-292206-5 (pbk)
ISBN: 978-0-429-13960-4 (ebk)

DOI: 10.1201/9781420073911

Visit the Taylor & Francis Web site at
http://www.taylorandfrancis.com

and the CRC Press Web site at
http://www.crcpress.com

All models are wrong, some are useful. (Box 1976)

Contents

List of Tables

List of Figures

Symbol Description

ACE	genetic model	M_0	generic symbol for a cumulative baseline hazard
AFT	accelerated failure time		
AIC	Akaike information criterion	$\log N(m, s^2)$	log-normal distribution with parameters m, s^2
AR	autoregressive process	MCEM	Markov Chain EM
BMI	body mass index	MCMC	Markov Chain Monte Carlo
BLUB	best linear unbiased predictor		
		ML	maximum likelihood
CAD	coronary artery disease	MZ	monozygotic
		NSCLC	non-small cell lung carcinoma
CSRF	corrected scale reduction factor		
		$\mathbf{P}(A)$	probability of event A
CHD	coronary heart disease	pdf	probability density function
cdf	cumulative density function		
		PH	proportional hazards
DIC	Bayesian information criterion	PPL	penalized partial likelihood
		PVF	power variance function
DZ	dizygotic	S	generic symbol for a survival function
$\mathbf{E}$	expectation		
EBCT	electron-beam computed tomography	t^+	truncation time
		TNM	classification of malignant tumours
ECOG	Eastern Cooperative Oncology Group		
		$\mathbf{V}$	variance
EM	expectation-maximization	$U(a, b)$	uniform distribution in the interval $[a, b]$
f	generic symbol for pdf	$N(\mu, \sigma^2)$	normal distribution with parameters μ, σ^2
F	generic symbol for cdf		
Γ	gamma function	$Exp(\lambda)$	exponential distribution with parameter λ
H_0	null hypothesis		
H_A	alternative hypothesis	$W(\lambda, \nu)$	Weibull distribution with parameters λ, ν
ICD	International Classification of Diseases		
		$G(\lambda, \varphi)$	Gompertz distribution with parameters λ, φ
iid	independent and identically distributed		
		$\Gamma(k, \lambda)$	gamma distribution with parameters k, λ
$\mathbf{L}$	Laplace transform		
L	likelihood function	$\log L(\nu, \kappa)$	log-logistic distribution with parameters ν, κ
μ	generic symbol for a hazard		
μ_0	generic symbol for a baseline hazard	$Ps(\alpha)$	positive stable distribution with parameter α
M	generic symbol for a cumulative hazard	$cP(\gamma, k, \lambda)$	compound Poisson distribution with parameters γ, k, λ

Preface

The analysis of lifetime data (or more exactly, time-to-event, event-history, or duration data) plays an important role in medicine, epidemiology, biology, demography, economics, engineering, actuarial science, and other fields. It has expanded rapidly in the last three decades, with works having been published in various disciplines in addition to statistics. But what distinguishes survival analysis from other fields of statistics? Why does survival data need a special statistical theory? The main problem is censoring, which means that, for some individuals in the study population, the researcher only has the information that the event of interest did not occur before a particular time point. To put it plainly, a censored observation contains only partial information about the random variable of interest. This kind of incomplete observation needs special methods. As a consequence of censoring, survival times are usually a mixture of discrete (censoring indicator) and continuous (event/censoring time) data that lend themselves to a different type of analysis from that used in the traditional discrete or continuous case. The mixture is the result of censoring and has an important effect on data analysis. The Kaplan–Meier estimator (Kaplan and Meier 1958) of the survival function is a major step in the development of suitable models for such kind of data. Furthermore, most evaluations are made conditionally on what is known at the time of the analysis, and this changes over time. Usually, as the population under study is changing, we only consider the individual risk to die for those who are still alive, but this means that many standard statistical approaches cannot be applied.

Models based on the hazard function have dominated survival analysis since the construction of the proportional hazards model by Cox (1972). One of the reasons this model is so popular is the ease with which technical difficulties such as censoring and truncation are handled. This is due to the appealing interpretation of the hazard as a risk that changes over time. Naturally, the concept allows for the entering of covariates in order to describe their influence and to model different levels of risk for different subgroups.

This book focuses on frailty models, a specific area in survival analysis. The concept of frailty provides a convenient way of introducing unobserved heterogeneity and associations into models for survival data. In its simplest form, frailty is an unobserved random proportionality factor that modifies the hazard function of an individual or related individuals. In essence, the concept goes back to the work of Greenwood and Yule (1920) on "accident proneness" with binary data. The first univariate frailty model was suggested by Beard (1959), considering different mortality models. The term *frailty* itself was introduced by Vaupel et al. (1979) in the univariate context. Its first applications to problems in multivariate survival analysis date from a seminal paper by Clayton (1978).

Ordinary methods in survival analysis implicitly assume that populations are homogenous, meaning that all individuals have the same risk of death. However, in general, it is impossible to include all relevant risk factors, perhaps because we have no information on individual values, which is often the case in demography. Furthermore, we may not know all relevant risk factors, or it is impossible to measure them without great financial costs, something that is common in medical and biological studies. The neglect of covariates leads to unobserved heterogeneity. That is, the population consists of subjects with different risks. As a consequence, it is important to consider the population as heterogeneous, i.e., as a mixture of individuals with different hazards. A frailty model is a random effects model for time-to-event data, where the random effect (frailty) has a multiplicative effect on the baseline hazard. It can be used for univariate (independent) lifetimes, i.e., to adjust for unobserved risk factors in a proportional hazards model (heterogeneity). The variability of event-time data is split into one part that depends on covariates and is thus theoretically predictable, and one part that is initially unpredictable, even knowing all relevant information at that time. There are advantages in separating these sources of variability: unobserved heterogeneity can explain some unexpected results or give an alternative interpretation, for example, crossing-over or leveling-off effects of hazards.

However, considering multivariate (dependent) duration times is especially interesting. The introduction of a common random effect – frailty – is a natural way of modeling the dependence of event times. The random effect explains the dependence in the sense that had we known the frailty, the event times would have been independent. In other words, because we do not know the frailty, the lifetimes are independent conditionally on the frailty. This approach can be used for survival times of related individuals such as twins or family members, where independence cannot be assumed, or for recurrent events in the same individual or for times to several events for the same individual, such as onset of different diseases, relapse, or death (competing risks). Different extensions of univariate frailty models to multivariate models are possible and will be considered in this book.

The standard assumption is to use a gamma distribution for frailty, but other distributions are also possible. The relationships between individual and observed survival characteristics play a key role in the statistical analysis of duration data in heterogeneous populations.

Various frailty models have been developed in the past. However, compared with standard mixed models, frailty models pose additional difficulties in developing inferential methods, caused by incomplete data due to censoring and truncation. Thus, inferential methods have been less developed here than in other mixed models.

To keep the book to a reasonable length, some topics are discussed only briefly, and references are given for further reading. Because the literature on frailty models is extensive (especially in the last few years), the choice of subject matter is difficult. The material discussed in detail is to some extent a reflection of the author's interest in this research field. However, my attempt has been to present a relatively comprehensive and complete overview of the fundamental approaches in the field of frailty models.

The present monograph is primarily aimed at the biostatistical community with applications from biomedicine, (genetic) epidemiology, and demography. Some efforts were also undertaken to include literature from other fields like econometrics if interesting methodological problems are raised. The practical use of models is a key issue in biostatistics, where the data at hand often are motivating for the development of new models. The language of this book is nontechnical and therefore it can be understood by nonspecialists. Nevertheless, some experience with survival analysis is an advantage.

Acknowledgments

I would like to express my sincere thanks to everyone who supported directly or indirectly this book; my former Ph.D. advisor Friedrich Liese (Rostock) for awakening my interest in statistical research, Anatoli Yashin and Konstantin Arbeev (Duke), Paul Janssen and Niel Hens (Hasselt), Catherine Legrand (Louvain-la-Neuve), Alexander Begun (Hamburg), Nicole Giard (Gütersloh), Kaare Christensen and Ivan Iachine (Odense), Isabella Locatelli (Lausanne), Slobodan Zdravkovic (Kopenhagen), Samuli Ripatti (Helsinki), Oliver Kuß (Halle), and Juni Palmgren (Stockholm) for many helpful discussions and fruitful collaboration. I take the opportunity to thank all my colleagues at the Institute for Medical Epidemiology, Biostatistics, and Informatics at the Medical Faculty of the Martin Luther University Halle-Wittenberg, especially Johannes Haerting as head of the institute, for providing an excellent research environment. I would like to thank the Danish and Swedish Twin Registries for making the unique twin data available. I extend my sincere thanks to the Max Planck Institute for Demographic Research (Rostock) and its founding director, James Vaupel, where I began to work on frailty models and where I returned several times as a guest researcher during the last years. Special thanks go to Luc Duchateau (Ghent) for careful reading an earlier version of the manuscript and giving many very helpful suggestions. Furthermore, I would like to thank my Ph.D. students Katharina Hirsch and Diana Pietzner (Halle) for many fruitful discussions and help in preparing the manuscript.

Finally, acknowledgments go to my family. To my parents Margit and Kurt Wienke for all their love and support. Also, to my sons Moritz, Jakob, and Finn, showing that there is a life beyond research and, finally, to my loving wife Kati Moeller, who always strongly encouraged me to finish this book.

Halle, June 2010   Andreas Wienke

Chapter 1

Introduction

1.1 Goals and Outline

Survival analysis is one of the core research methods used in many fields such as medicine, biology, epidemiology, demography, and engineering. Notion survival analysis reflects the origin of the methods in medical and demographic studies of mortality. Especially since the end of the 1970s, the empirical analysis of event history data has become widespread by the development of the proportional hazards model in the seminal paper by Cox (1972) and several extensions during the last three decades. The present monograph deals with one important direction of extensions in this field, namely frailty models. A frailty model is a multiplicative hazard model consisting of three components: a frailty (random effect), a baseline hazard function (parametric or nonparametric), and a term modeling the influence of observed covariates (fixed effects).

Only a few books exist on this subject, which contain short chapters devoted to frailty models. Ibrahim et al. (2001) consider parametric as well as semi-parametric shared frailty models based on a Bayesian approach. Klein and Moeschberger (2003) consider the application of the EM algorithm in semi-parametric shared frailty models. Aalen et al. (2008) take a process point of view dealing with different frailty models. The present book extends in two main directions the presentation of frailty models made in the seminal monographs by Hougaard (2000), Therneau and Grambsch (2000), and Duchateau and Janssen (2008). First, univariate frailty models with their focus on unobserved heterogeneity are covered in more detail compared to previous books. In univariate models all durations describe the time to the same type of event, and event times are considered as independent. Second, the main emphasis is placed on correlated frailty models as natural extensions of shared frailty models. Here, different strengths of association between clustered lifetimes are of special interest.

One of the main problems in the application of frailty models to real data is the limited availability of standard software in this area. Consequently, one aim of this monograph is to show which of the models considered can be applied to real data by using standard statistical packages such as R, SAS, and STATA. Here, the link to generalized linear mixed models will be exploited. Both parametric as well as semiparametric models are considered. Furthermore, models are fitted by the frequentist and Bayesian approaches. Most of the Bayesian analyses are performed with WinBUGS, but the new PROC MCMC in SAS opens new possibilities for the future.

In this first chapter we will introduce different data sets used throughout the book to illustrate modeling techniques and practical interpretations of the results. In Chapter 2 an introduction to basic and general concepts in survival analysis and a definition of common terminology are given. The topic is also covered by other books, for example, Miller (1981), Cox and Oakes (1984), Andersen et al. (1993), Lawless (2002), Kalbfleisch and Prentice (2002), Klein and Moeschberger (2003), Collett (2003), and Machin, Cheung, and Parmar (2006). The recent book by Finkelstein (2008) has a special focus on reliability but also covers a wide range of exiting topics in biostatistics and demography. Though, it is not necessary for people acquainted with this field to read it, it does contain notations and key results and lays the basis for the more advanced frailty models treated in the following chapters. After this preparatory chapter we deal with univariate frailty models (single spell data) in Chapter 3, discussing the broad range of possible frailty distributions with their specific features. Gamma distribution is the most often applied frailty distribution because frailties appearing in conditional likelihood can be integrated out, giving simple expressions of unconditional likelihood. Then, maximization of unconditional likelihood can be used for estimation. Here, the interpretation of frailty is as unobserved heterogeneity due to nonobserved covariates. The focus of Chapter 4 is on the shared frailty model, which has already been discussed in detail by other authors (Hougaard 2000, Therneau and Grambsch 2000, Duchateau and Janssen 2008). Shared frailty models are an important tool for analyzing multivariate (clustered) survival data. Hence, this chapter forms the basis of the correlated frailty model and its extensions considered in detail in Chapter 5. Advantages and limitations of the proposed models are discussed, and simulations show the properties of the parameter estimates for finite sample sizes. Different approaches and applications are presented to demonstrate the flexibility of the correlated frailty approach in modeling associations in clustered event times. Chapter 6 deals with copula models and analyzes similarities and dissimilarities between frailty and copula models. Chapter 7 gives an overview of different problems related to frailty models such as tests for homogeneity, identifiability aspects, and available software. The Appendix provides a series of technical mathematical results and background about genetic models used throughout the book.

The present monograph does not attempt to give a complete overview of the fast growing literature on frailty models; this would not be possible. The treatment of the topics covered are restricted to explaining the basic ideas in frailty modeling and statistical techniques, with focus on real data application and interpretation of the results. In many cases different models are applied to the same data to compare and discuss their advantages and limitations under varying model assumptions.

1.2 Examples

Different survival models are considered in this book. Most of them will be applied to real data, mainly using examples from research fields such as medicine, epidemiology, and demography. Survival analysis deals with the analysis of times until the occurrence of a well defined event. The occurrence of this event describes the transition from one state to another, for example, occurrence of a disease is the transition from the state of being healthy to the state of being sick. Sometimes the transition is of special interest (incidence of the disease), and in other cases the state (prevalence of the disease) is the target of the analysis. For such kind of analysis it is necessary to define the time scale and a starting time point zero. In many cases the time scale is the age of the individual. In clinical trials the starting point is often beginning of treatment. If the focus is on the development of a disease, the time of diagnosis is usually the starting point. In occupational cohort studies the starting point is often the beginning of employment or unemployment.

We first consider the univariate event times, which means data with no clustering. Such data set is given in Example 1.1, based on a prognostic study analyzing the value of electron-beam computed tomography (EBCT) derived calcium scores for risk stratification in symptomatic patients. Example 1.2 presents the malignant melanoma data. The models fitted to these data sets are parametric and semiparametric proportional hazard models. The most important goal of Chapter 3 is to analyze the effect of including unobserved heterogeneity on regression parameter estimates.

However, the main focus of this book is on multivariate frailty models, where event times are clustered. Example 1.3 will serve as an example of univariate as well as multivariate data. In the last situation the cancer-diagnosing units were considered as clusters. The cluster size differs from cluster to cluster, which is common in multicenter clinical trials. Here, frailty can describe center-to-center variations not explained by observed covariates. In addition to the problem of analyzing the effect of observed covariates, an important research problem is evaluating the dependence between event times in clusters. In genetic studies, correlations between family members are the basis of the analysis of heritability of specific traits, for example, the times of onset of breast cancer or cause of death specific lifetimes. We use Danish and Swedish twin data provided by the Danish Twin Registry at the University of Southern Denmark in Odense and the Swedish Twin Registry at the Karolinska Institute in Stockholm to emphasize the practical purpose of the frailty models with fixed and small cluster sizes. In Example 1.4, cause-specific lifetimes of Danish twins are considered. A subsample with additional covariate information is presented in Example 1.5. Example 1.6 provides data on the age of onset of breast cancer in Swedish twins, whereas Example 1.7 deals with current status data. The next section provides a brief description of these data.

Example 1.1 **Prognostic Study of the EBCT Calcium Score**

EBCT-derived calcium score is a measure of coronary arteriosclerotic plaque that can be used for more precise risk stratification in symptomatic patients (Schmermund et al. 2004). In the study presented here, it was investigated whether EBCT-derived calcium score can add prognostic information compared with clinical information derived from risk-factor assessment, exercise stress testing, and coronary angiography. Patients with recent (<3 months) onset of symptoms were retrospectively identified and examined for possible coronary artery disease (CAD) and underwent EBCT. Complete follow-up after 42 months was available for 255 patients with mean age at baseline of 58 years, who were finally included into the study.

Table 1.1:   Five patients in the EBCT study

id	time	status	risk group	calcium score	age
1	42	0	2	0	70
2	42	0	1	0	59
3	42	0	1	1	74
4	14	1	4	1	70
5	42	0	1	0	50

Four clinical risk groups with increasing evidence of CAD were constructed based on risk factor assessment, exercise stress testing, coronary angiographic anatomy, and revascularization at baseline. The main interest was in the occurrence of a combined event consisting of major adverse cardiac events such as myocardial infarction, cardiac death, and revascularization. The event was observed in 40 (16%) patients during the follow-up, the observations of the other patients are mainly censored after 42 months at the end of the study. The data for five patients are presented in Table 1.1.

Table 1.2:   Description of the EBCT study population

covariate	category	absolute frequency	relative frequency
risk group	1	79	31.0%
	2	78	30.6%
	3	42	16.5%
	4	56	21.9%
calcium score	< 100	150	58.8%
	≥ 100	105	42.2%
age (years)	$23 - 54$	85	33.3%
	$55 - 62$	79	31.0%
	$63 - 84$	91	35.7%

The first column gives the patient specific identification number, the observed event or censoring time in the second column is measured in months. The covariate of main interest in this study is the CAD risk divided into four prognostic groups (group 1 – no evidence of ischemia, ≤ 1 conventional risk factor; group 2 – evidence of ischemia and/or ≥ 2 conventional risk factors, no angiographic stenoses; group 3 – angiographic stenoses, no revascularization at baseline; group 4 – early revascularization). The dichotomous covariate calcium indicates an EBCT-derived calcium score larger than 100. There is no clustering in this data set. One of the research questions was to examine whether the EBCT-derived calcium score can add prognostic information compared with the clinical information summarized in the risk groups. Age (in years) was categorized into three groups with the youngest age group as the reference. The covariate frequencies are given in Table 1.2. ▯

Example 1.2 Malignant Melanoma Data

The data set contains observations of 205 patients with radical surgery for malignant carcinoma (skin cancer) at the University Hospital of Odense in Denmark during 1962–1977. Radical surgery means that the tumor was completely removed including the skin within a distance of about 2.5 cm around it. Patients were followed up until 1977 and 57 deaths from malignant melanoma, and 14 deaths due to other causes (coded as censored event times) were observed. The data of five patients are given in Table 1.3.

Table 1.3: Data of five patients of the malignant melanoma study

id	time	status	gender	age	thickness
1	10	0	1	76	676
2	30	0	1	56	65
3	35	0	1	41	134
4	99	0	0	71	290
5	185	1	1	52	1208

The first column provides the unique patient identification number. Variable time measures time since surgery in months and variable status indicates the occurrence of death caused by malignant melanoma. There are several covariates available in the data set; for ease of presentation we will restrict them in this application to the following three covariates: gender (0 = female, 1 = male), age at surgery (years), and tumor thickness (in 1/100 mm). This is a univariate data set without clustering. The data was first analyzed by Drzewiecki et al. (1980a,b) and later published and reanalyzed in more detail by Andersen et al. (1993). ▯

Example 1.3 Halluca Study

The Halle Lung Cancer (Halluca) study was a study investigating provision of medical care to lung cancer patients in the region of Halle and Dessau in the eastern part of Germany (Bollmann et al. 2004, Kuß et al. 2008). The study region covers about 1.5 million inhabitants and belongs to the State of Saxony-Anhalt. In cooperation with the regional clinical tumor registries, all lung cancer patients in the study region were recorded from April 1996 to September 1999, and follow-up was done until September 2000. A total of 1696 lung cancer patients were observed, and survival was defined as time from clinical, histological or cytological diagnosis to death. 1349 patients (79.5%) died until the end of follow-up; median survival in the study population was 9.3 months. To validate and complement survival information, the data from the Clinical Cancer Registry were compared to death certificates collected by the local health institutions and linked to the data from the Common Cancer Registry of Eastern Germany. Minimal follow-up time was 12 months, and the median follow-up time 33 months. To judge the influence of prognostic and risk factors on overall survival, five fixed-effects covariates, known to be important in the prognosis of survival regarding lung cancer, were included. The information for five patients is given in Table 1.4. The first column gives

Table 1.4:   Data of five patients in the Halluca study

id	time	status	unit	gender	age	type	ECOG	stage
1	54.74	1	1	1	75.02	1	0	4
2	6.68	1	1	1	63.60	1	0	5
3	0.33	1	1	1	52.68	2	.	.
4	24.28	1	2	1	55.14	.	0	.
5	15.46	0	2	0	79.28	2	0	1

the patient-specific id number, and the second column the survival time (in months). The third column contains the survival status (1 = death, 0 = alive) and the fourth column the cluster variable diagnosing unit. Lung cancer was diagnosed in 56 different diagnosing units with numbers of patients ranging from 1 to 392 (mean 30.3). The Halluca data is analyzed using univariate approaches in Chapters 2 and 3. In Chapter 4 the data is treated like from a multicenter study with the diagnosing unit as cluster variable. A cluster effect by diagnosing unit is indicated by Figure 1.1. In multicenter studies (with treatment center as cluster), despite the tight study protocols, often center-to-center variation occurs, which cannot be explained by covariates. Frailty models can be used to investigate this variation. The other columns represent variables gender (0 = female, 1 = male), age (years), histologic type (1 = small-cell lung cancer, 2 = non-small-cell lung cancer), ECOG status (range 0 to 4), and UICC stage (1 = I, 2 = II, 3 = IIIa, 4 = IIIb, 5 = IV).

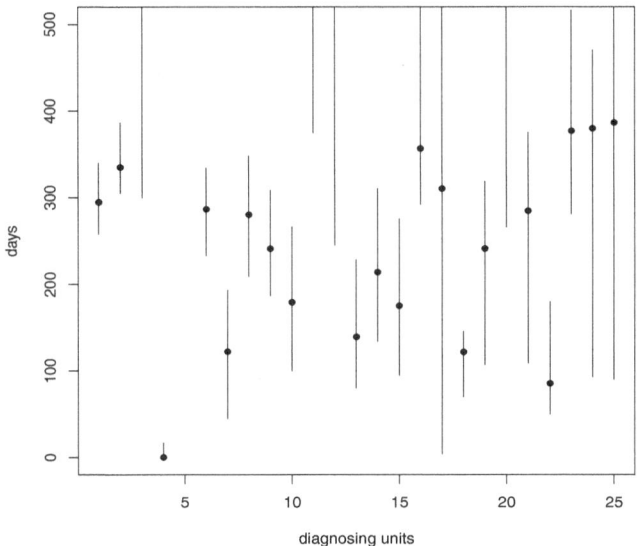

Figure 1.1: Median survival (95% CI) of 25 diagnosing units in Halluca

Dots indicate missing covariate values. It was initially decided to model these as separate categories despite the dangers of this procedure. Throughout the book, in the tables presenting the results, these missing categories are omitted.

Table 1.5: Description of the Halluca study population

covariate	category	absolute frequency	relative frequency
gender	male	1374	81.0%
	female	322	19.0%
histologic type	NSCLC	1183	69.8%
	SCLC	366	21.5%
	missing	147	8.7%
ECOG	ECOG 0-2	1366	68.7%
	ECOG 3-4	123	7.3%
	missing	407	24.0%
stage	I	185	10.9%
	IIa	79	4.7%
	IIb	195	11.5%
	III	280	16.5%
	IV	621	36.6%
	missing	336	19.8%

We further explicitly omitted the primary treatment as a covariate. This was to prevent unjustified treatment recommendations, which should only be derived from randomized trials and not from observational studies. The study population is described in Table 1.5. Mean age at diagnosis was 65 years. ☐

Example 1.4 Danish Twins Cause-Specific Mortality Data

The Danish Twin Registry was the world's first nation–wide twin registry, established in 1954 by Bent Harvald and Mogens Hauge. The older part of this population based registry includes all twins born in Denmark during the period 1870–1910 and all like-sex pairs born between 1911 and 1930 in which both partners survived to the age of six years. Pairs with deaths before the age of six were excluded because it turns out to be very difficult to obtain detailed information especially about the zygosity of such twin pairs. The birth registers from all 2200 parishes of Denmark during the relevant calendar years were manually scrutinized to identify multiple births. After such births were identified, a search was then carried out for the twins or, whenever needed, for their closest relatives in regional population registers (in operation since 1924) or other public sources, especially the archives of probate courts and censuses. As soon as a twin was traced, a questionnaire was sent to the twin (if she or he was alive) or to the closest relatives (if she or he was not alive). Questions about phenotypic similarities were included in the questionnaires to assess the zygosity by self-reported similarities. The reliability of this method was validated by comparison with the results of laboratory methods based on blood serum enzyme group determination in a subgroup of twins. The misclassification rate of this method was found to be less than 5% in the Danish twin data (Holm 1983). Similar results are known from the Swedish Twin Registry (Cederlöf et al. 1961) The follow-up procedure traced nearly all twins who did not die or emigrate before the age of six years. For further, more detailed information about the construction and the composition of the Danish Twin Registry see Hauge (1981).

The data provided by the Danish twin registry contain 8201 monozygotic (MZ) and dizygotic (DZ) twin pairs who were born between 1 January 1870 and 31 December 1930, and who were both still alive on 1 January 1943. As a consequence of this restriction, around two-thirds of the twin pairs born were excluded because of the high infant mortality of this period (1870–1930). Furthermore, twins have a higher infant mortality than singletons because of their lower birth weight. It was necessary to exclude early deaths because it was nearly impossible to obtain zygosity information when one or both twin partners died at young ages. Zygosity information is crucial to the application of the methods in twin research.

Table 1.6:   Data of three Danish twin pairs

id	time	status	pair	gender	zygosity	cause	birth
1	76.09	1	1	1	1	2	1889
2	76.02	1	1	1	1	2	1889
3	64.73	1	2	0	2	4	1908
4	94.75	1	2	0	2	1	1908
5	85.62	0	3	0	1	0	1881
6	68.61	1	3	0	1	2	1881

Observed covariates are gender, zygosity and year of birth. A total of 246 twin pairs with incomplete information about the cause of death were excluded, leaving a study population of 7955 twin pairs. Individuals were followed up through 31 December 1993, and those identified as deceased after that date have been classified here as living. Altogether, we have 1344 male MZ twin pairs and 2411 DZ twin pairs, and 1470 female MZ twin pairs and 2730 DZ twin pairs. In addition to the lifetimes, there is information about cause of death for all noncensored lifetimes, that is, for all individuals in the study population who died before 31 December 1993. For the present analysis, only the underlying cause of death was considered.

The data for the first six twins are given in Table 1.6. The first column gives the identification number of the individual, and the second one the survival or censoring time (in years). The third column contains the censoring indicator (1 = death, 0 = alive), the fourth column is the identification number of the twin pair (cluster), and the four other columns represent the covariates gender (0 = female, 1 = male), zygosity (1 = monozygotic, 2 = dizygotic), cause of death (0 = alive, 1 = cancer, 2 = coronary heart disease, 3 = stroke, 4 = respiratory diseases, 5 = other), and year of birth. For more detailed information about cause of death, gender, and zygosity of the study population see Table 1.7.

Table 1.7: Causes of death in the Danish twin population (number of individuals)

cause of death	males		females	
	MZ twins	DZ twins	MZ twins	DZ twins
cancer	440	809	423	823
coronary heart disease	666	1180	548	999
stroke	161	278	186	335
respiratory diseases	143	203	89	205
other causes	336	661	330	555
all causes together	1746	3131	1576	2917
alive	942	1691	1364	2543

Information regarding death status, age at death, and cause of death was obtained from the Central Person Register, the Danish Cancer Register, the Danish Cause–of–Death Register, and other public registries in Denmark. The main source for obtaining information on cause of death was the Death Register at the National Institute of Public Health. Information about cause of death is available from this register for individuals who died after 1942 (Juel and Helweg-Larsen 1999). Consequently, cause of death is included in the twin register only for twins who died after this year.

Table 1.8:   Cause of death groups by ICD number

cause of death	ICD revision 6 & 7	ICD revision 8
cancer	140 – 205	140 – 209
coronary heart disease	420	410 – 414
stroke	330 – 334	430 – 439
respiratory diseases	470 – 527	460 – 519

The validity of the twin register was checked on the basis of a comparison of information about year of death with the nationwide Danish Cancer Register. There was around 99% agreement, although both registries were independent. Further data corrections increased this level of agreement to almost 100%. Cause of death was coded following the sixth, seventh, and eighth edition of the International Classification of Diseases (ICD). Four different groups of main causes of death are considered in the present example: cancer, coronary heart disease (CHD), stroke, and diseases of the respiratory system. ICD codes in three revisions of the ICD for these broad cause-of-death groups are given in Table 1.8. Causes of death are a common example for competing risks.   ⬚

Example 1.5 Danish twins CHD mortality data with covariates

The data in this example is a subset of the cause-specific mortality data in the foregoing example. Here the main focus is on age at death with death caused by coronary heart disease and the influence of BMI and smoking on this outcome.

In 1966, a questionnaire including questions about smoking, height, and weight was mailed by the Danish Twin Registry to all Danish twins born in the period 1890–1920 who were alive and traceable on 1 January 1966. 3709 individuals answered the questionnaire (response rate 65%). Excluded from the study were 813 twins with nonresponding partners, four pairs with unknown zygosity, and 212 pairs with incomplete or uncertain information on height and weight. A total of 23 pairs were excluded because of incomplete information about the cause of death, resulting in a total study population of 1209 complete twin pairs.

Individuals were followed from 1 January 1966 to 31 December 1993. Those persons identified as deceased after the follow-up period are classified for our purposes as censored. At the end of follow-up period, approximately 40% of the twins were still alive, resulting in the right censored data. Altogether, there were 210 male monozygotic twin pairs and 316 dizygotic twin pairs, and 273 female monozygotic twin pairs and 410 dizygotic twin pairs. The data for the first six twins in the study population are given in Table 1.9. The first column provides the unique identification number of the twin, the second column the observation time (in years). The third column contains the

Table 1.9: Data of three Danish twin pairs with covariates

id	time	status	pair	gender	zygosity	birth	BMI	smoking
1	74.23	1	1	0	2	1893	1	1
2	81.52	0	1	0	2	1893	2	2
3	72.58	1	2	0	2	1912	2	4
4	54.89	1	2	0	2	1912	1	2
5	57.31	0	3	1	1	1897	3	3
6	83.79	1	3	1	1	1897	1	4

censoring indicator (1 = death by CHD, 0 = censored (including non-CHD deaths)), the fourth column the number of the twin pair (cluster), and the following five columns represent the covariates gender (0 = female, 1 = male), zygosity (1 = monozygotic, 2 = dizygotic), year of birth, body mass index (1 if $BMI < 22\text{kg/m}^2$, 2 if $22\text{kg/m}^2 \leq BMI \leq 28\text{kg/m}^2$, 3 if $28\text{kg/m}^2 < BMI$), and smoking (1 = nonsmoker, 2 = cigarette smoker, 3 = other smoker (pipe smoker, cigar smoker, etc.), 4 = former smoker). More detailed information about the distribution of gender, smoking, and BMI in the study population is given in Table 1.10.

Table 1.10: Study population (number of individuals) by gender, BMI, and smoking

	non-smokers	former smokers	other smokers	cigarette smokers	total
males					
BMI < 22	11	12	45	31	99 (9.4%)
BMI 22–28	78	141	333	208	760 (72.2%)
BMI > 28	24	35	91	43	193 (18.3%)
Total	113	188	469	282	
	(10.7%)	(17.9%)	(44.6%)	(26.8%)	
females					
BMI < 22	105	46	47	99	297 (21.7%)
BMI 22–28	350	138	134	171	793 (58.1%)
BMI > 28	157	40	37	42	276 (20.2%)
Total	612	224	218	312	
	(44.8%)	(16.4%)	(16.0%)	(22.8%)	

Altogether, 562 CHD deaths occurred in the population during follow-up. CHD is grouped as ICD 420 in the sixth and seventh revision, and as ICD 410–414 in the eighth ICD revision. The same data set (with minor differences) was used by Herskind et al. (1996a) with focus on total mortality. ▯

Example 1.6 Swedish twins breast cancer data

First established in the late 1950s to study the influence of smoking and alcohol consumption on cancer and cardiovascular diseases while controlling for genetic propensity to disease, the Swedish Twin Registry has developed into a unique source. Since its establishment, the registry has been expanded and updated on several occasions, and the focus has similarly been broadened to include most common complex diseases. Today it contains around 70,000 twin pairs born between 1886 and 1990. Nearly 400 papers have been published based on data from the Swedish Twin Registry.

When the twin registry was initiated, the church registers from all parishes of the period 1886–1925 were checked manually to identify all multiple births. Between 1959 and 1961, questionnaires were sent to all twins, including a question about phenotypic similarities between partners to assess zygosity: 'Were you as children as alike as two peas in a pod?' When both partners agreed, they were defined as monozygotic twins. If both responded 'not alike', they were classified as dizygotic. If the twins did not agree, or if only one member of the pair answered the question, the pair was classified as of unknown zygosity. This classification was compared with laboratory methods (serological markers) and the misclassification rate was found to be very low (Cederlöf et al. 1961), similar to the Danish data (Holm 1983).

At present, the Swedish Twin Registry contains information about three cohorts of Swedish twins referred to as the 'old', 'middle', and 'young' cohort. Here the focus is on the old cohort consisting of all like-sex pairs born between 1886 and 1925 where both members in a pair were alive and living in Sweden in 1959. The data for the first six twins are given in Table 1.11.

Table 1.11:   Data of three Swedish twin pairs

id	time	status	pair	gender	zygosity	birth	age
1	76.09	1	1	1	1	1889	23
2	76.02	0	1	1	1	1889	26
3	64.73	0	2	0	2	1908	0
4	94.75	0	2	0	2	1908	23
5	85.62	0	3	0	1	1887	25
6	68.61	1	3	0	1	1887	29

The first column gives the identification number of the individual, and the second column the age at diagnosis of breast cancer or censoring (in years). The third column contains the censoring indicator (1 = onset of breast cancer, 0 = no onset of breast cancer), the fourth column the identification number of the twin pair (cluster), and the other columns represent gender (0 = female, 1 = male), zygosity (1 = monozygotic, 2 = dizygotic), year of birth, and age at giving first birth (in years). Zero indicates nulliparous women.

The summary for the old cohort is given in Table 1.12, stratified according to the censoring status. The event under study is the onset of breast cancer. If a woman did not develop breast cancer or if she died from other causes during the follow-up, the corresponding observation is censored. Age at onset of breast cancer ranges from 36 years to 93 years.

The data set was created by merging the Swedish Twin Registry with the Swedish Cancer Registry maintained by the National Board of Health and Welfare. At the time of record linkage of the data used here, the Swedish Cancer Registry contained all cases of cancer that were diagnosed during the period 1959 through 2000, and 715 cases of breast cancer were identified during follow-up.

Table 1.12: Breast cancer in Swedish twins (old cohort)

	number of twin pairs			
	both censored	one censored	none censored	total
MZ twin pairs	1767	218	18	2003
DZ twin pairs	3420	407	27	3854
total	5187	625	45	5857

In another analysis, without considering the covariate age at first birth, the twins from the old and the middle cohort are combined. The middle cohort comprises all twins born between 1926 and 1967 who were alive and living in Sweden in 1970. Altogether, 1096 breast cancer cases were observed during the follow-up until 2000 in both cohorts. The data structure is the same as in Table 1.11 (but without covariate age). Summary statistics for both cohorts combined are given in Table 1.13.

Table 1.13: Breast cancer in Swedish twins (old & middle cohort)

	number of twin pairs			
	both censored	one censored	none censored	total
MZ twin pairs	4304	335	33	4672
DZ twin pairs	7236	625	35	7896
total	11540	960	68	12568

For a comprehensive description of the Swedish Twin Registry database at the Karolinska Institute (Stockholm) with focus on the recent data collection efforts and a review of the principal findings that have come from the registry, see Lichtenstein et al. (2002). □

Example 1.7 **Cross-Sectional Multisera Data on Hepatitis A and B**
Viral hepatitis is a serious health problem throughout the world. To obtain a clear picture of the prevalence of hepatitis A, B, and C, a sero-epidemiological study was undertaken in 1993/1994 in Flanders (Belgium). From the 4058 blood samples drawn from a study population representative of the Flemish population, the main focus is on complete cases specifically with respect to hepatitis A and B, resulting in 3787 blood samples. These blood samples were then tested for the presence of antibodies for the different infections and, using prespecified cut-off values, were classified as either positive or negative. Together with the patient's age and the assumption of lifelong immunity, these data constitute current status data on whether or not past infection took place. Hepatitis C was not considered here because of its low prevalence (less than 1%). More details about this data can be found in Beutels et al. (1997). It would be interesting to look at the heterogeneity in acquisition of either infection and the correlation between the acquisition of both infections. While age-dependent seroprofiles reflect the age-specific risk of infection, the proper assessment of heterogeneity has direct implications with respect to the two key quantities in infectious disease epidemiology, the basic reproduction number, and their associated critical vaccination coverage (Farrington et al. 2001). Estimating the correlation could indicate transmission through similar routes (correlation near one) or could reflect to what extent a latent process, such as the social or hygienic behavior of people, drives the more general infection process. Note that the main transmission route for hepatitis A is foodborne or feco-oral, and for hepatitis B it is sexual or bloodborne, reflecting hygienic behavioral conduct of individuals. Moreover, joint infections caused by more than one pathogen are an aggravating factor in disease progression for virtually all infections and thus of interest to be quantified. The variable

Table 1.14: Data of five patients of the hepatitis study

id	time	status A	status B
1	6	0	0
2	17	1	1
3	35	0	1
4	56	0	0
5	12	1	1

id is the identification number of the probands, who are the clusters. Time refers to age of the probands when the sample was taken and is given in years. Consequently, time denotes monitoring time and not event time. Status A and B refer to the presence of antibodies with respect to the hepatitis A and B virus, respectively. The data of five probands are given in Table 1.14. □

Chapter 2

Survival Analysis

2.1   Basic Concepts in Survival Analysis

This section describes basic statistical aspects of univariate survival data, and therefore might be skipped by experienced readers. However, it contains notation and important results that form the basis of specific points considered in later chapters. We will use the traditional approach to survival analysis and refer the reader interested in the approach based on counting processes and martingale theory (Aalen 1978) to the well-known books of Fleming and Harrington (1991), Andersen et al. (1993), Martinussen and Scheike (2006), and Aalen et al. (2008).

First we come back to the questions from the preface: What distinguishes survival analysis from other fields of statistics? Why does survival data need a special statistical theory? The reason is that time is the response variable, and time is not measured like other variables. First, survival times are usually a mixture of discrete and continuous data that require a different type of analysis than in the traditional discrete or continuous case. The mixture is the result of censoring and has an important effect on data analysis. Second, most evaluations are made conditionally on the knowledge available at the time of the analysis, and this changes over time. Usually, as the population under study is changing, we only consider the individual risk of death for those who are still alive. However, this means that many standard statistical approaches cannot be applied. This special feature of survival data is called conditioning and is discussed in detail in the books by Hougaard (2000) and Duchateau and Janssen (2008).

We consider a random variable T^*. Specifically, let T^* be nonnegative, representing the time from a well-defined specific starting point until the occurrence of an event. If the event is death, T^* is the survival time, which gives the field its name. The term survival time is also used with other events such as the onset of disease, complications after surgery, healing, or relapse in the medical field. In demography, death as well as leaving home of young adults, pregnancy, marriage, giving birth, migration, or divorce are of special interest. In engineering, the event is typically the failure of a technical unit, often consisting of different subunits. In economics, it can denote the acceptance of jobs by the unemployed or early retirement, major investments, end of strikes or training programs. In consumer economics, durations are studied until the purchase of a durable or storable product. In macroeconomic research, the durations of business cycles are of special interest. Considering convicted criminals, the event of recidivism is of great interest in making conclusions about the efficiency of punishments. The occurrence of mastitis in diary cow udders is analyzed in veterinary sciences and is an important economic factor. In political sciences, events such as international conflicts or cabinet transitions are considered. We will use survival time, lifetime, event time, time to event, and duration time as synonyms.

Usually, the event time T^* is assumed to follow a continuous distribution, and we will mainly focus on this case in the present book with only a few exceptions considered later. All functions of the event time distribution are defined over the interval $[0, \infty)$ if not stated otherwise in the following. The probability density function (p.d.f.) is denoted by f. The distribution of a random variable is completely and uniquely determined by its probability density function. Other useful functions exist that can be obtained from the probability density function. The most important one is

$$F(t) = \mathbf{P}(T^* \le t) = \int_0^t f(s)\, ds,$$

the cumulative distribution function (c.d.f.) of T^*, where $\mathbf{P}(A)$ denotes the probability that event A occurs. In survival analysis, one is more interested in the probability of an individual to survive time t, which is given by the survival function

$$S(t) = 1 - F(t) = \mathbf{P}(T^* > t) = \int_t^\infty f(s)\, ds.$$

The major concept in survival analysis is the hazard function. This function is also called (depending on the field of application) mortality rate, incidence rate, mortality curve, failure rate, or force of mortality. The hazard function is defined by

$$\mu(t) = \lim_{\epsilon \to 0} \frac{\mathbf{P}(t < T^* \le t + \epsilon | T^* > t)}{\epsilon} = \frac{f(t)}{1 - F(t)}. \tag{2.1}$$

The hazard function characterizes the hazard of death changing over time (or age, depending on which time scale is used). It specifies the instantaneous failure rate at time t, given that the individual survives until time t. It is also called the exit rate to stress the fact that it means exit out of the state of interest. Sometimes, it is useful to deal with the cumulative (or integrated) hazard function

$$M(t) = \int_0^t \mu(s)\, ds.$$

For the topic covered by this monograph, the concept of the Laplace transform **L** of a random variable is crucial to inference in this research area:

$$\mathbf{L}(u) = \mathbf{E}e^{-uT^*} = \int_0^\infty e^{-ut} f(t)\, dt.$$

All the functions f, F, S, μ, M, and **L** provide equivalent specifications of the distribution of the nonnegative random variable T^*. We use f, F, S, μ, M and **L** as generic symbols without index, and their arguments make evident which random variable is considered.

It is easy to derive relations between the different notions; for example, (2.1) implies that

$$M(t) = \int_0^t \mu(s)\, ds = \int_0^t \frac{f(s)}{1 - F(s)}\, ds = -\ln(1 - F(t))$$

and consequently

$$S(t) = 1 - F(t) = e^{-\int_0^t \mu(s)\, ds} = e^{-M(t)}. \tag{2.2}$$

This equation is the main exponential formula of survival analysis. It presents a characterization of the distribution and survival function via the hazard function. It turns out that the hazard function is often more convenient to deal with compared to the density or distribution and survival function because of its meaningful probabilistic interpretation and its simplicity in likelihood expressions considered later on.

Example 2.1
Suppose that the random variable T^* follows a distribution with probability density function

$$f(t) = \lambda \nu t^{\nu-1} e^{-\lambda t^\nu}, \qquad t \geq 0, \tag{2.3}$$

where λ, ν are one-dimensional nonnegative parameters. This is a Weibull distribution, discussed in more detail in the next section. We consider it here to illustrate the foregoing formulas. The following relations hold, starting from the density (2.3).

$$
\begin{aligned}
\text{probability density function} \quad & f(t) = \lambda \nu t^{\nu-1} e^{-\lambda t^\nu} \\
\text{survival function} \quad & S(t) = e^{-\lambda t^\nu} \\
\text{hazard function} \quad & \mu(t) = \lambda \nu t^{\nu-1} \\
\text{cumulative hazard function} \quad & M(t) = \lambda t^\nu.
\end{aligned}
$$

As mentioned before, the concept of hazard function is particularly useful in survival analysis. That is, properties of the distribution of event times are generally discussed in terms of properties of the hazard function. It describes the way in which the instantaneous probability of failure for an individual changes with time. Applications often contain qualitative information about the hazard function, which is helpful in selecting a model with good fit. For example, there may be biological reasons to restrict the analysis to models with increasing hazards or with hazard functions that have other well-defined characteristics.

The hazard function can take very different shapes. It can be increasing (for example, a Weibull distribution with shape parameter $\nu > 1$), decreasing (Weibull distribution with $\nu < 1$), constant (Weibull distribution with $\nu = 1$), J-, U- or bell-shaped (log-normal distribution). Models with these and other shapes of the hazard function are all useful in practice: In demography, for example, for following humans from birth to death, a J-shaped hazard function is often appropriate. After an initial period in which deaths result primarily from birth defects and infant diseases, the death rate drops and remains relatively constant until the age of 30 years or so, after which it increases again with age. This pattern is also observed in many other populations, including those consisting of technical items. For example, during a run-in phase, the hazard of failure of technical items often decreases, followed by a period with relatively constant hazard. After some time the hazard function starts to increase again. Such pattern can be described, for example, by a U-shaped hazard function. Models with increasing hazards are used most often. This is because interest often centers on periods in the life of individuals in which measurable aging takes place (for example, old ages in humans). Models with a constant hazard function have a simple structure, as we will see in the next section. They can be extended to piecewise constant hazard models, which are much more flexible and easy to handle. Less common are models with a decreasing hazard, but they are sometimes used in reliability to describe failure times of electronic devices, at least over a fairly long initial period of use. Furthermore, mortality rates of patients who have recently undergone a serious surgery (for example, a transplantation) are usually declining starting from the surgery. This is because patients experiencing complications often die shortly after the surgery, leaving the patients without such complications in the study population.

The main points to remember here are that the hazard function represents an aspect of the probability distribution of a nonnegative random variable that has a direct physical meaning, and that qualitative information about the form of the hazard function is useful in selecting an appropriate (parametric) model for the situation under investigation.

Furthermore, from a more practical point of view, models based on the hazard function can easily handle censoring and truncation often occurring in survival data. These specific and common problems of time to event data are discussed in the following two sections in more detail.

2.2 Censoring and Truncation

Censoring is what distinguishes survival analysis from other fields of statistics. Basically, a censored observation is an incomplete observation; it contains only partial information about event time. That means the patient is followed up for some time, but the event does not occur during this period. It is only known that the true event time exceeds the observed censoring time. There are different types of censoring; here we consider type I right censoring only because this type of censoring is the most common one in real data applications of survival analysis.

Let $T_1^*, T_2^*, \ldots, T_n^*$ be i.i.d. survival times with cumulative distribution function F and let $C_1, C_2, \ldots, C_n$ be i.i.d. censoring times with cumulative distribution function G. Throughout the book, we assume that F, and G are absolutely continuous. Furthermore, let f and g be probability density functions with respect to F and G. We are only able to observe the bivariate data $(T_1, \Delta_1), (T_2, \Delta_2), \ldots, (T_n, \Delta_n)$, where $T_i = \min\{T_i^*, C_i\}$ denotes the observation time and

$$\Delta_i = \begin{cases} 1 & : \quad \text{if } T_i^* \leq C_i, \quad \text{that is, } T_i \text{ is not censored} \\ 0 & : \quad \text{if } T_i^* > C_i, \quad \text{that is, } T_i \text{ is censored.} \end{cases}$$

Censoring is a common problem arising in many applications, for example, in clinical trials. Here, patients may enter the study at different times; then each is treated with one of several possible drugs or therapies. We are interested in observing their event times, but for some patients censoring occurs in one of the following forms:

- **Loss to follow-up.** The patient may move elsewhere; she or he is never seen again.

- **Drop out.** The treatment may have such strong side effects that it is necessary to stop the therapy. Or the patient may refuse to continue the treatment.

- **Termination of study.** The study ends at a predefined point of time. This type of censoring is called administrative censoring.

- **Competing risks.** The event of interest cannot be observed because of the occurrence of a competing event (for example, death by accident).

In Figure 2.1 the event times of patients 2, 4, and 5 are completely observed. The event times of patients 1 and 3 are censored because of loss to follow-up, drop out, or competing risks. Event times of patients 6 and 7 are censored because of termination of study.

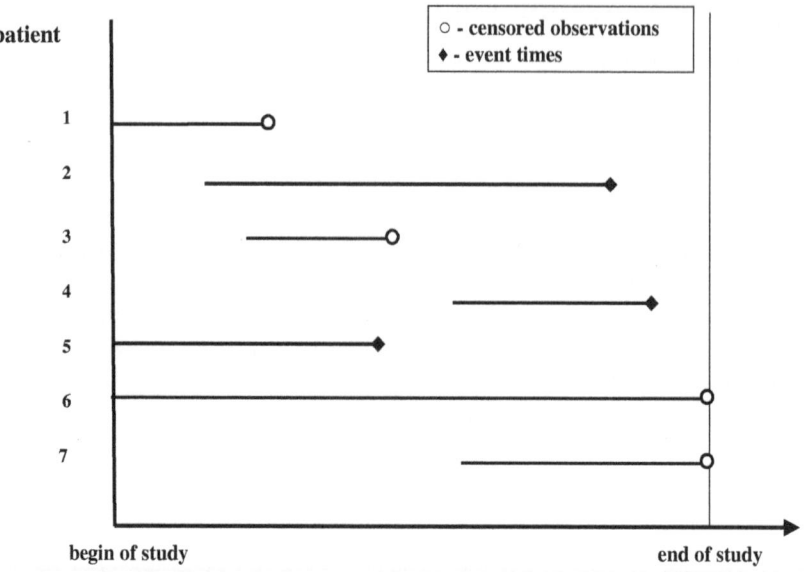

Figure 2.1:   Event and censoring times of patients in a clinical trial.

In the subsequent part we use T^* and C, without subscripts, as shorthand for all the T_i^* and C_i lifetime and censoring variables, respectively, and denote by H the distribution function of the observation time $T = \min\{T^*, C\}$. Then the following relation can easily be derived:

$$
\begin{aligned}
H(t) &= \mathbf{P}(\min\{T^*, C\} \le t) \\
&= 1 - \mathbf{P}(\min\{T^*, C\} > t) \\
&= 1 - \mathbf{P}(T^* > t, C > t).
\end{aligned}
$$

Assuming independence between event time T^* and censoring time C implies the simplification

$$
\begin{aligned}
H(t) &= 1 - \mathbf{P}(T^* > t)\mathbf{P}(C > t) \\
&= 1 - (1 - \mathbf{P}(T^* \le t))(1 - \mathbf{P}(C \le t)) \\
&= 1 - (1 - F(t))(1 - G(t)).
\end{aligned}
$$

This underlines the importance of the independence assumption regarding event and censoring times usually made in survival analysis.

Remark: The cumulative distribution function of the noncensored data (discarding the censored observations) is **not** F!

$$\mathbf{P}(T \leq t, \Delta = 1) = \mathbf{P}(T^* \leq t, T^* \leq C)$$

$$= \int\limits_{t^* \leq t, t^* \leq c} \int f(t^*)g(c)\, dt^*\, dc$$

$$= \int\limits_{t^* \leq t} f(t^*)\left(\int\limits_{t^* \leq c} g(c)\, dc\right) dt^*$$

$$= \int\limits_{t^* \leq t} f(t^*)(1 - G(t^*))\, dt^* \neq F(t) \qquad (2.4)$$

Consequently, ignoring the censored event times implies biased estimates.

THEOREM 2.1

The probability density function of the survival data (T, Δ) is

$$f(t, \delta) = \big(f(t)(1 - G(t))\big)^{\delta} \big(g(t)(1 - F(t))\big)^{1-\delta}. \qquad (2.5)$$

Proof: Denote by H_0 and H_1 subdistribution functions of the observation time T, and by h_0 and h_1 their subdensities. It holds that

$$H_1(t) = \mathbf{P}(T \leq t, \Delta = 1) = \int\limits_{t^* \leq t} f(t^*)(1 - G(t^*))\, dt^*,$$

see (2.4). Furthermore,

$$\bar{H}_0(t) = \mathbf{P}(T \leq t, \Delta = 0) = \mathbf{P}(C \leq t, C < T^*)$$

$$= \int\limits_{c \leq t, c < t^*} \int f(t^*)g(c)\, dt^*\, dc$$

$$= \int\limits_{c \leq t} g(c)\left(\int\limits_{c < t^*} f(t^*)\, dt^*\right) dc = \int\limits_{c \leq t} g(c)(1 - F(c))\, dc.$$

Consequently, $h_0(t) = \frac{dH_0(t)}{dt} = g(t)(1 - F(t)), h_1(t) = \frac{dH_1(t)}{dt} = f(t)(1 - G(t))$ and

$$f(t, \delta) = \delta h_1(t) + (1 - \delta)h_0(t)$$
$$= h_1(t)^{\delta} h_0(t)^{1-\delta}$$
$$= \big(f(t)(1 - G(t))\big)^{\delta} \big(g(t)(1 - F(t))\big)^{1-\delta}.$$

This completes the proof. ∎

In the following paragraph the likelihood function is derived based on results of Theorem 2.1 given earlier. Here a parametric situation is considered, which means the distribution of survival time is assumed to be known up to a finite dimensional unknown parameter vector $\boldsymbol{\theta}$. A parametric model for survival data is the exponential distribution. It is very rare that survival data follow this distribution because it is not very flexible as an one-parameter family. But for understanding all other survival distributions, the exponential model is of great importance. Other parametric approaches such as the Weibull model (often used in reliability) and the Gompertz model (preferred in actuarial and demographic settings) contain the exponential distribution as a special case. In biostatistical applications the piecewise exponential distribution becomes more and more popular. We will consider all these, emphasizing similarities and differences. The distributions are studied in the most simple case of independent and identically distributed random variables. Furthermore, semi-parametric and nonparametric approaches will be considered later on.

Here and in the following text, in addition to the independence between event and censoring times, we assume noninformative censoring. That means that the censoring distribution must not depend on the parameter vector $\boldsymbol{\theta}$ of the survival distribution. Otherwise the censoring distribution would contain information on the parameters of interest, which is, for example, the case in the Koziol–Green Model (Koziol and Green 1976). Furthermore, we do not aim to estimate parameters of the censoring distribution. Hence, the terms $g(t)$ and $G(t)$ in the density function (2.5) become additive constants independent of $\boldsymbol{\theta}$ in the log likelihood function. These additive constants drop from the derivative of the log-likelihood function and can therefore be dropped from the likelihood of the data. As a consequence of this and formula (2.5), the contribution of right-censored survival data (t_i, δ_i) $(i = 1, \ldots, n)$ to the likelihood function simplifies to

$$L_i(\boldsymbol{\theta}) = f(t_i; \boldsymbol{\theta})^{\delta_i} S(t_i; \boldsymbol{\theta})^{1-\delta_i}. \tag{2.6}$$

For complete observations, the likelihood is their density, as is the case in standard situations. Censored observations provide the information that the unknown survival time exceeds the observed censored time. Consequently, the second term in (2.6) reflects the probability to survive at least until t_i. Formula (2.6) can easily be expressed in terms of the hazard function

$$L_i(\boldsymbol{\theta}) = \mu(t_i; \boldsymbol{\theta})^{\delta_i} e^{-\int_0^{t_i} \mu(s; \boldsymbol{\theta}) \, ds}.$$

If we consider a sample of independent lifetimes $(t_1, \delta_1), \ldots, (t_n, \delta_n)$, the likelihood function of the data is

$$L(\boldsymbol{\theta}) = \prod_{i=1}^{n} L_i(\boldsymbol{\theta}) = \prod_{i=1}^{n} \mu(t_i; \boldsymbol{\theta})^{\delta_i} e^{-\int_0^{t_i} \mu(s; \boldsymbol{\theta}) \, ds} \tag{2.7}$$

because of the independence between the observed times (univariate model).

To underline the importance of the common assumption about independent censoring in survival analysis, the following example is provided, which deals with the case of dependent censoring. A joint distribution of lifetimes and the censoring times is assumed. It turns out that the likelihood function in the case of dependent censoring is the product of derivatives of the joint survival function of lifetimes and censoring times.

Example 2.2
Denote by (T, Δ), $T = \min\{T^*, C\}$, $\Delta = 1(T^* \leq C)$ censored observations under the assumption of dependent censoring. Let $S(t^*, c)$ and $f(t^*, c)$ be the joint survival and probability density function of T^* and C, respectively. Consequently, the subdistribution functions needed for the construction of the likelihood function can be derived by

$$
\begin{aligned}
H_1(t) &= \mathbf{P}(T \leq t, \Delta = 1) \\
&= \mathbf{P}(T^* \leq t, T^* \leq C) \\
&= \int \int_{\{t^* \leq t, t^* \leq c\}} f(t^*, c) \, dc \, dt^* \\
&= -\int_0^t S_1(t^*, t^*) \, dt^*
\end{aligned}
$$

with $S_1(t, c) = \frac{\partial S(t,c)}{\partial t}$. This implies that the subdensity of a noncensored ($\delta = 1$) observation is a derivative of the subdistribution function

$$
h_1(t) = \frac{dH_1(t)}{dt} = -S_1(t, t).
$$

Similar calculations yield the subdistribution and subdensity functions in the case of a censored observation ($\delta = 0$):

$$
\begin{aligned}
H_0(t) &= \mathbf{P}(T \leq t, \Delta = 0) \\
&= \mathbf{P}(C \leq t, C < T^*) \\
&= \int \int_{\{c \leq t, c < t^*\}} f(t^*, c) \, dt^* \, dc \\
&= -\int_0^t S_2(c, c) \, dc
\end{aligned}
$$

with

$$
S_2(t^*, c) = \frac{\partial S(t^*, c)}{\partial c} \quad \text{and} \quad h_0(t) = \frac{dH_0(t)}{dt} = -S_2(t, t).
$$

Consequently, the likelihood in case of a parametric model with $\boldsymbol{\theta}$ as the vector of unknown parameters is a composition of the subdensity functions

$S_1(t, t; \boldsymbol{\theta}) = S_1(t, t)$ and $S_2(t, t; \boldsymbol{\theta}) = S_2(t, t)$. For a sample $(t_1, \delta_1), \dots, (t_n, \delta_n)$ the likelihood function can be written as

$$L(\boldsymbol{\theta}) = \prod_{i=1}^{n} \left(-S_1(t_i, t_i; \boldsymbol{\theta}) \right)^{\delta_i} \left(-S_2(t_i, t_i; \boldsymbol{\theta}) \right)^{1-\delta_i}.$$

In the case of independent censoring with $S(t, c; \boldsymbol{\theta}) = \left(1 - F(t; \boldsymbol{\theta})\right)\left(1 - G(c)\right)$ this expression simplifies to (2.7).   ⬜

Up to now, only the situation of right-censored event time data was considered in the present monograph. However, in some cases, event times are only known to lie in a specific interval. This situation especially arises when study subjects are not under continuous observation, such as, for example, patients visiting their doctor at predetermined times (or times that are convenient to them), where the occurrence of the event can be diagnosed knowing that the event had not occurred at the time of the previous visit. Another situation is inspection times of technical equipment, where events can happen between two inspection times. Hence, it is only known that the event occurred between two visits or inspections but not the exact time point. This kind of censoring is called interval censoring and was considered in detail by Sun (2006). In general, right censoring is a special case of interval censoring and some of the methods for right censored data can be directly, or with minor changes, applied to interval censored data. However, most of the approaches for right-censored data are not appropriate for interval-censored data because the censoring mechanism behind interval censoring is much more complicated than in the case of right censoring.

An important special case of interval-censored data are so called current status data. The term *current status data* originates from applications in the field of demography (Diamond et al. 1986). It means the observation on each individual survival time interval includes either zero or infinity. Such kind of data usually occur when each study subject is observed only once, and the only available information for the event under study is whether the event has occurred before the observation was taken. Consequently, current status data are given in the form (T, Δ), where T denotes the monitoring time (which is not the time when the event happens!) and Δ is the indicator whether the event already occurred before the monitoring or not. In the parametric case, the likelihood function of a sample $(t_1, \delta_1), \dots, (t_n, \delta_n)$ with unknown parameter vector $\boldsymbol{\theta}$ to be estimated can be written in the form (Sun 2006)

$$L(\boldsymbol{\theta}) = \prod_{i=1}^{n} \left(1 - S(t_i; \boldsymbol{\theta})\right)^{\delta_i} S(t_i; \boldsymbol{\theta})^{1-\delta_i}, \tag{2.8}$$

with components depending on whether the event already occurred before the monitoring times ($\delta_i = 1$) or not ($\delta_i = 0$).

In the following paragraphs we shall take truncation into account. Truncation is, besides censoring, another important feature of event time data, requiring specific adaptation of the parameter estimation procedures. Censoring is a mapping of the original event times and censoring times, whereas truncation results in conditional distributions of the observations. Here we discuss only the most common truncation type, that is, left truncation. Furthermore, let us assume that truncation is nonrandom. Nonrandom left-truncation occurs when individuals are observed only from some known time after the natural origin of the event under study. That means individuals who failed before the truncation time in question are not recorded.

For example, the first patient in Figure 2.2 cannot be observed because of death before the study started. That means the researcher carrying out the study would not be aware of that observation. Patients 2, 3, and 4 are observable because their observation time T exceed their truncation time t^+ (shown in detail for patient 3 in the figure). In other words, truncation is sampling from a conditional distribution. That means an unknown number of subjects who experienced the event under study before the observation started are missing in the study sample.

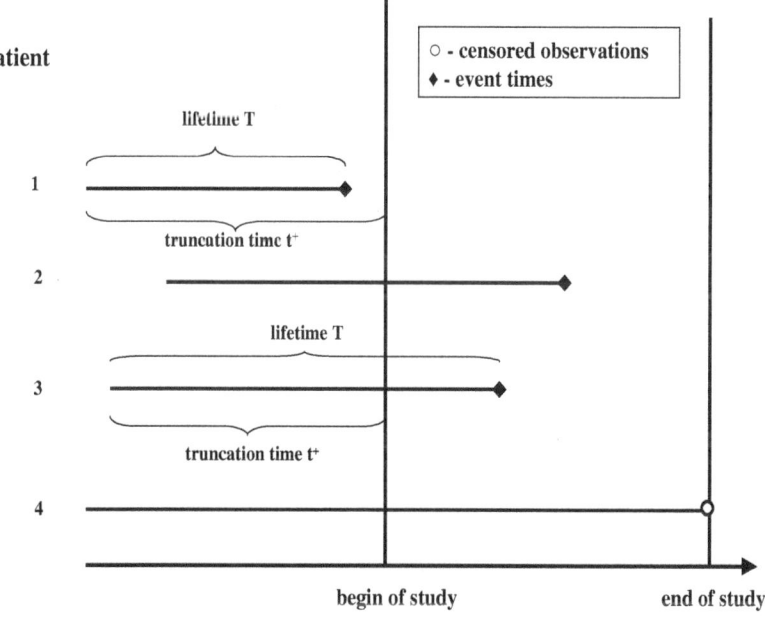

Figure 2.2: Event times of patients in a clinical trial with truncation.

Denote by (T^+, Δ^+) the observed truncated data following the distribution of the original data under the condition $(T > t^+)$ with t^+ as known (nonrandom) truncation time. So we get

$$
\begin{aligned}
\mathbf{P}(T^+ > t, \Delta^+ = \delta) &= \mathbf{P}(T > t, \Delta = \delta | T > t^+) \\
&= \frac{\mathbf{P}(T > t, \Delta = \delta)}{\mathbf{P}(T > t^+)} \\
&= \frac{\mathbf{P}(T > t, \Delta = \delta)}{(1 - F(t^+))(1 - G(t^+))}
\end{aligned}
$$

and the density of the (nonrandom) left-truncated and independent right-censored observations is given by the expression

$$
f(t, \delta, t^+) = \frac{\left(f(t)(1 - G(t))\right)^\delta \left(g(t)(1 - F(t))\right)^{1-\delta}}{(1 - F(t^+))(1 - G(t^+))}.
$$

As a consequence of this result, the likelihood function of univariate survival data $(t_1, \delta_1, t_1^+), \ldots, (t_n, \delta_n, t_n^+)$ with (nonrandom) left truncation times t_i^+ ($i = 1, \ldots, n$) in the parametric case with $\mu(t) = \mu(t; \boldsymbol{\theta})$ and $\boldsymbol{\theta}$ as the vector of parameters to be estimated can be written in the form

$$
L(\boldsymbol{\theta}) = \prod_{i=1}^n \mu(t_i; \boldsymbol{\theta})^{\delta_i} \exp\left(-\int_{t_i^+}^{t_i} \mu(s; \boldsymbol{\theta}) \, ds\right).
$$

Here, similar to the case of no truncation the distribution of the censoring times disappears from the likelihood function because of the independent and noninformative censoring assumption.

Truncation, alternatively called late entry, has enormous consequences for the approach to time to event data. It turns out that survival function and density function are changed by truncation at time t^+, which means by conditioning on $T > t^+$. This shows the advantage of the hazard function, which, unlike the other quantities, is not changed by truncation. This is because the hazard is already conditioned on survival time t. Therefore, it makes no difference if conditioning is also on smaller survival times than t. More details can be found in Turnbull (1976).

Truncation is a common problem in register data. Usually, a register is founded at a specific time point, and data collection starts from this time onward. Subjects who fail before this date are usually truncated, which means they are not included in the study population. For example, Swedish twins are only included in the Swedish Twin Registry if they were alive in 1959 when the register was established. Information about cancer is available for Danish people from 1943 onwards, the year in which the Danish Cancer Registry was founded. This problem will be discussed later on in a bivariate data situation in more detail.

2.3 Parametric Models

Now we will briefly consider some probability distributions that are helpful in the field of survival analysis. Naturally, any distribution of nonnegative random variables can be used to describe durations. In parametric event time models the baseline hazard is specified by a small number of one-dimensional parameters. The survival distributions to be discussed here in more detail are continuous with one exception – the piecewise constant hazard function. Throughout the literature on survival analysis, certain parametric models have been used repeatedly, such as exponential, Weibull, and Gompertz. These distributions have closed-form expressions for survival, density, and hazard functions. Gamma and lognormal distributions are computationally less convenient but applied frequently. To avoid model validity issues, the nonparametric approach, based on the Kaplan–Meier estimator (Kaplan and Meier 1958), is usually the preferred course. However, this alternative is often inefficient, as noted by Miller (1983). In particular, standard errors of parameter estimates in parametric models will tend to be smaller than in nonparametric models. However, the adequacy of the chosen distribution has to be checked. The pros and cons of different parametric, semiparametric and nonparametric models and methodology for statistical inference in event time data can be found in the monographs by Kalbfleisch and Prentice (1980), Miller (1981), Lawless (1982), Cox and Oakes (1984), Andersen et al. (1993), Parmar and Machin (1995), Smith (2002), Klein and Moeschberger (2003), Collett (2003), Tableman and Kim (2004), and Aalen et al. (2008). Keiding and Andersen (2006) provide a concise overview of important topics in survival analysis in the form of an encyclopedia.

Now we discuss some of the parametric standard failure time models for homogeneous populations. The properties and theoretical bases of these distributions are considered here only briefly. For a more detailed overview of lifetime distributions, the interested reader is referred to the book by Marshall and Olkin (2007). In this and the following sections the random variable T denotes the time until the occurrence of the event, which we are interested in making inferences about. Only the simplest case of independent and identically distributed event times $T_1, T_2, \ldots, T_n$ is considered here. How to overcome this restriction will be the topic of the following chapters. In general, we will use capital letters for random variables and lowercase letters for their realizations.

We will start with the exponential distribution in the next section as the fundamental one in survival analysis even if it is relatively rare that event time data follow this one-parameter distribution. However, the exponential distribution helps to understand the main issues of many other typical survival distributions.

2.3.1   Exponential distribution

The exponential model $(T \sim Exp(\lambda))$ is the simplest parametric lifetime model. It has only one single parameter λ. The model assumes a constant risk over time, which reflects the property of the distribution appropriately called *lack of memory*. The probability of failure within a particular time interval depends only on the length but not on the location of this interval. This means that the distribution of $T - t$ conditional on $T > t$ is the same as the original distribution. In other words, it holds that

$$\mathbf{P}(t < T \le t + \epsilon | T > t) = \mathbf{P}(T \le \epsilon)$$

for any positive ϵ. As a consequence, the exponential distribution as the only one is not influenced by the definition of time point zero. This property makes the exponential model a poor choice for modeling human survival or age at onset of diseases except over short time intervals. The parameter λ can take all positive values, and the distribution with $\lambda = 1$ is called the unit or standard exponential. Therefore, the following formulas can be derived by some simple algebraic calculations:

$$
\begin{aligned}
\text{probability density function} \quad & f(t) = \lambda e^{-\lambda t} \quad\quad (\lambda > 0) \\
\text{survival function} \quad & S(t) = e^{-\lambda t} \\
\text{hazard function} \quad & \mu(t) = \lambda \\
\text{cumulative hazard function} \quad & M(t) = \lambda t \\
\text{expectation} \quad & \mathbf{E}T = \frac{1}{\lambda} \\
\text{variance} \quad & \mathbf{V}(T) = \frac{1}{\lambda^2}
\end{aligned}
$$

Exponential distribution was widely used in early work on the reliability of electronic components and technical systems. The distribution of cT with a positive constant c is again exponentially distributed with parameter λ/c. The minimum of n independent exponential random variables with parameter λ is still exponential with parameter $n\lambda$:

$$\mathbf{P}(\min\{T_1, \ldots, T_n\} > t) = \prod_{i=1}^{n} \mathbf{P}(T_i > t) = \prod_{i=1}^{n} e^{-\lambda t} = e^{-n\lambda t}.$$

Exponential distribution is a special case of all the Weibull, Gompertz, gamma, and piecewise constant distributions to be described in the following sections. The simple form of the density implies a very easy and explicit maximum likelihood estimate for the parameter λ, which is shown in Example 2.3. It turns out that the maximum likelihood estimate is the reciprocal of the number of total person years of exposure. Methods in epidemiology based on person years in fact implicitly assume an exponential distribution. Software for planning sample size in clinical trials also often uses the assumption of exponential failure times.

Example 2.3

Let $T_1, T_2, \ldots, T_n$ be independent and identically distributed survival times with cumulative distribution function $F(t) = 1 - e^{-\lambda t}$. The question arises: How do we estimate the unknown parameter λ of interest when using the maximum likelihood method?

First step: Under the assumption of independent censoring, the likelihood function can be derived using (2.7) and $\boldsymbol{\theta} = \lambda$:

$$L(\lambda) = \prod_{i=1}^{n} \mu(t_i; \lambda)^{\delta_i} e^{-\int_0^{t_i} \mu(s;\lambda)\, ds}$$

$$= \prod_{i=1}^{n} \lambda^{\delta_i} e^{-\lambda t_i}.$$

Taking the logarithm yields

$$\log L(\lambda) = \log(\lambda) \sum_{i=1}^{n} \delta_i - \lambda \sum_{i=1}^{n} t_i.$$

Second step: Maximization of the log-likelihood function with respect to the unknown parameter λ:

$$\frac{\partial \log L(\lambda)}{\partial \lambda} = \frac{1}{\lambda} \sum_{i=1}^{n} \delta_i - \sum_{i=1}^{n} t_i$$

$$\frac{1}{\lambda} \sum_{i=1}^{n} \delta_i - \sum_{i=1}^{n} t_i = 0$$

$$\hat{\lambda} = \frac{\sum_{i=1}^{n} \delta_i}{\sum_{i=1}^{n} t_i}$$

The estimator has a straightforward interpretation, as $\hat{\lambda}$ is just the ratio of the number of events and the total observation time. □

The model is very sensitive to even a modest variation because it has only one adjustable parameter. The inverse of parameter λ is both mean and standard deviation. Recent works have overcome this limitation by using more flexible distributions, which are introduced in the following sections.

One interesting extension of the exponential model is the piecewise constant hazard model. In this model the hazard function is constant within some prespecified time intervals, meaning, that for each time interval, a separate exponential model is assumed. Consequently, results from the exponential distribution can be used by considering each interval separately. The main advantage of this model is its flexibility, depending on the number and length of time intervals used in the analysis. On the other hand, each additional interval implies an additional parameter to be estimated, which practically restricts the number of intervals depending on the sample size. The main disadvantage of the model is that it is not continuous. There are jumps at each interval end. One interesting special case is the equidistant case where all intervals are of the same length. Liu and Huang (2008) recommend the use of piecewise constant hazard functions especially in frailty models because of the ease of implementation. Simulations show the very good performance of this method compared to semiparametric methods. An interesting extension of the model is the use of piecewise linear functions. At the cost of an additional slope parameter per time interval, the model can be extended to a continuous model. Of course, this model is also much more difficult to fit. Further extensions in this direction deal with splines of higher order that yield a smooth hazard function.

2.3.2 Weibull distribution

The Weibull model was introduced by Waloddi Weibull (1939) and is a popular generalization of the exponential model with two positive parameters. The second parameter ν allows great flexibility to the model and different shapes of the hazard function. The convenience of the Weibull model is due, on the one hand, to this flexibility and, on the other hand, the simplicity of the hazard and survival functions. The expressions of expectation and variance contain the gamma function and are not of simple form. We abbreviate the distribution as $W(\lambda, \nu)$. In the case of $\nu = 1$, the exponential distribution is obtained as a special case. For the Weibull distribution the following formulas can be derived

$$
\begin{aligned}
\text{probability density function} \quad & f(t) = \lambda \nu t^{\nu-1} e^{-\lambda t^{\nu}} \qquad (\lambda > 0, \nu > 0) \\
\text{survival function} \quad & S(t) = e^{-\lambda t^{\nu}} \\
\text{hazard function} \quad & \mu(t) = \lambda \nu t^{\nu-1} \\
\text{cumulative hazard function} \quad & M(t) = \lambda t^{\nu} \\
\text{expectation} \quad & \mathbf{E}T = \lambda^{-\frac{1}{\nu}} \Gamma(1 + \frac{1}{\nu}) \\
\text{variance} \quad & \mathbf{V}(T) = \lambda^{-\frac{2}{\nu}} \left(\Gamma(1 + \frac{2}{\nu}) - \Gamma(1 + \frac{1}{\nu})^2 \right),
\end{aligned}
$$

where Γ is the gamma function with $\Gamma(k) = \int_0^\infty s^{k-1} e^{-s} \, ds \quad (k > 0)$.

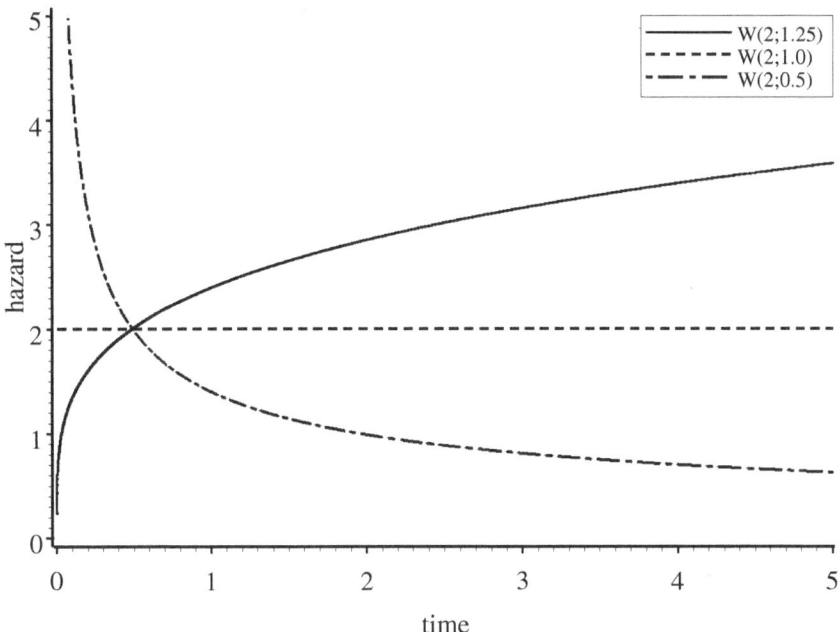

Figure 2.3: Weibull hazard functions with different shape parameters.

The hazard function decreases monotonously for $\nu < 1$, is constant for $\nu = 1$, and it monotonously increases for $\nu > 1$, which is illustrated by Figure 2.3.

If $T \sim W(\lambda, \nu)$, then it holds that $cT \sim W(\lambda c^{-\nu}, \nu)$, when c is a positive constant. Furthermore, the minimum of n i.i.d. random variables is $W(n\lambda, \nu)$ distributed (minimum-stable distribution property). Weibull distribution can also be generated as the limiting distribution of the minimum of a sample from a continuous distribution on $[0, u)$ for some u ($0 < u < \infty$). Due to this extreme value property, Weibull distribution is appropriate for modeling the distribution of individual time to death. Different causes of death compete with each other, and the first one to strike will cause the death of the individual.

The Weibull model seems to be the most widely applied parametric lifetime model. It has been used in a wide range of biostatistical problems; for example, it has been derived theoretically for studies of time until occurrence of cancer in laboratory animals by Pike (1966) and Peto et al. (1972). In medical applications time to death by lung cancer is modeled by Weibull distribution (Whitthemore and Altshuler 1976, Berry 2007). It is unknown whether it has similar relevance for other diseases. Weibull distribution is inappropriate for hazard functions that are unimodal or bathtubshaped. A generalization of Weibull distribution to include such shapes was proposed by Mudholkar et al. (1996). A comprehensive overview about the Weibull distribution is given in Murthy et al. (2003).

2.3.3   Log-logistic distribution

An alternative to the foregoing Weibull distribution is log-logistic distribution. Log-logistic distribution is fairly flexible with two parameters, denoted by $\log L(v, \kappa)$. It is one of the parametric survival-time models in which the hazard is decreasing for $\kappa \leq 1$ and hump-shaped for $\kappa > 1$ (Figure 2.4). The distribution imposes the following functional forms on the density, survival, hazard, and cumulative hazard function:

$$\text{probability density function} \quad f(t) = \frac{v\kappa(vt)^{\kappa-1}}{(1 + (vt)^{\kappa})^2} \quad (v > 0, \kappa > 0)$$

$$\text{survival function} \quad S(t) = \frac{1}{1 + (vt)^{\kappa}}$$

$$\text{hazard function} \quad \mu(t) = \frac{v\kappa(vt)^{\kappa-1}}{1 + (vt)^{\kappa}}$$

$$\text{cumulative hazard function} \quad M(t) = \ln(1 + (vt)^{\kappa})$$

The general shape of the hazard function of a log-logistic distribution is very similar to that of log-normal distribution which will be introduced in a later section.

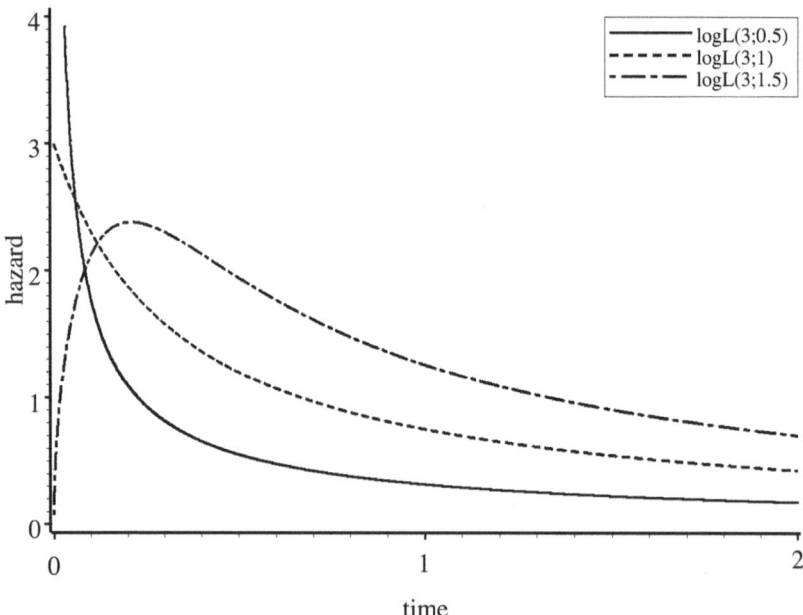

Figure 2.4:   Log-logistic hazard functions with different parameters.

2.3.4 Gompertz distribution

In 1825 the British actuary Benjamin Gompertz made the observation that a law of exponential progression gives a good description of large portions of different tables of mortality for humans. The simple formula he derived describes the exponential rise in death rates between sexual maturity and old age. It is commonly referred to as the Gompertz equation – a formula that remains a valuable tool in demography and other scientific disciplines. Gompertz's observation of a mathematical regularity in human life tables made him believe in the presence of a law of mortality that explained common age patterns of death. It has been widely used, especially in actuarial and biological applications and in demography. A random variable T follows a Gompertz distribution with parameters λ and φ ($T \sim G(\lambda, \varphi)$), if one of the following relations holds:

$$\text{probability density function} \quad f(t) = \lambda e^{\varphi t} e^{-\frac{\lambda}{\varphi}(e^{\varphi t}-1)} \quad (\lambda > 0)$$

$$\text{survival function} \quad S(t) = e^{-\frac{\lambda}{\varphi}(e^{\varphi t}-1)}$$

$$\text{hazard function} \quad \mu(t) = \lambda e^{\varphi t}$$

$$\text{cumulative hazard function} \quad M(t) = \frac{\lambda}{\varphi}(e^{\varphi t}-1)$$

The hazard function is increasing starting from λ at time zero (Figure 2.5). For parameter values $\varphi < 0$, the hazard function is decreasing, and the cumulative hazard converges to the constant $-\lambda/\varphi$ for $t \to \infty$ so that not all individuals in the population experience the event under study. This situation is discussed in more detail in so-called cure models later on in this monograph. Obviously, exponential distribution is a special case of Gompertz distribution in the case of $\varphi = 0$. The Gompertz model (Gompertz 1825) was generalized to the Gompertz–Makeham distribution (Makeham 1860) by adding a constant c to the hazard function

$$\mu(t) = \lambda e^{\varphi t} + c.$$

Here the additional parameter c describes a nonaging aspect in the study population that is independent of time t, whereas the Gompertz part in the formula still represents the age-dependent aspect with an exponential form. The parameters λ and c are not identifiable in the case of $\varphi = 0$; only their sum can be estimated.

The Gompertz–Makeham distribution describes the age dynamics of human mortality rather accurately in the age range of about 30 – 80 years. At more advanced ages the death rates do not increase as fast as predicted by this mortality law – a phenomenon known as the late-life mortality deceleration. This phenomenon was one of the starting points for developing univariate frailty models.

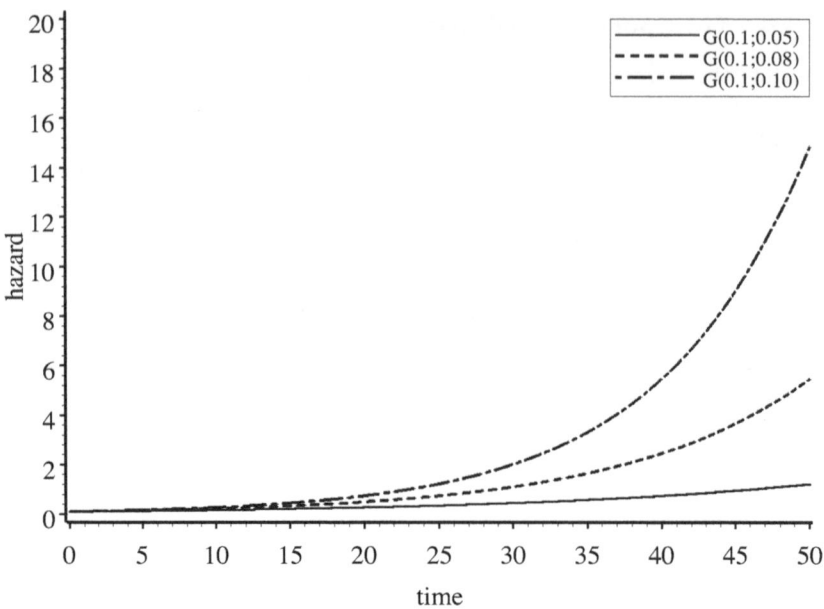

Figure 2.5: Gompertz hazard functions with different parameters.

2.3.5　Log-normal distribution

In the log-normal model ($T \sim \log\mathrm{N}(m, s^2)$), the natural logarithm $\log(T)$ (or more exactly $\ln(T)$) of event time T is assumed to be normally distributed with mean m and variance s^2. The product of a large number of independent and identically distributed random variables follows asymptotically a log-normal distribution. This is similar to the fact that a normal distribution results if a variable is the sum of a large number of independent and identically distributed random variables (Central Limit Theorem). The following relations hold for log-normal distribution:

$$\text{probability density function} \quad f(t) = \frac{1}{\sqrt{2\pi}st}e^{-\frac{(\log t - m)^2}{2s^2}}$$

$$\text{survival function} \quad S(t) = 1 - \Phi\left(\frac{\log t - m}{s}\right)$$

$$\text{hazard function} \quad \mu(t) = \frac{\frac{1}{st}\phi\left(\frac{\log t - m}{s}\right)}{1 - \Phi\left(\frac{\log t - m}{s}\right)}$$

$$\text{expectation} \quad \mathbf{E}T = e^{m + \frac{s^2}{2}}$$

$$\text{variance} \quad \mathbf{V}(T) = e^{2m + s^2}\left(e^{s^2} - 1\right)$$

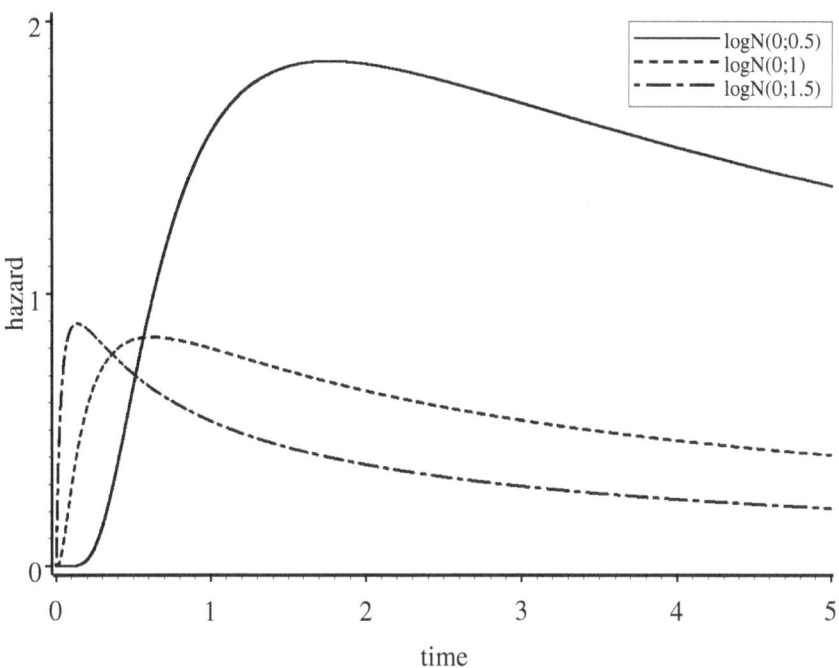

Figure 2.6: Log-normal hazard functions with different parameters.

In the formulas used above $\phi(x) = \frac{1}{\sqrt{2\pi}}e^{-\frac{x^2}{2}}$ denotes the probability density function, and $\Phi(x)$ the cumulative distribution function, of the standard normal distribution $N(0,1)$.

Log-normal distribution may be convenient to use with noncensored data, but when this distribution is applied to censored event times computations quickly become challenging. Unfortunately, the hazard function has a strange form: it takes value zero at $t = 0$, increases to a maximum, and then decreases, approaching zero as t heads to infinity (Figure 2.6). Because of the decreasing form of the hazard function for older ages, the distribution seems implausible as a lifetime model in most real situations. Nevertheless, it makes sense if interest is focused on time periods of younger ages. Despite its unattractive features, log-normal distribution has been widely used as failure distribution in diverse situations such as the analysis of electrical insulation or for modeling repair times in engineering systems. In medicine log-normal distribution is often used for modeling latent times, for example, time from infection until the occurrence of the first symptoms of infectious diseases (Sartwell 1966). Around two third of the 86 examples reviewed by Kondo (1977) in this research field appear to follow approximately a log-normal distribution.

2.3.6 Gamma distribution

Gamma distribution is another exciting extension of exponential distribution. It is of limited use in survival analysis because the gamma models do not have closed-form expressions for survival and hazard functions. Both include the incomplete gamma integral

$$I_k(x) = \frac{\int_0^x s^{k-1}e^{-s}\,ds}{\Gamma(k)}.$$

Consequently, traditional maximum likelihood estimation is not simple and requires the calculation of incomplete gamma integrals, imposing numerical problems in parameter estimation. If variable T follows a gamma distribution with shape parameter k and inverse scale parameter λ ($T \sim \Gamma(k, \lambda)$), then the following relations hold

$$
\begin{array}{ll}
\text{probability density function} & f(t) = \dfrac{\lambda^k t^{k-1} e^{-\lambda t}}{\Gamma(k)} \qquad (k > 0, \lambda > 0) \\[3ex]
\text{survival function} & S(t) = 1 - I_k(\lambda t) \\[2ex]
\text{hazard function} & \mu(t) = \dfrac{\lambda^k t^{k-1} e^{-\lambda t}}{(1 - I_k(\lambda t))\Gamma(k)} \\[3ex]
\text{expectation} & \mathbf{E}T = \dfrac{k}{\lambda} \\[3ex]
\text{variance} & \mathbf{V}(T) = \dfrac{k}{\lambda^2} \\[3ex]
\text{Laplace transform} & \mathbf{L}(u) = \mathbf{E}e^{-Tu} = (1 + \dfrac{u}{\lambda})^{-k}
\end{array}
$$

If $k = 1$, gamma distribution is reduced to exponential distribution. With integer k, gamma distribution is often called a special Erlangian distribution. It can be derived as the distribution of the waiting time until the kth emission from a Poisson source with intensity parameter λ. Consequently, the sum of k independent exponential variables with parameter λ has a gamma distribution with parameters k and λ (see Example 2.4) and can be used to model lifetimes of technical systems with repeated repairing after failure.

Example 2.4
Let $T_1, T_2, \ldots, T_k$ denote k i.i.d. random variables with $T_i \sim Exp(\lambda)$ and introduce T by $T = T_1 + \ldots + T_k$. Then it holds that

$$\mathbf{L}(u) = \mathbf{E}e^{-Tu} = \mathbf{E}e^{-(T_1+\ldots+T_k)u} = \prod_{i=1}^{k} \mathbf{E}e^{-T_i u} = \prod_{i=1}^{k}(1 + \frac{u}{\lambda})^{-1} = (1 + \frac{u}{\lambda})^{-k},$$

which is the Laplace transform of a gamma distribution with parameters k and λ. Here $T_1, T_2, \ldots, T_k$ denote times between repairing. $\square$

2.3.7 Pareto distribution

Pareto distribution was introduced by Vilfredo Pareto (1897) to explain the distribution of income of a given population at the end of the 19th century. The distribution is skewed and heavy-tailed with two parameters $\omega > 0$ and $\zeta > 0$. The kth moment of the Pareto distribution is finite if the restriction $\zeta > k$ applies. The hazard is monotone declining. Here we consider a shifted version of the Pareto distribution.

$$\text{probability density function} \quad f(t) = \frac{\zeta}{\omega}\left(\frac{\omega}{\omega + t}\right)^{\zeta + 1} \quad (\omega > 0, \zeta > 0)$$

$$\text{survival function} \quad S(t) = \left(\frac{\omega}{\omega + t}\right)^{\zeta}$$

$$\text{hazard function} \quad \mu(t) = \frac{\zeta}{\omega + t}$$

$$\text{cumulative hazard function} \quad M(t) = -\zeta \log\left(\frac{\omega}{\omega + t}\right)$$

$$\text{expectation} \quad \mathbf{E}T = \frac{\omega}{\zeta - 1} \quad (\zeta > 1)$$

Pareto distribution can be seen as a gamma mixture of exponential distributed lifetimes. It is often applied in areas including city population distributions, stock price fluctuations, oil-field locations, and socioeconomic studies. Pareto distribution is also a standard distribution for the purposes of reinsurance, taking care of the largest claims of a portfolio. It can be extended to the generalized Pareto distribution with hazard function $\mu(t) = \frac{\zeta}{\omega + t} + c$. More details about the generalized Pareto distribution can be found in Davis and Feldstein (1979).

Example 2.5
We would like to derive the expectation of Pareto distribution under the assumption $\zeta > 1$.

$$\begin{aligned}
\mathbf{E}T &= \int_0^\infty t f(t)\, dt \\
&= \int_0^\infty S(t)\, dt \\
&= \int_0^\infty \left(\frac{\omega}{\omega + t}\right)^{\zeta} dt \\
&= -\frac{\omega}{\zeta - 1}\left(\frac{\omega}{\omega + t}\right)^{\zeta - 1}\Big|_0^\infty \\
&= \frac{\omega}{\zeta - 1}
\end{aligned}$$

Here assumption $\zeta > 1$ is important, otherwise the expectation is infinite. □

2.4   Estimation of Survival and Hazard Functions

In the case of parametric inference, it is necessary to make assumptions about
the distribution of failure times. In some circumstances this makes sense,
especially when additional information about the nature of the underlying
aging or disease process is available. If such information is not available,
it is common to use nonparametric models. The simplest nonparametric
estimate of a distribution function is the empirical distribution function. That
means, even in the case of a continuous distribution, the estimate is discrete.
Major steps in the development of appropriate nonparametric and semiparametric techniques in survival analysis with censored observations were the
introduction of the Kaplan–Meier estimator (Kaplan and Meier 1958) and its
extension to the case of truncated lifetimes (Turnbull 1976, Tsai et al. 1987).
Another important milestone in this field was the semiparametric proportional
hazards regression model (Cox 1972).

Whether to use a parametric or a nonparametric model is an important
question. An advantage of nonparametric models is their flexibility and the
resulting ability to deal with any probability distribution. However, there is a
high price to pay. First, nonparametric methods need much more data to get
reasonable results. Second, it is hard to get estimates of the hazard function,
which is often an interesting and relevant information. For this, it is necessary
to smooth out the discrete point masses of the Kaplan–Meier estimator, for
example, by kernel function smoothing. In contrast, parametric models often
allow closed-form expressions of the hazard and survival function depending
on the chosen model. Parametric models can be described by the values of a
few parameters. They often give good results even in the case of small sample
size. If the assumed model is correct, the estimation is more efficient than in
a nonparametric estimation procedure.

2.4.1   Kaplan–Meier estimator

A useful way of characterizing survival in a group of individuals is to compute
and graph the empirical survival function. If there are no censored observations in the sample, the empirical survival function at time t is the ratio of
survivors at time t and the sample size n. This step function decreases by
$\frac{1}{n}$ just after each observed failure (for ease of presentation we first assume
no ties here). In practical situations, however, some of the observations are
censored. Consequently, a methodology for handling this with convenience is
required. Remember that we observe the pairs $(T_1, \Delta_1), \ldots, (T_n, \Delta_n)$, where
$T_i = \min\{T_i^*, C_i\}$ and $\Delta_i = 1(T_i^* \leq C_i)$. Let $T_{(1)} < T_{(2)} < \ldots < T_{(n)}$ be the
order statistics of $T_1, T_2, \ldots, T_n$, and with an abuse of notation define $\Delta_{(i)}$ to
be the value of Δ that is associated with $T_{(i)}$, that is, $\Delta_{(i)} = \Delta_j$ if $T_{(i)} = T_j$.
Note that the $\Delta_{(1)}, \Delta_{(2)}, \ldots, \Delta_{(n)}$ are not ordered.

The Kaplan–Meier estimator (sometimes called product limit estimator) was introduced by Kaplan and Meier (1958) as

$$\hat{S}(t) = \prod_{i:t_{(i)}<t} \left(1 - \frac{\delta_{(i)}}{n - i + 1}\right).$$

Assuming a continuous event time distribution, only one death will be observed at most at each time t_i with probability one. In practice, ties can occur, for example, because of coarse measurement. To deal with ties, let t_i denote the r distinct observation times $t_1 < t_2 < \ldots < t_r$ with $r \leq n$. Taking this into account, the Kaplan–Meier estimator is

$$\hat{S}(t) = \prod_{i \in R(t)} \left(1 - \frac{d_i}{\#R(t_i)}\right)$$

with d_i the number of events at time t_i. $R(t)$ denotes the set of indices of all individuals at risk at time t, meaning all individuals alive just before t. $\#R(t)$ denotes the number of individuals in the risk set at time t. The Kaplan–Meier estimator is a decreasing step function, changing only at time of an event. A problematic point is that $\hat{S}$ is not defined after the largest observation time if the last observation is a censored one. In this case, $\hat{S}(t)$ is usually left unspecified after the largest observation time. One consequence of this is that the mean lifetime cannot be estimated. A solution to this problem is to assume that the survival function is zero after the largest time, which results obviously in a biased estimate. A better solution is to consider the median survival time.

Figure 2.7 illustrates the Kaplan–Meier method by presenting the estimates of the survival curves of different patient groups in the EBCT study presented in detail in Example 1.1. Here time from baseline investigation of patients with coronary artery disease until the occurrence of a major adverse cardiac event is the duration of interest. Consequently, in this application the notion of survival is used in the more general sense of being free of well defined major cardiac events. The patients were grouped according to four levels of evidence of coronary artery disease. This allows a comparison of the event times in these groups. It is easy to see that group is a very strong predictor of event time; for example, individuals presenting with the lowest evidence level in group 1 have around 98% chance to be event free compared to only 50% chance in group 4, which is the group of highest level of disease evidence. Furthermore, jumps can be found at each event time point in the survival curve estimates.

Throughout the book we assume continuous survival times preventing ties. However, in many real-data applications, the researcher will be faced with observations at the same time point. Different methods exist to handle ties, which can produce different results. The exact method computes the exact conditional probability under the proportional hazards assumption for

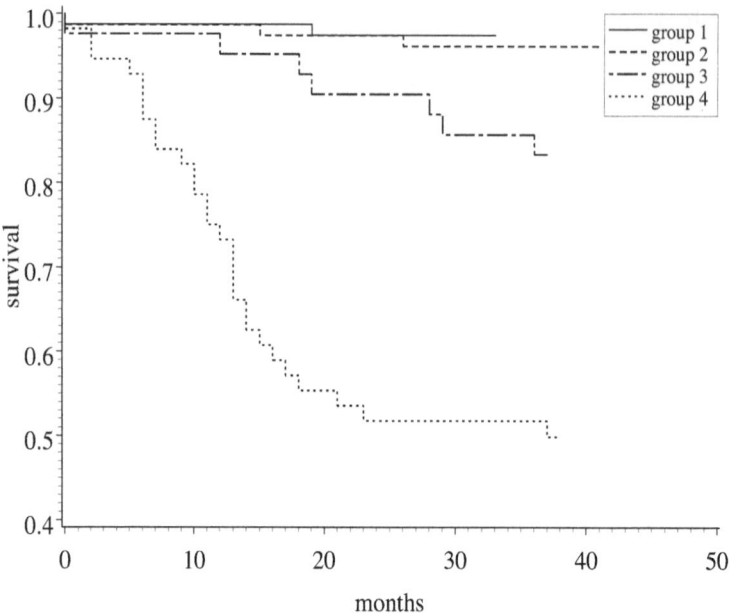

Figure 2.7: Kaplan–Meier curves for different patient groups in the EBCT study.

all tied events occurring before censored observations of the same or larger time. This is equivalent to summing all terms of the marginal likelihood that are consistent with the observed data. The method assumes that ties are due to lack of precision in measuring survival times and computes all possible orderings of tied event times (Kalbfleisch and Prentice 1980). The exact method needs abundant of computer resources for large data sets with many ties. The discrete method assumes that events occurred at exactly the same time and computes probabilities for events occurring to a set of observations with tied event times. It consumes less computer resources than the exact method. The most common method to handle ties is that by Breslow (1974) using an approximate likelihood. Another method suggested later by Efron (1977) also uses an approximate likelihood. If ties are not extensive, the methods by Breslow and Efron provide satisfactory approximations to the exact method for the continuous time-scale model. In general, Efron's approximation gives results that are much closer to the exact method results than Breslow's approximation does. If there are no ties, all three methods result in the same likelihood and yield identical estimates. The Breslow method is the most efficient one when there are no ties. With the exception of the R package, nearly all statistical software use the Breslow method as default. Throughout the book we have used this method.

For the variance of the Kaplan–Meier estimate, the Greenwood formula (Greenwood 1926) given by the expression

$$\mathbf{V}(\hat{S}(t)) = \hat{S}^2(t) \sum_{i \in R(t)} \frac{d_i}{\#R(t_i) - d_i}$$

is commonly used. Peterson (1977) shows that the Kaplan–Meier estimator is consistent, and Breslow and Crowley (1974) show its asymptotic normality.

Efron (1967) suggested an interesting procedure to obtain the Kaplan–Meier estimator (called redistribute-to-the-right algorithm): Start with an ordinary estimate of S, which assumes point mass $\frac{1}{n}$ at each observed time (survival or censoring times). Start at the first observation $t_{(1)}$, go to the right to the first censored observation, and redistribute the mass of this observation equally among the following times. Now go to the next censored observation and distribute its mass again among the following observed times. Treating the other censored times in a similar manner results in the Kaplan–Meier estimator.

2.4.2 Nelson–Aalen estimator

Consider the problem of estimating the cumulative hazard function $M(t)$. The Nelson–Aalen estimator was suggested by Nelson (1972) in a reliability context and rediscovered by Aalen (1978) who derived the estimator using modern counting process techniques. It is an estimator of the cumulative hazard function $M(t) = \int_0^t \mu(s) \, ds$ and of the form

$$\hat{M}(t) = \sum_{i \in R(t)} \frac{d_i}{\#R(t_i)}$$

with notations similar to the Kaplan–Meier estimator in the previous section. Intuitively, this expression is estimating the hazard at each distinct death time as the ratio of the number of deaths to the number at risk. Cumulative hazard is just the sum of all hazards at all death times up to time t, and has a nice interpretation as the expected number of deaths in $(0, t]$ per unit at risk. The variance of the Nelson–Aalen estimate can be evaluated by (Aalen 1978)

$$\mathbf{V}(\hat{M}(t)) = \sum_{i \in R(t)} \frac{d_i}{(\#R(t_i))^2}.$$

Figure 2.8 shows Nelson–Aalen plots of the four different levels of evidence for coronary artery disease in the EBCT study of Example 1.1. In agreement with the Kaplan–Meier curves, patients of group 1 show a good prognosis, whereas patients in groups with higher levels of evidence of the disease are faced with an increasing risk of major cardiac events.

The Nelson–Aalen estimator is often used in choosing between different parametric models. For this, one plots the estimator using a transformed

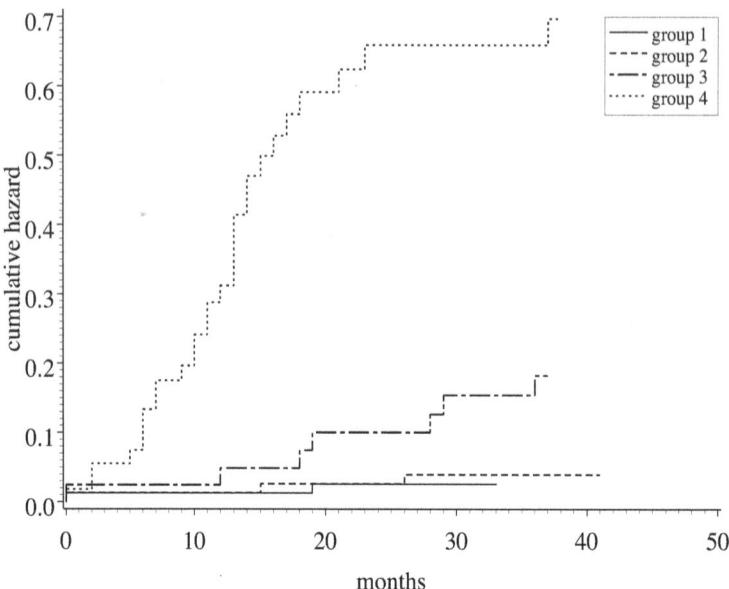

Figure 2.8: Nelson-Aalen curves for different patient groups in the EBCT study.

scale so that, if a given parametric model fits the data, the resulting graph should be approximately linear. For example, a plot of $\hat{M}(t)$ versus t will be approximately linear in the case of an exponential distribution. Checking the adequacy of a Weibull model, $\ln(\hat{M}(t))$ versus $\ln(t)$ should be approximately linear. The event times of the different groups in Figure 2.8 follow the exponential model reasonably, with some deviations at later times in group 4.

Similar to the Kaplan–Meier plots, there are only jumps at event times. In the case of continuous event times the functions $S(\cdot)$ and $M(\cdot)$ are related by $S(t) = e^{-M(t)}$ (see (2.2)). Consequently, it seems reasonable to consider $\bar{S}(t) = e^{-\hat{M}(t)}$ as an estimator of the survival function, which is different from the Kaplan–Meier estimator and was suggested by Breslow in the discussion of the paper by Cox (1972). Fleming and Harrington (1991) recommend it as an interesting alternative and have pointed out that it has a slightly smaller mean-squared error in some situations. Estimators for the hazard function μ can be derived from the Nelson–Aalen estimator based on kernel estimators. The formal derivations of the Kaplan–Meier and Nelson–Aalen estimators and their asymptotic properties are performed in the framework of counting processes (Aalen 1978, Fleming and Harrington 1991, Andersen et al. 1993, Martinussen and Scheike 2006, Aalen et al. 2008). Both estimators are asymptotically equivalent and quite close to each other, particularly when the number of deaths is small relative to the number of individuals at risk.

2.5 Regression Models

2.5.1 Proportional hazards model

The models presented so far deal with the simplest case of independent and identically distributed variables. This implies a homogeneous population. However, in most practical applications, the population under study is not homogeneous. For example, individuals in epidemiological studies may differ in age, gender, socioeconomic status, education, blood pressure, body mass index, smoking habits, nutrition, physical activity, heart rate, family status, genetic predisposition, and other factors. Perhaps some of these covariates are of special interest, such as the effect of a treatment in a clinical trial, or they are confounders which effect needs to be adjusted for in the analysis. In both cases, we will use the notion covariate for these variables. The proportional hazards model introduced by Cox (1972) is a regression model with event time as dependent variable. It allows the inclusion of information about known (observed) covariates in models of survival data in an easy way and is the most applied model in this area.

Let $\mu(t|\mathbf{X})$ denote the hazard of an individual at time t with covariate vector $\mathbf{X}' = (X_1, \ldots, X_k)$. Here $\mathbf{X}'$ denotes the transpose of the column vector $\mathbf{X}$. The proportional hazards model specifies that

$$\mu(t|\mathbf{X}) = \mu_0(t)h(\mathbf{X}) \qquad (2.9)$$

where $\mu_0(t)$ is the baseline hazard function and $h(\cdot)$ some positive function. The model assumes a baseline hazard (risk of death or other event) that all individuals in the study population have in common. This assumption can be relaxed but keeps presentation easy. The parameters of primary interest are contained in $h(\mathbf{X}) = h(\boldsymbol{\beta}, \mathbf{X})$, often

$$h(\mathbf{X}) = e^{\boldsymbol{\beta}'\mathbf{X}},$$

with $\boldsymbol{\beta}' = (\beta_1, \beta_2, \ldots, \beta_k)$ denoting the vector of regression parameters. In this model, the covariates act multiplicatively on the baseline hazard, adding further risks, as determined by the individuals' prognostic information. This allows the model a simple and easy interpretation. It is assumed that all individual variation in the hazard can be characterized by a finite-dimensional vector of observed covariates (explanatory variables, risk factors, predictive factors, and regressors). The main idea behind it is the separation of the time effect in the baseline hazard function on the one hand and the effect of the covariates in an exponential term on the other. In essence, this assumption says that the hazards of two individuals at time t is related by a proportionality constant that does not depend on t. The simple two-sample situation is obtained by restricting to a single ($k = 1$) binary covariate X in the model with $X = 0$ or $X = 1$, depending on group membership. In this case, the method is truly nonparametric, and e^{β} denotes the hazard ratio between the two groups. However, if X is continuous, a parametric form of $h(\cdot)$ is required. Inference is now dependent on that parametric form but still independent of $\mu_0(t)$, and the model is called a semiparametric model because of the parametric nature of the covariate term and the nonparametric baseline hazard function. The survival function given the covariates $\mathbf{X}$ is

$$S(t|\mathbf{X}) = S_0(t)^{e^{\beta'\mathbf{x}}},$$

where $S_0(t) = e^{-\int_0^t \mu_0(s)\,ds}$ denotes the baseline survival function and the components of the vector $\boldsymbol{\beta}$ are unknown regression parameters. That means the survival function of an individual with covariate vector $\mathbf{X}$ is a power of the baseline survival function. The class of distributions generated by this procedure is sometimes called Lehmann alternatives.

Two different approaches are possible with the proportional hazards model. Sometimes it occurs that covariates have skewed distributions, for example, when only a small fraction of the individuals are exposed to the risk factor of interest. It is also very common that a large fraction of lifetimes is censored. Especially in large cohort studies analyzing the effect of a rare exposition on an event, the number of exposed cases may be very small. One may then question the validity of inference based on asymptotic results. In the parametric case, the baseline hazard is chosen from the class of parametric lifetime distributions. For example, starting from (2.7), the likelihood function in the Weibull model with $\boldsymbol{\theta} = (\lambda, \nu)$ is of the form

$$L(\boldsymbol{\beta}, \boldsymbol{\theta}) = \prod_{i=1}^{n} \left(\lambda\nu t_i^{\nu-1} e^{\boldsymbol{\beta}'\mathbf{X}_i}\right)^{\delta_i} e^{-\lambda t_i^{\nu} e^{\boldsymbol{\beta}'\mathbf{X}_i}} \qquad (2.10)$$

and looks like

$$L(\boldsymbol{\beta}, \boldsymbol{\theta}) = \prod_{i=1}^{n} \left(\lambda e^{\varphi t_i} e^{\boldsymbol{\beta}'\mathbf{X}_i}\right)^{\delta_i} e^{-\frac{\lambda}{\varphi}(e^{\varphi t_i}-1)e^{\boldsymbol{\beta}'\mathbf{X}_i}} \qquad (2.11)$$

with $\boldsymbol{\theta} = (\lambda, \varphi)$ in the Gompertz model.

Example 2.6
Table 2.1 gives the results for the parametric proportional hazards model with the Weibull, exponential, and Gompertz baseline hazard, respectively, analyzing the Halluca data from Example 1.3.

Analysis was performed using PROC NLMIXED in SAS by maximizing the likelihood function given (2.10) and (2.11). The likelihood in the exponential model is obtain from (2.10) with $\nu = 1$. Both the Weibull and the Gompertz model provide a much better fit compared to the exponential model based on the values of the log-likelihood function. The cost of the better fit is an additional parameter. The exponential model is nested in the Weibull

Table 2.1: Parametric proportional hazards models for Halluca data.

parameter	Weibull	exponential	Gompertz
age (in years)	0.010 (0.003)	0.010 (0.003)	0.010 (0.003)
sex (females)	-0.166 (0.071)	-0.173 (0.071)	-0.151 (0.071)
type (NSCLC)	-0.136 (0.067)	-0.162 (0.066)	-0.114 (0.067)
ECOG (3 & 4)	0.612 (0.103)	0.619 (0.104)	0.595 (0.104)
stage II	0.455 (0.168)	0.431 (0.172)	0.418 (0.171)
stage IIIa	0.606 (0.131)	0.661 (0.130)	0.596 (0.132)
stage IIIb	0.970 (0.120)	1.043 (0.120)	0.971 (0.120)
stage IV	1.358 (0.110)	1.466 (0.109)	1.357 (0.110)
λ	0.029 (0.007)	0.018 (0.004)	0.023 (0.006)
ν	0.859 (0.019)		
φ			0.022 (0.003)
log-likelihood	-4858.672	-4883.351	-4858.707

as well as Gompertz models. Consequently, the two models can be compared by means of the likelihood ratio test, which yields a test statistic $\chi^2 = -2(-4883.351+4858.672) = 49.358$ (Weibull vs. exponential model) and $\chi^2 = -2(-4883.351 + 4858.707) = 49.288$ (Gompertz vs. exponential model). Both test statistics follow asymptotically an χ^2-distribution with one degree of freedom, resulting in p-values less than 0.001. Hence, the additional parameter in the Weibull and Gompertz distributions cause a significant improvement in the fit to the data. The Gompertz model show a similar value of the log-likelihood function compared to the Weibull model, with both models having the same number of parameters.

Age (in years) is the only continuous variable in the model. An increase in age by 10 years results, for an example, in an increased risk of $e^{0.1}$=1.1. Females show a reduced risk of $e^{-0.166}$=0.85 compared to males (using the results from the Weibull model). Patients with non-small-cell lung carcinoma have a reduced risk of $e^{-0.136}$=0.87 compared to patients with small-cell lung carcinoma. Patients with bad performance status (ECOG 3 or 4) at baseline face a higher risk ($e^{0.612}$=1.84) compared to patients with ECOG status less or equal to 2. We see an increasing risk with higher disease stage. For example, the hazard ratio of patients in stage IV is $e^{1.358} = 3.89$ times higher compared to patients with stage I who serve as reference group. □

The parameter estimates depend on the parametric assumption about the baseline hazard. This limits the applicability of the parametric proportional hazards model because more detailed investigations about the shape of the baseline hazard are necessary. The Weibull model is the only one that is a proportional hazards model as well as an accelerated failure time (AFT) model. Parameters can easily be transformed from one model to the other and back. Similar to the proportional hazards model the AFT model allows an easy and natural interpretation of the parameter estimates and is discussed in Section 2.5.2. However, the main focus of the present book is on extensions of the proportional hazards model, the AFT model is considered here for completeness only.

It turns out that the parametric approach is much more important in frailty models than in proportional hazards models without random effects because of additional technical estimation problems in the frailty approach. Other choices are of course possible, but in the sequel we will mainly use the Weibull and Gompertz baseline hazard functions in parametric models.

In the common semiparametric case (without parametric specification of the baseline hazard function), the model is natural and sufficiently flexible to suit many purposes. Since $e^{\beta' \mathbf{X}}$ is always positive, the individual hazard $\mu(t|\mathbf{X})$ is automatically nonnegative for all t and all values of β. One additional reason for considering this model is that censoring and competing risks are easily accommodated within this formulation. Since the likelihood contains the unspecified hazard function, the use of the traditional maximum likelihood method becomes problematic. Therefore, we need an adapted version of the likelihood that contains sufficient information about the parameter vector β but not the unspecified baseline hazard. Cox (1972, 1975) suggested using a partial likelihood approach. In this particular case, the technical problems of statistical inference have a simple solution if the baseline hazard is considered an infinite-dimensional nuisance parameter. Denote the observed data with sample size n by $(t_i, \delta_i, \mathbf{X}_i)$ $(i = 1, \ldots, n)$ and assume no ties for ease of presentation. The likelihood of the survival data is given in (2.7) and can now be written in the form

$$\prod_{i=1}^{n} \left(\mu_0(t_i) e^{\beta' \mathbf{X}_i} \right)^{\delta_i} \exp \left(- M_0(t_i) e^{\beta' \mathbf{X}_i} \right). \tag{2.12}$$

Based on arguments from nonparametric maximum likelihood estimation, a discrete version of the baseline hazard $\mu_0(\cdot)$ is assumed, which is zero except for the times t_i at which an event takes place (similar to the Nelson–Aalen estimator). This leads to a discrete version of the cumulative baseline hazard function

$$M_0^d(t) = \sum_{t_j \leq t} \mu_0(t_j).$$

Plugging this discrete cumulative baseline hazard function into the likelihood (2.12) results in

$$\prod_{i=1}^{n} \left(\mu_0(t_i) e^{\beta' \mathbf{X}_i} \exp \left(- \mu_0(t_i) \sum_{j \in R(t_i)} e^{\beta' \mathbf{X}_j} \right) \right)^{\delta_i}, \tag{2.13}$$

where $R(t)$ denotes the risk set at time t containing all individuals (more exactly their indices) that are still at risk of experiencing the event of interest at time t. This is a modified likelihood function that can be used to find estimates of the (discrete) baseline hazard function. Taking the logarithm and the partial derivative with respect to $\mu_0(t_i)$ of expression (2.13) we get

$$\frac{1}{\mu_0(t_i)} - \sum_{j \in R(t_i)} e^{\boldsymbol{\beta}' \mathbf{X}_j}.$$

Equating these partial derivatives to zero implies

$$\hat{\mu}_0(t_i) = \frac{\delta_i}{\sum\limits_{j \in R(t_i)} e^{\boldsymbol{\beta}' \mathbf{X}_j}}. \tag{2.14}$$

Plugging in this solution into expression (2.13), a likelihood function for the regression parameters is obtained:

$$L(\boldsymbol{\beta}) = \prod_{i=1}^{n} \left(\frac{e^{\boldsymbol{\beta}' \mathbf{X}_i}}{\sum\limits_{j \in R(t_i)} e^{\boldsymbol{\beta}' \mathbf{X}_j}} \right)^{\delta_i}. \tag{2.15}$$

This expression is called *partial likelihood* and does not depend on the baseline hazard $\mu_0(t)$, which simplifies parameter estimation. It is used to estimate the regression coefficients in the semiparametric proportional hazards model. The second derivative of the partial likelihood function is well behaved in the sense that the negative of the second derivative is always positive definite (or semidefinite). This is in contrast to the behavior of general likelihoods, which are only known to fulfill this property locally around the parameter estimate. The second derivative of the partial likelihood can be used to evaluate the (asymptotic) variance.

Inference for the Cox estimator is almost exclusively based on asymptotic results (Andersen and Gill 1982). The validity of these large sample properties have been found acceptable with moderately large sample sizes, moderate amount of censoring, and balanced covariates. This semiparametric model is the most often applied one in survival analysis. It is implemented in all statistical packages, is very easy to handle, and results allow an easy and intuitive interpretation.

Expression (2.14) forms the basis for the well-known Breslow estimator of the cumulative hazard function

$$\hat{M}_0(t) = \sum_{i=1}^{n} \frac{1(t_i \leq t)\delta_i}{\sum\limits_{j \in R(t_i)} e^{\boldsymbol{\beta}' \mathbf{X}_j}}.$$

The Breslow estimator of the cumulative hazard function can be used to create a corresponding estimator for the survival function. It is based on the exponential formula (2.2)

$$\hat{S}(t|\mathbf{X}) = e^{-\hat{M}_0(t) e^{\boldsymbol{\beta}' \mathbf{X}}}.$$

Hypothesis testing in the Cox model for a single regression parameter, usually for testing the null hypothesis $H_0 : \beta_j = \beta_0$ (with β_0 as specified value, often zero) versus the alternative hypothesis $H_A : \beta_j \neq \beta_0$, can be performed in three different ways. The first one is a likelihood ratio test based on the partial likelihood $L(\cdot)$, treating it as an ordinary likelihood function. Under the null hypothesis, the test statistic

$$T = -2\Big(\log \frac{L(\beta_0)}{L(\hat{\beta}_j)} \Big)$$

is asymptotically χ^2 distributed with one degree of freedom. Here $\hat{\beta}_j$ denotes the maximum likelihood estimate of regression parameter β_j. Alternatively, if several regression parameters need to be tested jointly in one test procedure, the test statistic is again asymptotically χ^2 distributed and the number of parameters tested defines the number of degrees of freedom.

A simple alternative to the likelihood ratio test is the Wald test with test statistic

$$T = \Big(\frac{\hat{\beta}_j - \beta_0}{se(\hat{\beta}_j)} \Big)^2,$$

which is also asymptotically χ^2 distributed with one degree of freedom under the null hypothesis. Here, the standard error se of the parameter estimate is found from the inverse of the second derivatives of the partial likelihood function.

A third but less frequently used possibility for parameter testing is the score test with test statistic

$$T = -\frac{l_1^2}{l_2}$$

where

$$l_1 = \frac{\partial \log L(\boldsymbol{\beta})}{\partial \beta_j}\Big|_{\beta_j = \hat{\beta}_j}$$

and

$$l_2 = \frac{\partial^2 \log L(\boldsymbol{\beta})}{\partial \beta_j^2}\Big|_{\beta_j = \hat{\beta}_j}$$

are the first- and second-order derivatives of the logarithm of the partial likelihood function under the alternative hypothesis. Similar to the other two tests the test statistic follows under the null hypothesis asymptotically a χ^2 distribution with one degree of freedom.

Example 2.7

In the following the Cox model is applied to the data from the Halluca study. In Table 2.2 the parameter estimates of the (semiparametric) Cox model are given. For comparison, the parameter estimates from the Weibull proportional hazards model are given as well. Despite the fact that the baseline hazard in

Table 2.2: Proportional hazards models for Halluca data.

parameter	Weibull PH	Cox model
age (in years)	0.010 (0.003)	0.009 (0.003)
sex (females)	-0.166 (0.071)	-0.162 (0.071)
type (NSCLC)	-0.136 (0.067)	-0.125 (0.067)
ECOG (3 & 4)	0.612 (0.103)	0.610 (0.104)
stage II	0.455 (0.168)	0.455 (0.169)
stage IIIa	0.606 (0.131)	0.594 (0.131)
stage IIIb	0.970 (0.120)	0.947 (0.120)
stage IV	1.358 (0.110)	1.345 (0.110)
λ	0.029 (0.007)	
ν	0.859 (0.019)	

the parametric approach is modeled by a Weibull distribution, the parameter estimates and standard errors in both models are very similar. The interpretation of the parameters is similar in both models, and the hazard ratios e^β are usually interpreted as relative risks. Estimates in the Weibull model depend on the correctness of the assumption of the baseline hazard. ☐

The partial likelihood depends only on the ranking of the observations, that is, the order in which the events happen, but not on the actual times. This can be illustrated by varying observations, keeping the ranks unchanged. Then there is no change in the parameter estimate, but if the ranks are changed, the estimate is changed. In this sense, the parameter estimator is a step function and not a continuous function. This underlines the importance of measuring event times as accurately as possible (for example, in days) to get the ranks right and to prevent tied observations. If this is impossible because of important measurement error in the event times (as with cancer diagnosis), it might be preferable to use a parametric Cox model to avoid discontinuities in the likelihood function.

Samuelsen (2003) investigates advantages and limitations of exact inference in the proportional hazards regression model and compares it with logistic and conditional logistic regression.

Note that covariate vector **X** could vary with time, but this is beyond the scope of this book.

2.5.2 Accelerated failure time model

The second important regression model in survival analysis is the accelerated failure time (AFT) model (Lawless 1982, Kalbfleisch and Prentice 2002). The Cox model and its various generalizations are mainly used in the medical and biostatistical field, while the AFT model is primarily applied in reliability theory and industrial experiments and as an alternative if the proportional hazards assumption does not hold. The hazard of the AFT regression model can be written in the form

$$\mu(t|\mathbf{X}) = \mu_0(te^{\boldsymbol{\beta}'\mathbf{X}})e^{\boldsymbol{\beta}'\mathbf{X}}, \tag{2.16}$$

with $\mu_0(\cdot)$ as baseline hazard. Due to computational difficulties AFT models are mainly used based on parametric approaches with log-normal, gamma, and inverse Gaussian baseline hazards. In contrast to the proportional hazards model, the AFT model can best characterized and interpreted in terms of the survival function. Assuming a model with only one single binary covariate X (for example, indicating treatment (X=1) and control group (X=0) in a randomized clinical trial) for the survival function, the relation

$$S(t|X = 1) = S(e^{\beta}t|X = 0)$$

holds. The hazard function (2.16) of an individual in the control group is then the baseline hazard $\mu(t|0) = \mu_0(t)$. The factor e^{β} is called acceleration factor, meaning that the probability to survive time point t in the treatment group is similar to the probability to survive time point te^{β} in the control group. This means, for example, that the median survival time of a patient in the treatment group is e^{β} times that of a patient in the control group. In fact, the same argument holds for any percentile of the event time distribution. Hence, individuals age e^{β}-times faster in some biological sense in the control group compared to the treatment group, which allows a very simple and, especially for clinicians, attractive and natural interpretation of the model parameters.

The AFT model will not be treated in detail here in this book, but we would like to mention that these models offer a number of advantages. In particular, they provide a wide variety of shapes of baseline hazard functions since the family includes unimodal hazards such as the one in the log-normal distribution. Furthermore, the loglinear formulation of such models underlines that the roles of regression and dispersion parameters are clearly separated (Keiding et al. 1997).

Example 2.8

In the present analysis, PROC LIFEREG from SAS is used to apply Weibull, exponential, and log-logistic AFT models to the Halluca lung cancer data from Example 1.3. The results are given in Table 2.3. As already mentioned in the paragraph about the parametric proportional hazards model, the model with a parametric Weibull baseline hazard function is also an AFT model,

Table 2.3: Parametric AFT models for Halluca data

parameter	Weibull	exponential	log-logistic
age (in years)	-0.011 (0.003)	-0.010 (0.003)	-0.014 (0.004)
sex (females)	0.193 (0.083)	0.178 (0.071)	0.182 (0.092)
type (NSCLC)	0.161 (0.078)	0.159 (0.067)	0.048 (0.088)
ECOG (3 & 4)	-0.705 (0.121)	-0.638 (0.103)	-1.210 (0.150)
stage II	-0.532 (0.196)	-0.488 (0.169)	-0.545 (0.201)
stage IIIa	-0.707 (0.152)	-0.646 (0.131)	-0.766 (0.156)
stage IIIb	-1.131 (0.140)	-1.037 (0.120)	-1.205 (0.144)
stage IV	-1.584 (0.128)	-1.463 (0.109)	-1.662 (0.130)
intercept	4.139 (0.278)	4.022 (0.239)	4.030 (0.297)
ν	0.859 (0.019)		
κ			0.848 (0.020)
log-likelihood	-2766.666	-2791.216	-2786.161

and parameters can be transformed from one model to the other. Denoting the regression parameters in the AFT model by β^* for the parameters of the proportional hazards model hold $\beta = -\nu\beta^*$ with ν from the Weibull baseline hazard. Parameter λ is given by $\lambda = \exp(-\nu \times \text{intercept})$. The interpretation of the regression parameters in both models is completely different. Note the opposite sign of the model parameters in the proportional hazards and AFT models. The hazard ratio of patients with disease stage IV is around $e^{1.358}$=3.89 times higher compared to patients with stage I (reference group) in the proportional hazards model, interpreted as relative risk. In the AFT model the expression $e^{-1.584} = 0.21$ indicates a reduction of survival time by this factor, meaning that patients in stage group IV experience the event around five times faster than patients in risk group I.

Similar to the parametric proportional hazards model, the Weibull model shows a significant improvement compared to the exponential model. The exponential AFT model is not nested in the log-logistic AFT model. Hence, for comparison of the two models the Akaike Information Criterion (AIC) should be used (Akaike 1974). The AIC statistic is given by the expression -2(log-likelihood+ #parameters), where #parameters denote the number of model parameters. Consequently, the AIC value is 8.11 for the comparison of the exponential and log-logistic model. This favors the log-logistic compared to the exponential model, which is not a proportional hazards model. Because of the same number of parameters in both the Weibull as well as log-logistic models the Weibull model performs better based on the log-likelihood. The AFT model is more robust with respect to unobserved covariates compared to the proportional hazards model (Hougaard et al. 1994, Hougaard 1999). Orbe et al. (2002) compare Cox and AFT models in detail and discuss their advantages and limitations.　　　　　　　　　　　　　　　　　　　　　　　　　□

2.6   Identifiability Problems

The assumption of independent censoring is made in numerous applications of lifetime experiments. Of course, for a number of reasons, one can assume some of the risks to be acting independently, namely, the end of study censoring, patients moving to another location for reasons unrelated to the treatment, accidental deaths, etc. But in some situations this convenient independence assumption is of doubtful validity. Especially, different causes of death such as cancer and heart diseases are usually not independent. Hence, a need for methods in survival analysis in dependent censoring arises. Unfortunately, the observed data (T, Δ) with $T = \min\{T^*, C\}$ and $\Delta = 1(T^* \leq C)$ provides not sufficient information to determine the joint distribution of the vector (T^*, C). Cox (1959) discussed this identifiability problem first. It turns out that there exist both an independent and one or even more dependent models for (T^*, C) that generate the same joint distribution for (T, Δ) (Tsiatis 1975). It turns out that these "equivalent" independent and dependent joint distributions may have quite different marginal distributions as demonstrated by the following simple example, which is based on a two-dimensional version of the exponential distribution.

Example 2.9

(Tsiatis 1975) Let T^* and C be nonnegative random variables with joint cumulative distribution function

$$H(t^*, c) = 1 - e^{-\lambda t^*} - e^{-\mu c} + e^{-\lambda t^* - \mu c - \vartheta t^* c}.$$

The distribution of the observed data (T, Δ) is uniquely determined by the two subdistributions $H_0(t) = \mathbf{P}(T < t, \Delta = 0)$ and $H_1(t) = \mathbf{P}(T < t, \Delta = 1)$. Denote by $h(t^*, c) = \frac{\partial^2 H(t^*, c)}{\partial t^* \partial c}$ the probability density function of (T, Δ) and let $H_{t^*}(t^*, c) = \frac{\partial H(t^*, c)}{\partial t^*}$ and $H_c(t^*, c) = \frac{\partial H(t^*, c)}{\partial c}$. Then it follows for the subdistribution functions

$$
\begin{aligned}
H_0(t) &= \int\limits_{\{c < t, c < t^*\}} \int h(t^*, c)\, dt^*\, dc \\
&= \int_0^t H_c(\infty, c) - H_c(c, c)\, dc \\
&= \int_0^t (\mu + \vartheta c) e^{-\lambda c - \mu c - \vartheta c^2}\, dc
\end{aligned}
$$

and in a similar way

$$H_1(t) = \int\int\limits_{\{t^*<t,t^*\le c\}} h(t^*,c)\,dt^*dc$$

$$= \int_0^t H_{t^*}(t^*,\infty) - H_{t^*}(t^*,t^*)\,dt^*$$

$$= \int_0^t (\lambda + \vartheta t^*)e^{-\lambda t^* - \mu t^* - \vartheta(t^*)^2}\,dt^*.$$

Let $\bar{T}^*$ and $\bar{C}$ be independent random variables with cumulative distribution functions

$$F(t^*) = 1 - e^{-\lambda t^* - \frac{1}{2}\vartheta(t^*)^2} \text{ and } G(c) = 1 - e^{-\mu c - \frac{1}{2}\vartheta c^2}.$$

Using the foregoing notation it holds that $\bar{T} = \min\{\bar{T}^*, \bar{C}\}$ and $\bar{\Delta} = 1(\bar{T}^* \le \bar{C})$. Consequently,

$$\bar{H}_0(t) = \mathbf{P}(\bar{T} < t, \bar{\Delta} = 0)$$

$$= \int\int\limits_{\{c<t,c<t^*\}} f(t^*)g(c)\,dt^*\,dc$$

$$= \int_0^t (1 - F(c))g(c)\,dc$$

$$= \int_0^t (\mu + \vartheta c)e^{-\lambda c - \mu c - \vartheta c^2}\,dc$$

and

$$\bar{H}_1(t) = \mathbf{P}(\bar{T} < t, \bar{\Delta} = 1)$$

$$= \int\int\limits_{\{t^*<t,t^*\le c\}} f(t^*)g(c)\,dt^*\,dc$$

$$= \int_0^t (1 - G(t^*))f(t^*)\,dt^*$$

$$= \int_0^t (\lambda + \vartheta t^*)e^{-\lambda t^* - \mu t^* - \vartheta(t^*)^2}\,dt^*.$$

That means $H_0(t) = \bar{H}_0(t)$ and $H_1(t) = \bar{H}_1(t)$. Hence, the distributions of the observable random variables (T, Δ) and $(\bar{T}, \bar{\Delta})$ are equal. It is impossible to distinguish between the dependent and the independent model based on the observed data (T, Δ). One possibility to circumvent this problem is the inclusion of observed covariates into the model. □

Chapter 3

Univariate Frailty Models

This chapter focuses on the analysis of univariate data, for example, event times of unrelated individuals. Basic survival models deal with the simplest case of independent and identically distributed data. This is based on the assumption that the study population is homogeneous up to some observed covariates. Such kind of models were considered in the last chapter. However, it is a basic observation that individuals differ greatly, for example, with respect to the effects of a drug, a treatment, or the influence of various explanatory variables. This heterogeneity is often referred to as variability, and it is one of the important sources of variability in medical, epidemiological and biological applications. The issue of this chapter is unobserved heterogeneity in survival analysis. This heterogeneity may be difficult to assess, but it is nevertheless of great importance. In recent decades, a large amount of papers on frailty models have appeared. The key idea of these models is that individuals have different frailties, and that the most frail will die earlier than the less frail. Consequently, systematic selection of robust individuals takes place, which biases what is observed. When mortality rates are estimated, one may be interested in how they change over time or age. Quite often, they rise at the beginning of the observation period, reach a maximum, and then decline (unimodal hazard) or level off. This, for example, is typical for death rates of cancer patients, meaning that the longer the patient lives beyond diagnosis and treatment, the better her or his chances of survival are. But it is often an open question whether this reflects changes in the individual hazard. It is likely that unimodal hazards are often the result of selection and that they do not reflect an underlying development on the individual level. The population hazard starts to decline simply because high-risk individuals have already died, but the hazard of a given individual might well continue to increase.

If covariates are observed, then they can be included in the analysis, for example, by using the proportional hazards model. However, it is nearly impossible to include all important risk factors, perhaps because the researcher has little or no information on the individual level. This applies, for example, to population studies where often the only known variables are sex and age. Furthermore, we may not know the relevance of the risk factor or even that the factor exists. In other cases it may be impossible to measure the risk factor without great financial cost or time effort. In such cases it is useful to consider two sources of variability in duration data: variability accounted for by observable risk factors included in the model (and therefore theoretically predictable) and heterogeneity caused by unknown covariates and which is thus theoretically unpredictable. It is the latter that is of specific interest in the present chapter, and the subject of observable covariates is treated here only for completeness. Following Hougaard (1991), there are advantages in considering these two sources of variability separately: heterogeneity may explain some unexpected results or gives an alternative explanation of some results, for example, nonproportional or decreasing hazard functions. If some individuals experience a higher risk of failure, then the remaining individuals tend to form a more or less selected group with lower risk. An estimate of the individual hazard rate without taking into account the unobserved frailty will thus underestimate the hazard function to an increasingly greater extent as time goes by. Here the reader is referred to Aalen et al. (2008).

To be aware of such selection effects, mixture models could be used. That means the population is assumed to be a mixture of individuals with at least partly unknown different risks. The nonobservable risks are described by the mixture variable, which is called *frailty* in survival analysis. It is a random variable that is assumed to follow some distribution. The precise nature of the relationship between individual and population aging depends on the frailty distribution among individuals. Different choices of distributions for the unobserved covariates are possible. The general characteristics of the frailty distributions are studied in Section 3.1. Of special interest is how the effect of the frailty on the survival and hazard function can be deduced from the Laplace transform of the frailty distribution. Section 3.2 considers the discrete frailty model, including binary frailty, in detail. The gamma and log-normal distributions are discussed in Sections 3.3 and 3.4. The popularity of the log-normal frailty model stems mainly from the link with generalized mixed models, where the standard assumption is that the random effects (which are the log frailties) follow a normal distribution. Section 3.5 deals with inverse Gaussian frailty. In Sections 3.6 and 3.7 the positive stable and the power variance function (PVF) frailty models are considered. The positive stable distribution has some interesting features such as absence of finite moments. It transfers the proportional hazards condition from the conditional to the unconditional model. The PVF family contains the gamma, positive stable, and inverse Gaussian distributions as special cases. The compound Poisson frailty model is discussed in Section 3.8. It allows a subpopulation to be not at risk for the event under study. Section 3.9 considers distributions based on the concept of quadratic hazard, whereas Sections 3.10 and 3.11 discuss frailty generated by the Lévy processes and log-t frailty models. Cure models as a specific type of frailty models are discussed in Section 3.12. The frailty approach to modeling unobserved covariates is the topic of Section 3.13. Based on the choice of frailty distribution, the variance in frailty determines the degree of unobserved heterogeneity and deals as an indicator for important risk factors missing in the proportional hazards model.

3.1   The Concept of Univariate Frailty

Before starting to study specific frailty distributions in detail, we collect a few results that hold for all these distributions in general. Special focus is on the Laplace transform of the frailty because unconditional survival and hazard functions can be easily expressed using this Laplace transform. Hence, the likelihood function can also be expressed by means of the Laplace transform. This is the reason why frailty distributions with easy Laplace transforms are so popular; they allow for traditional maximum likelihood methods in parameter estimation.

To address the problem of unobserved heterogeneity in event times resulting from unobserved covariates, first Beard (1959) (in a long-time unrecognized paper) and later Vaupel et al. (1979) and Lancaster (1979) independently suggested a random effects model for durations. Beard (1959) used the term *longevity factor* rather than *frailty*. The purpose of introducing the random effect was to improve the fit of mortality models in populations. Vaupel et al. (1979) introduced the concept of frailty to the biostatistical community and applied it to population mortality data. Lancaster (1979) dealt with times of unemployment and introduced the model to the econometric literature, where the model is known as the mixed proportional hazards model (MPH). First we will consider the frailty model without observed covariates to focus on the main aspects of univariate frailty modeling. The classical and most frequently applied model assumes a proportional hazards structure that is conditional on the random effect (frailty). To be more specific, the hazard function of an individual depends on an unobservable, time-independent random variable Z. In the multiplicative hazards framework that we will focus on throughout this book, Z acts multiplicatively on the baseline hazard function μ_0

$$\mu(t|Z) = Z\mu_0(t). \tag{3.1}$$

Here, Z is considered a nonnegative random mixture variable, varying across the population. Note that a scale factor common to all subjects in the study population maybe absorbed into the baseline hazard function $\mu_0(t)$, so that frailty distributions are standardized to $\mathbf{E}Z = 1$ if the expectation of frailty distribution exists. Otherwise, another standardization has to be used as will be discussed in the positive stable model. The variance $\sigma^2 = \mathbf{V}(Z)$ (if it exists) is interpretable as a measure of heterogeneity across the population in baseline risk. When σ^2 is small, the values of Z are closely located around one. If σ^2 is large, then values of Z are more dispersed, inducing greater heterogeneity in the individual hazards $Z\mu_0(t)$. Frailty changes the individual hazard and is sometimes called *liability* or *susceptibility* in other settings. All individuals, apart from the individual frailty variable Z, are assumed to follow the same mortality pattern.

The problem is that what can be observed in a study population is not the conditional hazard but the net result for all the individuals with different values of the random variable Z. The individual frailty variable Z is assumed to be constant over time throughout the book. Approaches that relaxes this restriction are discussed in Section 7.7.

It is quite clear that a multiplicative frailty model such as (3.1) represents a rather simplified view of how heterogeneity might act. Nevertheless, simple mathematical models represent one way of understanding the consequences of heterogeneity. The assumptions that the frailty is timeindependent and that it acts multiplicatively on the underlying baseline hazard function are arbitrary, but they have been taken as the basis for much subsequent work on unobserved heterogeneity in survival analysis.

Only for the sake of completeness would we want to mention other cases of frailty models that are not based on the proportional hazards assumption. For example, the additive frailty model where frailty acts additively on the baseline hazard function. For more details of this model, see Rocha (1996), Silva and Amaral-Turkman (2004), and Tomazella et al. (2006). A more general model, including the additive as well as the multiplicative frailty model as special cases, is considered by Gupta and Gupta (2009). Proportional odds frailty models are covered in detail by Lam et al. (2002) and Lam and Lee (2004). Murphy et al. (1997) point out the link between proportional odds models and frailty models. AFT frailty models are dealt with, for example, by Anderson and Louis (1995), who use the model in bivariate survival with parametric and nonparametric frailty distributions. Keiding et al. (1997) focus on the effect of heterogeneity caused by omitted covariates and found the AFT model more stable than the proportional hazards model in the presence of heterogeneity. Klein et al. (1999) consider a normal regression model based on log-normal frailty distribution. Pan (2001) proposes a model for correlated failure times by modeling the error term of the AFT model with a frailty approach. Because of instability problems in Pan's EM algorithm, Zhang and Peng (2007) suggest a semiparametric estimation procedure based on M-estimates and the EM algorithm. Xu and Zhang (2010) develop a more stable estimation procedure in the semiparametric gamma frailty AFT model. Lambert et al. (2004) study a parametric AFT model with an additive frailty term. Further interesting papers in this direction are Schnier et al. (2004), Chang (2004) and Komárek et al. (2007). Sankaran and Gleeja (2008) suggest the use of proportional reversed hazards frailty models, which are of interest in the case of left-truncated event time data.

It is natural to introduce observed covariates into model (3.1) similar to the Cox model by

$$\mu(t|\mathbf{X}, Z) = Z\mu_0(t)e^{\boldsymbol{\beta}'\mathbf{X}} \tag{3.2}$$

with $\mathbf{X} = (X_1, \ldots, X_k)$ and $\boldsymbol{\beta} = (\beta_1, \ldots, \beta_k)$ as covariates and regression parameters, respectively. Consequently, a frailty model is a generalization of the well-known proportional hazards model. The proportional hazards model is obtained if the frailty distribution degenerates to Z=1 for all individuals. The likelihood of the data $(T_i, \Delta_i, \mathbf{X}_i, Z_i)\,(i = 1, 2, \dots, n)$ is similar to the expression (2.12) given by

$$\prod_{i=1}^{n} \left(Z_i \mu_0(t_i) e^{\boldsymbol{\beta}' \mathbf{X}_i}\right)^{\delta_i} \exp\left(- Z_i M_0(t_i) e^{\boldsymbol{\beta}' \mathbf{X}_i}\right), \tag{3.3}$$

but now conditional on the unobserved frailty variables $Z_1, Z_2, \dots, Z_n$. This likelihood forms the basis for further parameter estimation. The random effect (frailty) can be integrated out (in closed form or by numerical or stochastical integration, depending on the frailty distribution) to get a likelihood function not depending on unobserved quantities. Estimation procedures now depend on whether a parametric or a semiparametric model is chosen. Inference for the semiparametric frailty model with results about uniform consistency and weak convergence are established under mild regularity assumptions for all parameters, including the baseline hazard function, in Kosorok et al. (2004). The paper is restricted to the case of one-parameter frailty distributions, which covers most of the common frailty distributions used. If the model is correctly specified, its method is efficient, achieving the semiparametric information bound for all parameter components. Detailed results are also given for the case of misspecified frailty distribution.

For the sake of simplicity, we will restrict our treatment to the model (3.1) sometimes in order to focus on the main ideas of frailty models. Let $S(t|Z)$ denote the survival function of an individual conditional on the frailty Z:

$$S(t|Z) = e^{- \int_0^t \mu(s|Z)\,ds} = e^{-Z \int_0^t \mu_0(s)\,ds} = e^{-Z M_0(t)}. \tag{3.4}$$

Here $M_0(t) = \int_0^t \mu_0(s)\,ds$ denotes the cumulative baseline hazard function, and equation (3.4) is a generalization of relation (2.2). Up to now, the model has been described at the individual (conditional) level. However, data for this individual model are not observable. Consequently, it is necessary to consider the population level where the frailty term is integrated out. The population survival function is the weighted mean of the conditional survival functions with weights given by the density function of the frailty distribution. The population survival function is obtained from the conditional survival function $S(t|Z)$ by integrating out the frailty. It can be viewed as the (unconditional) survival function of an individual randomly drawn from the study population, and corresponds to what can actually be observed:

$$S(t) = \mathbf{E}S(t|Z) = \mathbf{E}e^{-Z M_0(t)} = \mathbf{L}(M_0(t)). \tag{3.5}$$

This is based on relation (3.4) and underlines the important role of the Laplace transform in frailty models. The derivatives of the Laplace transform can be used to obtain general results about unconditional survival distribution. For example, density and hazard function of the event times and expectation and variance of the frailty can be characterized by the Laplace transform of the frailty distribution and their derivatives

$$f(t) = -\mu_0(t)\mathbf{L}'(M_0(t))$$
$$\mu(t) = -\mu_0(t)\frac{\mathbf{L}'(M_0(t))}{\mathbf{L}(M_0(t))}$$
$$\mathbf{E}Z = -\mathbf{L}'(0)$$
$$\mathbf{V}(Z) = \mathbf{L}''(0) - (\mathbf{L}'(0))^2, \tag{3.6}$$

assuming the existence of the foregoing expressions. For example, in the case of a positive stable distribution the moments do not exist. Here, $\mathbf{L}'$ and $\mathbf{L}''$ denote the first and second derivative of the Laplace transform. Thus, if the Laplace transform has a simple form, performing this calculation is easy. The connection with the Laplace transform was first pointed out and exploited by Hougaard (1984, 1986a,b). It follows that, when seeking distributions for the frailty variable Z, it is natural to use those which have explicit Laplace transforms. This simplifies parameter estimation.

Frailty distribution describes the frailty in the population at the start of the follow-up. Frailty is assumed to be fixed for each individual over time, but the composition of the population changes as time goes by. On average, the more frail individuals die earlier. Due to this fact the frailty distribution in the population at risk changes over time. The following theorem points on this fact and establishes the link between the conditional and the unconditional model.

THEOREM 3.1
(Vaupel et al. 1979) Assume a frailty model given by formula (3.1). The population hazard $\mu(t) = \frac{f(t)}{S(t)}$ is generally $\mu(t) = \mathbf{E}(\mu(t|Z)|T > t)$, or more specifically,

$$\mu(t) = \int_0^\infty \mu(t|z)f(z|T > t)\,dz$$
$$= \mu_0(t)\int_0^\infty zf(z|T > t)\,dz, \tag{3.7}$$

where $f(z|T > t)$ represents the frailty density among the survivors of time point t.

Proof: Starting with relation (3.1) we get

$$\mu(t|z) = \frac{f(t|z)}{S(t|z)} = z\mu_0(t)$$

$$f(t|z) = z\mu_0(t)S(t|z)$$

$$f(t,z) = z\mu_0(t)S(t|z)f_Z(z)$$

$$f(t) = \mu_0(t)\int_0^\infty zS(t|z)f_Z(z)\,dz$$

with f_Z as p.d.f. of the frailty distribution. Hence,

$$\mu(t) = \frac{\mu_0(t)\int_0^\infty zS(t|z)f_Z(z)\,dz}{S(t)}.$$

Because survival of time point t implies a death time that is greater than t, it holds that

$$f(z, T > t) = \int_t^\infty f(z,s)\,ds$$

$$= f_Z(z)\int_t^\infty z\mu_0(s)S(s|z)\,ds$$

$$= f_Z(z)S(t|z)$$

$$f(z|T > t) = \frac{f_Z(z)S(t|z)}{S(t)}. \tag{3.8}$$

This completes the proof. ■

The hazard of the population is thus interpreted as the weighted mean of individual hazards among the survivors (see formula (3.7)). The weights are determined by the frailty distribution. Frail individuals with high values of Z will tend to die first. For example, an individual with frailty equal to two is twice as likely to die as a standard individual with frailty equal to one. An individual with frailty equal to 0.5 experiences only half of the risk to die compared to a standard individual. Thus, the average frailty of the surviving cohort $\int_0^\infty zf(z|t)\,dz$ will decline with time, or more generally, the frailty distribution of the survivors is changing. Consequently, equation (3.7) implies that the hazard for individuals increases more rapidly than for the cohort to which the individuals belong. In this sense, individuals age faster than their cohort (see Figure 3.1). An illustrative example is given in the paper by Manton and Stallard (1981), describing the different mortality patterns of heterogeneous populations. The frailty was introduced in order to interpret mortality data more appropriately. The proposed model is a univariate model where each subject owns it individual frailty value, thus allowing for individual differences in hazard functions. The main objective of Vaupel et al. (1979) and Manton and Stallard (1981) was to point out that the population hazard does not reflect the hazard of individuals from that population as shown earlier.

This kind of leveling-off effects in population hazard functions are reported by Vaupel et al. (1998) for different populations such as humans, med flies, fruit flies, nematodes, yeast, and automobiles. Vaupel et al. (1979) used the frailty approach to derive the individual hazard function based on the population hazard function obtained from life tables. Finkelstein (2008) analyzes the asymptotic behavior of unconditional (mixed) hazard functions. It can be shown that, in some special cases, even for increasing conditional hazards the unconditional hazard function asymptotically decreases to zero. Furthermore, the asymptotic behavior of the unconditional hazard depends only on the behavior of the frailty distribution in the neighborhood of the left end point of its support and not on the whole frailty distribution.

Equation (3.8) gives the distribution of the frailty among the survivors at time point t, which will be used in the EM algorithm for parameter estimation later on. The frailty distribution of those individuals who die at time point t is a result of Bayes' formula:

$$f(z|t) = \frac{f(z,t)}{f(t)} = \frac{f(t|z)f(z)}{f(t)}. \tag{3.9}$$

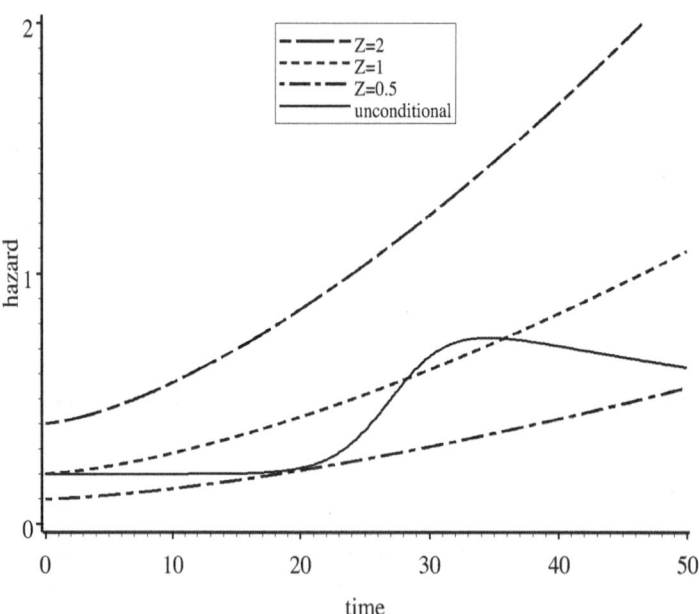

Figure 3.1:   Conditional and unconditional hazard functions of a fictive heterogeneous population.

To prove the existence of unobserved heterogeneity in a population, stress experiments with laboratory animals (e.g., insects, worms) were suggested. The idea of using data from stress experiments for testing the heterogeneity assumption is based on the belief that the same exposure to stress produces different survival outcomes in heterogeneous and homogeneous populations after the exposure to stress. During the exposure, the heterogeneous study population will experience higher selection (since the frailer individuals die first). In the homogenous group, mortality is driven by randomness and not by selecting the frailer individuals. Hence, after exposure to stress, mortality of the stress group should be lower than that of the control group. Frailty models focus only on aspects of unobserved heterogeneity, which is of course a simplification. For example, the concept of adaptation is not included in the frailty models considered here. Adaptation means that individuals can adapt to stress after exposition to moderate stress. Debilitation is the opposite effect after stress exposure. Both effects are not included in the frailty concept because frailty in statistical modeling is usually assumed to be time constant, excluding the time-dependent effects of adaptation or debilitation. For more details see a series of discussion papers, for example, Khazaeli et al. (1995), Drapeau et al. (2000), Mueller et al. (2003), Wu et al. (2006), Rose et al. (2006), and Rockwood and Mitnitski (2007).

Under model (3.2), the unconditional hazard function can be expressed as the expectation of the hazard function (Nielsen et al. 1992) conditional on being at risk at time t and covariate vector $\mathbf{X}$; that is,

$$\mu(t|\mathbf{X}) = \mu_0(t)e^{\boldsymbol{\beta}'\mathbf{X}}\mathbf{E}(Z|T > t, \mathbf{X}).$$

Taking the expectation above represents an averaging over all individuals in the population. Since the expectation is conditional on being at risk at time point t, it implies averaging over a subset of the original population. Hence, relative weights for hazards with high frailty become smaller as time goes by, corresponding to high mortality. An important implication is that studies of human aging based on cohort mortality data may be systematically biased or based on erroneous functional forms. The precise nature of the relationship between individual and cohort aging depends on the distribution of the frailty among individuals. Different choices for the frailty distribution are possible. Some main results can be found in Vaupel and Yashin (1985). Note that a parametric specification of the frailty distribution is a matter of mathematical convenience, and we will follow this line. However, this parametric specification is not necessary. Especially in the econometric field this is a topic of research. For example, Heckman and Singer (1984a) estimate the frailty distribution nonparametrically but under parametric assumptions on the baseline hazard. Horowitz (1999) proposes strategies to estimate both the frailty distribution and the baseline hazard nonparametrically. It turns out, that it is very difficult to estimate the frailty distribution in real data applications, see Heckman and Taber (1994), Kortram et al. (1995), and

Horowitz (1999). For an extensive overview of identifiability results regarding frailty models with unspecified frailty distribution, see van den Berg (2001). A short summary of the most important identifiability results related to the different univariate and multivariate frailty models considered in this book is given in Section 7.8. However, analytical results are sparse and in many situations simulations are the only way to deal with this often overlooked problem.

Assigning a probability distribution to frailty implies that frailty can be integrated out in the likelihood function. After this integration the likelihood can be maximized in the usual way if an explicit form of it exists. Otherwise, more sophisticated approaches like numerical integration or Markov Chain Monte Carlo methods need to be applied. In the following sections different frailty distributions are discussed. The most often used frailty distributions are the gamma and the log-normal distribution. The positive stable and the inverse Gaussian distribution are also common. Using a larger distribution family provides for a better fit but at the cost of additional parameters and more complex models. We will consider the power variance function (PVF) distribution as an example of such a large mixing distribution family, which includes the gamma and inverse Gaussian distributions as special cases. Only very few results are published in the literature on comparing models with different frailty distributions; much more research is needed in this important research area. In the following we will compare different frailty distributions and discuss their specific advantages and limitations in applications to real data examples.

The term *frailty* originates from gerontology where it is used to indicate the susceptibility to mortality and morbidity. However, there is a lack of agreement as to what determines the medical and gerontological concept of frailty (Rockwood 2005, Rockwood and Mitnitski 2007 and references therein). In the fields of biostatistics and demography, frailty is interpreted as a random effect. This statistical definition of frailty is different from the frailty used in the fields of gerontology and medicine, and the two concepts should not be mixed. Frailty in biostatistics and demography is usually assumed to be constant over time for an individual (for a few exceptions, see Section 7.7) with an interpretation as a random effect. In the medical and gerontological context frailty is assumed to be changing, usually increasing over time. Univariate frailty models in biostatistics are often used to model the effect of unobserved heterogeneity (unobserved covariates), whereas in the medical context the main objective is to find surrogate measures (specific scores, for example, with respect to the activity of daily living) for frailty to identify frail individuals. In contrast, determining which individuals are frail seems to be of less importance for frailty models in biostatistics and demography.

A deeper discussion of the variety of frailty concepts from a medical and gerontological point of view is beyond the scope of this book. For more details see Morley et al. (2002) and references therein.

3.2 Discrete Frailty Model

As a simple introduction and explanation of univariate frailty models, the study population is considered as consisting of two subpopulations. Both subpopulations are assumed to be homogeneous with different risks. This model is called the *binary frailty model*. This could, for example, correspond to the presence/nonpresence of a specific disease genotype. If no detailed information on the disease genotype of each individual exists, it is impossible to include the genotype in the analysis such as an observed covariate. Instead we have to consider the genotype as unobserved covariate. Let us assume that the proportion of individuals carrying the disease genotype η_1 is π. Hence, a randomly selected person from the population carries the genotype with probability π. Naturally, this leads to an increased variation in the response time when compared to the case where the genotype is known. Furthermore, assume that $\mathbf{P}(Z = \eta_1) = \pi$ and $\mathbf{P}(Z = \eta_2) = 1 - \pi$. In this case, it holds for the Laplace transform $\mathbf{L}$ and their derivatives

$$\mathbf{L}(u) = \pi e^{-u\eta_1} + (1 - \pi)e^{-u\eta_2}$$
$$\mathbf{L}'(u) = -\pi\eta_1 e^{-u\eta_1} - (1 - \pi)\eta_2 e^{-u\eta_2}$$
$$\mathbf{L}''(u) = \pi\eta_1^2 e^{-u\eta_1} + (1 - \pi)\eta_2^2 e^{-u\eta_2}.$$

The expectation and variance of a binary-distributed frailty variable can now be obtained from the derivatives of the Laplace transform (3.6)

$$\mathbf{E}Z = \pi\eta_1 + (1 - \pi)\eta_2$$
$$\mathbf{V}(Z) = \pi\eta_1^2 + (1 - \pi)\eta_2^2 - (\pi\eta_1 + (1 - \pi)\eta_2)^2$$
$$= \pi(1 - \pi)(\eta_1 - \eta_2)^2.$$

The survival and density function can now be easily derived from the Laplace transform by using (3.5)

$$S(t) = \mathbf{L}(M_0(t)) = \pi e^{-\eta_1 M_0(t)} + (1 - \pi)e^{-\eta_2 M_0(t)}$$

and

$$f(t) = \pi\eta_1\mu_0(t)e^{-\eta_1 M_0(t)} + (1 - \pi)\eta_2\mu_0(t)e^{-\eta_2 M_0(t)}.$$

This implies the hazard

$$\mu(t) = \frac{\pi\eta_1 e^{-\eta_1 M_0(t)} + (1 - \pi)\eta_2 e^{-\eta_2 M_0(t)}}{\pi e^{-\eta_1 M_0(t)} + (1 - \pi)e^{-\eta_2 M_0(t)}}\mu_0(t). \tag{3.10}$$

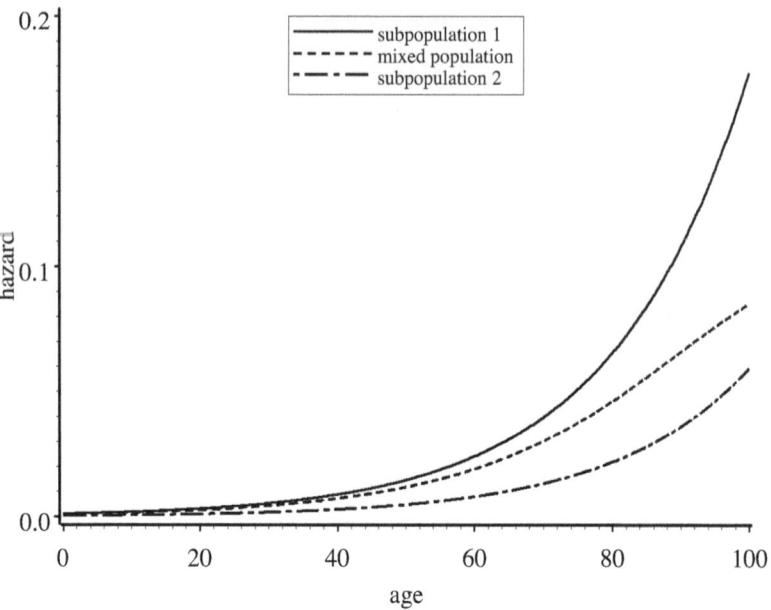

Figure 3.2: Mortality hazards of two populations with Gompertz hazard $\mu_0(t) = 0.001e^{0.05t}$ and their mixed hazard. The frailty values are $\eta_1 = 1.2$ and $\eta_2 = 0.4$ for the two subpopulations. At birth, the mixed population contains 75% of subpopulation 1 and 25% of subpopulation 2. The mortality of the mixed population is given by expression (3.10). The change in the proportion of the two subpopulations is shown in Figure 3.3.

To fulfill the standardization condition $\mathbf{E}Z = 1$ in the binary frailty model, it holds $\pi\eta_1 + (1 - \pi)\eta_2 = 1$, yielding the relation

$$\eta_2 = \frac{1 - \pi\eta_1}{1 - \pi}. \tag{3.11}$$

Consequently, the model contains, with π and η_1, two additional parameters compared to the model without binary frailty. Note that the condition $\mathbf{E}Z = 1$ is not necessary in the binary frailty model, but is used here to make models comparable. Using (2.7) and highlighting the dependence of the baseline hazard distribution on parameter vector $\boldsymbol{\theta}$, the likelihood function in the binary frailty model with $\eta = \eta_1$ is of the form

$$L(\boldsymbol{\theta}, \eta, \pi) = \prod_{i=1}^{n} \left(\frac{\pi\eta e^{-\eta M_0(t_i;\boldsymbol{\theta})} + (1 - \pi\eta)e^{-\frac{1-\pi\eta}{1-\pi} M_0(t_i;\boldsymbol{\theta})}}{\pi e^{-\eta M_0(t_i;\boldsymbol{\theta})} + (1 - \pi)e^{-\frac{1-\pi\eta}{1-\pi} M_0(t_i;\boldsymbol{\theta})}} \mu_0(t_i; \boldsymbol{\theta}) \right)^{\delta_i} \tag{3.12}$$

$$\times \left(\pi e^{-\eta M_0(t_i;\boldsymbol{\theta})} + (1 - \pi)e^{-\frac{1-\pi\eta}{1-\pi} M_0(t_i;\boldsymbol{\theta})} \right).$$

Denote by $\pi(t)$ the proportion of individuals with the disease genotype (subpopulation 1) at time point t (e.g., $\pi = \pi(0)$). Consequently, $1 - \pi(t)$ denotes the proportion of the second subpopulation without the disease genotype. Here, special focus is on the proportion $\pi(t)$. This quantity changes over time as a result of the selection process. Selection takes place if the lifetimes of different subpopulations follow different mortality patterns. To calculate $\pi(t)$, we introduce the conditional survival function for individuals with the disease genotype and without the disease genotype. Conditioning is with respect to the event $\{J = j\}$, meaning that the individual belongs to subpopulation j $(j = 1, 2)$: $\mathbf{P}(T > t|J = j) = e^{-\eta_j M_0(t)}$. By using the Bayesian formula we can now write the proportion of the fraction in the form

$$
\begin{aligned}
\pi(t) = \mathbf{P}(J = 1|T > t) &= \frac{\mathbf{P}(T > t, J = 1)}{\mathbf{P}(T > t)} \\
&= \frac{\mathbf{P}(T > t|J = 1)\mathbf{P}(J = 1)}{\mathbf{P}(T > t|J = 1)\mathbf{P}(J = 1) + \mathbf{P}(T > t|J = 2)\mathbf{P}(J = 2)} \\
&= \frac{\pi e^{-\eta_1 M_0(t)}}{\pi e^{-\eta_1 M_0(t)} + (1 - \pi)e^{-\eta_2 M_0(t)}}.
\end{aligned}
\tag{3.13}
$$

The binary frailty is sometimes also called two-point frailty. Nickell (1979) used this model to account for heterogeneity in unemployment spell data. The population was divided into groups of motivated and nonmotivated searchers of a job. Furthermore, this frailty distribution was used by Vaupel and Yashin (1985) to discuss ideas of the heterogeneity and selection concept in detail, and by Schumacher et al. (1987) to model heterogeneity in clinical trials. A special case of binary frailty is dividing the population into a proportion that is at risk and a proportion that is never at risk. The terminology to describe the never-at-risk group varies from field to field. It includes "long-term survivors" (Farewell 1982) or "cured" in epidemiology (Price and Manatunga 2001), "nonsusceptibles" in toxicology (Pack and Morgan 1990), "stayers" in finite Markov transition models of occupational mobility (Blumen et al. 1955), the "nonfecundable" in fertility models (Heckman and Walker 1990), and "non-recidivists" among convicted criminals (Schmidt and Witte 1989, Maller and Zhou 2002). We will use the term *cure model* to describe such models and come back to this problem later on in Section 3.12 and Section 5.8.

Example 3.1
In Table 3.1 the results are given for the parametric binary frailty model with Weibull baseline hazard analyzing the Halluca lung cancer data. For comparison, the results of the parametric proportional hazards model with Weibull baseline hazard are given as well. The analysis was performed using PROC NLMIXED in SAS by specifying the likelihood function given in (3.12), substituting the expressions $\mu_0(t_i)$ and $M_0(t_i)$ with their regression counterparts $\mu_0(t_i)e^{\boldsymbol{\beta}'\mathbf{X}_i}$ and $M_0(t_i)e^{\boldsymbol{\beta}'\mathbf{X}_i}$, respectively. The two-point frailty model

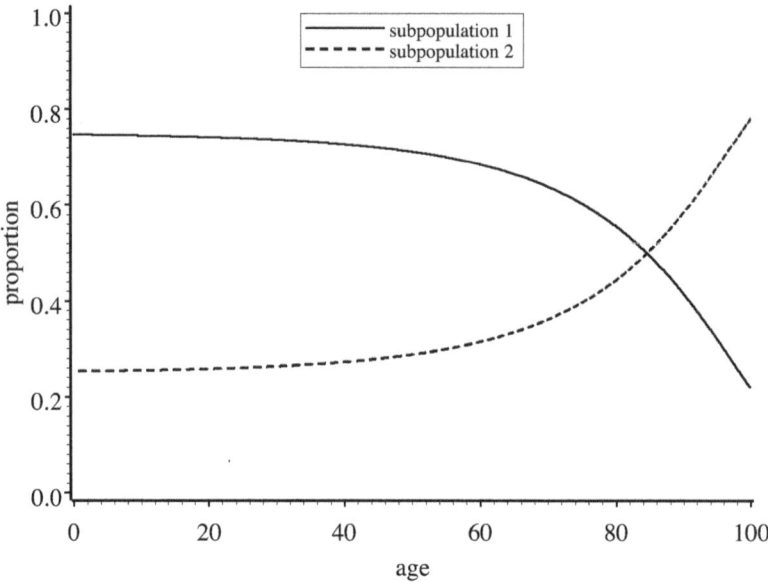

Figure 3.3: Age trajectories of the proportions of the two subpopulations in the mixing of the two Gompertz populations described in Figure 3.2. The proportions are given by (3.13). The first population (with higher mortality) dies faster over time. For this reason the hazards of the mixed population and the second subpopulation converge at older ages in Figure 3.2.

with Weibull baseline hazard provides a better fit compared to the Weibull proportional hazards model based on the comparison of the log-likelihood (see Table 3.1). Both mass points η_1, η_2 of the frailty are very different from each other. The model detects a very small subgroup of individuals with extremely high risk of death. Further detailed analysis shows that this group consists of patients in whom lung carcinoma was detected after death in the pathology (cluster 4 in Figure 1.1). Hence, for these patients, the event time is zero. The standard error for η_2 is not given because it is not a free parameter in the model (see (3.11)). ⬜

Obviously, the binary frailty model can be extended with no additional efforts to the finite discrete distribution of frailty Z (k-point distribution). In this case the hazard function is

$$\mu(t|\mathbf{X}, Z) = Z\mu_0(t)e^{\beta'\mathbf{X}}$$

with

$$\mathbf{E}Z = \sum_{j=1}^{k} \mathbf{P}(Z = \eta_j)\eta_j = 1.$$

Table 3.1: Parametric binary frailty model for Halluca data

parameter	Weibull PH	two-point frailty
age (in years)	0.010 (0.003)	0.010 (0.003)
sex (females)	-0.166 (0.071)	-0.159 (0.072)
type (NSCLC)	-0.136 (0.067)	-0.159 (0.067)
ECOG (3 & 4)	0.612 (0.103)	0.568 (0.107)
stage II	0.455 (0.168)	0.461 (0.170)
stage IIIa	0.606 (0.131)	0.620 (0.131)
stage IIIb	0.970 (0.120)	0.990 (0.120)
stage IV	1.358 (0.110)	1.388 (0.110)
λ	0.029 (0.007)	0.200 (0.080)
ν	0.859 (0.019)	0.920 (0.022)
π		0.987 (0.034)
$1 - \pi$		0.013 ($-$)
η_1		0.118 (0.168)
η_2		66.22 ($-$)
log-likelihood	-4858.672	-4844.373

Similar to the binary frailty model denote by $\pi_j(t)$ the size of the fraction of subpopulation j at time point t (e.g., $\sum_{j=1}^{k} \pi_j(t) = 1$) and $\pi_j = \pi_j(0)$. We are now interested in the behavior of $\pi_j(t)$. To calculate this function we introduce the conditional survival function. Again, conditioning is with respect to the event $\{J = j\}$, meaning that the individual belongs to the subpopulation j $(j = 1, 2, \ldots, k)$.

$$S_j(t) = \mathbf{P}(T > t | J = j) = e^{-\eta_j M_0(t)} = e^{-\eta_j \int_0^t \mu_0(s)ds}$$

Now we can write the proportion of subpopulation j on the whole population using the Bayes' formula in the form

$$\begin{aligned}
\pi_j(t) &= \mathbf{P}(J = j | T > t) \\
&= \frac{\mathbf{P}(T > t, J = j)}{\mathbf{P}(T > t)} \\
&= \frac{\mathbf{P}(T > t | J = j)\mathbf{P}(J = j)}{\sum_{i=1}^{k} \mathbf{P}(T > t | J = i)\mathbf{P}(J = i)} \\
&= \frac{\pi_j e^{-\eta_j M_0(t)}}{\sum_{i=1}^{k} \pi_i e^{-\eta_i M_0(t)}}.
\end{aligned}$$

Obviously, this is a simple generalization of relation (3.13). The proportion of subpopulation j changes over time, calculated by

$$\frac{\pi_j(t)}{dt} = -\frac{\pi_j \eta_j \mu_0(t) e^{-\eta_j M_0(t)}}{\sum_{i=1}^{k} \pi_i e^{-\eta_i M_0(t)}} + \frac{\pi_j e^{-\eta_j M_0(t)} \sum_{i=1}^{k} \pi_i \eta_i \mu_0(t) e^{-\eta_i M_0(t)}}{\left(\sum_{i=1}^{k} \pi_i e^{-\eta_i M_0(t)} \right)^2}$$

$$= \frac{\pi_j \mu_0(t) e^{-\eta_j M_0(t)}}{\sum_{i=1}^{k} \pi_i e^{-\eta_i M_0(t)}} \left(-\eta_j + \frac{\sum_{i=1}^{k} \pi_i \eta_i e^{-\eta_i M_0(t)}}{\sum_{i=1}^{k} \pi_i e^{-\eta_i M_0(t)}} \right)$$

$$= \pi_j(t) \mu_0(t) \left(\sum_{i=1}^{k} \pi_i \eta_i - \eta_j \right)$$

$$= \pi_j(t) \mu_0(t) (1 - \eta_j),$$

which holds because of $\mathbf{E}Z = \sum_{i=1}^{k} \mathbf{P}(Z = \eta_i)\eta_i = \sum_{i=1}^{k} \pi_i \eta_i = 1$. Hence, the proportion of subpopulations with frailty larger than one is decreasing because mortality is higher compared to subpopulations with smaller frailty.

In genetic studies, for example, the grouping factor is the genotype, and in most medical studies this is not directly observable. However, under a single-locus model with two alleles, A and a, three genotypes will occur; AA, Aa, and aa, with allelic frequencies of π (for A) and $1 - \pi$ (for a), respectively. Under the Hardy–Weinberg equilibrium, the expected proportions of the three unobservable genotypes are $\pi^2, 2\pi(1 - \pi)$, and $(1 - \pi)^2$. Thus, three latent classes with known expected proportions with parameter π to be estimated are assumed. If alleles are codominant, then the location of the heterozygote Aa will be midway between AA and aa. If A is dominant, then genotypes AA and Aa will coincide, and the model collapses to a two class problem. Where A is recessive, Aa and aa will coincide.

Example 3.2

In addition to binary frailty, a three-point as well as a four-point frailty distribution with Weibull baseline hazard function was applied to the Halluca data. The results are given in the third and fourth column of Table 3.2. Again, the small subgroup with extreme high risk as in the two-point frailty model can be found. Furthermore, the log-likelihood indicates a further improvement in the model by additional mass points in the discrete frailty distribution. It turns out that a five-point frailty model does not provide further significant improvement in the fit to the Halluca data (results are not shown). ⬚

We would like to point out that, in the literature, this model with a fixed number of discrete mass points is sometimes called a nonparametric frailty model, which is of course a misleading name. The notion of nonparametric (discrete) frailty should be reserved for models where the number of mass points is a random variable, which means the number of mass points is an additional parameter to be estimated (Heckman and Singer 1982b, dos Santos

Table 3.2: Discrete frailty models for Halluca data

parameter	2-point frailty	3-point frailty	4-point frailty
age (in years)	0.010 (0.003)	0.013 (0.004)	0.014 (0.004)
sex (females)	-0.159 (0.072)	-0.151 (0.086)	-0.204 (0.103)
type (NSCLC)	-0.159 (0.067)	-0.083 (0.082)	-0.160 (0.104)
ECOG (3 & 4)	0.568 (0.107)	1.034 (0.168)	1.085 (0.180)
stage II	0.461 (0.170)	0.498 (0.198)	0.592 (0.198)
stage IIIa	0.620 (0.131)	0.703 (0.151)	0.904 (0.190)
stage IIIb	0.990 (0.120)	1.096 (0.144)	1.360 (0.184)
stage IV	1.388 (0.110)	1.591 (0.131)	1.972 (0.194)
λ	0.200 (0.080)	0.201 (0.082)	0.322 (0.153)
ν	0.920 (0.022)	1.055 (0.040)	1.251 (0.080)
π_1	0.987 (0.034)	0.833 (0.065)	0.649 (0.052)
π_2	0.013 (–)	0.016 (0.004)	0.018 (0.004)
π_3		0.151 (–)	0.239 (0.065)
π_4			0.094 (–)
η_1	0.118 (0.168)	0.071 (0.024)	0.075 (0.032)
η_2	66.22 (–)	60.07 (12.95)	55.14 (10.65)
η_3		0.011 (–)	0.014 (0.008)
η_4			0.002 (–)
log-likelihood	-4844.373	-4824.343	-4820.123

et al. 1995, Lindstrom 1996). Furthermore, the standard errors in these models do not reflect uncertainty with respect to the true number of mass points. It is common to use an iterative procedure, starting with one mass point and increasing the number until the likelihood fails to show a significant improvement. Often, two or three points of support provide a sufficient fit (Guo and Rodriguez 1992). Macdonald (1999) applied two- and four-point frailty distributions to model the impact of genetics on insurance problems. Parametric proportional hazards frailty models to allow a negative binomial, Poisson, geometric or other discrete distribution of the frailty variable are considered recently by Caroni et al. (2010).

If it is known to which of the k subpopulations the individuals belong, then this can be included in the model as an observed covariate (fixed effects). This becomes problematic if the number of subpopulations and consequently the number of model parameters is large. Another possible approach is the use of different baseline hazards (stratified analysis). Here it is assumed that each subpopulation j ($j = 1, 2 \ldots, k$) has its own hazard function instead of using a common baseline in the population: $\mu(t|\mathbf{X}) = \mu_{0j}(t)e^{\beta'\mathbf{X}}$. This approach also is only applicable if the number of subpopulations is small compared to the sample size in each subpopulation. More complex designs, for example, in the context of multicenter clinical trials, are considered by Legrand et al. (2005, 2006). Their method is based on multivariate frailty models with a two-dimensional frailty distribution.

3.3   Gamma Frailty Model

The gamma distribution has been widely applied as a mixture distribution (Greenwood and Yule 1920, Beard 1959, Vaupel et al. 1979, Congdon 1995, dos Santos et al. 1995, Hougaard 2000, Duchateau and Janssen 2008). From a computational and analytical point of view, it fits very well as a mixture distribution to failure data. It is easy to derive the closed-form expressions of unconditional survival, cumulative density, and hazard function, which is due to the simplicity of the Laplace transform. This is also the reason why this distribution has been used in most applications published to date. The gamma distribution $\Gamma(k, \lambda)$ is a flexible distribution that takes a variety of shapes as k varies: when $k = 1$, it is identical to the well-known exponential distribution; when k is large, it takes a bell-shaped form reminiscent of a normal distribution (see Figure 3.4).

Despite these advantages, it is necessary to mention that no biological reason exists that makes the gamma distribution more preferable than other frailty distributions. Nearly all arguments in favor of the gamma distribution are based on mathematical and computational aspects. The paper by Abbring and van den Berg (2007) rationalizes the use of the gamma distribution for

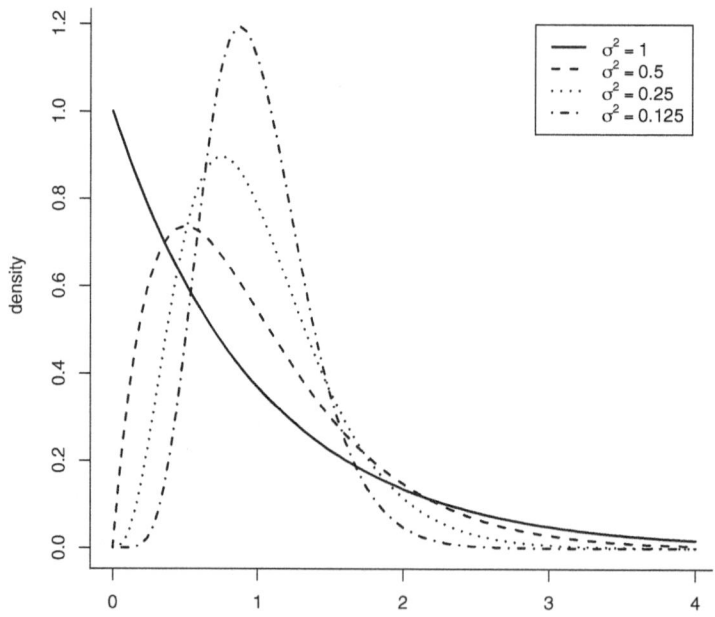

Figure 3.4:   Probability density functions of gamma distributions with expectation 1 and variances 1, 0.5, 0.25, and 0.125

frailties in time-to-event data analysis. The authors show that, in a large class of univariate frailty models, the distribution of the frailty among the survivors converges to a gamma distribution as time goes to infinity under mild regularity assumptions.

Frailty cannot be negative, and the gamma distribution is, along with the log-normal distribution, one of the most commonly used distributions to model variables that are nonnegative. The density of a gamma-distributed random variable is given by (see Section 2.3.6)

$$f(z) = \frac{1}{\Gamma(k)} \lambda^k z^{k-1} e^{-\lambda z}.$$

Consequently, for the Laplace transform it holds that

$$\begin{aligned}
\mathbf{L}(u) &= \frac{1}{\Gamma(k)} \lambda^k \int e^{-uz} z^{k-1} e^{-\lambda z} \, dz \\
&= \frac{\lambda^k}{(\lambda+u)^k} \frac{1}{\Gamma(k)} (\lambda+u)^k \int z^{k-1} e^{-(\lambda+u)z} \, dz \\
&= (1 + \frac{u}{\lambda})^{-k}.
\end{aligned}$$

Here, the equivalence of the second and third line is a consequence of the integration over the density of a gamma distribution with parameters k and $\lambda + u$. The first and second derivatives of the Laplace transform are

$$\mathbf{L}'(u) = -\frac{k}{\lambda}(1 + \frac{u}{\lambda})^{-k-1} \tag{3.14}$$

$$\mathbf{L}''(u) = \frac{k(k+1)}{\lambda^2}(1 + \frac{u}{\lambda})^{-k-2}. \tag{3.15}$$

Evaluating these derivatives at $u = 0$ implies

$$\mathbf{E}Z = \frac{k}{\lambda}$$

$$\mathbf{V}(Z) = \frac{k(k+1)}{\lambda^2} - \frac{k^2}{\lambda^2} = \frac{k}{\lambda^2}$$

To make sure that the model is identifiable, the restriction $k = \lambda$ is used for the gamma distribution, which results in $\mathbf{E}Z = 1$. Denote by $\sigma^2 := \frac{1}{\lambda}$ the variance of the frailty variable. The density of a gamma-distributed random variable $Z \sim \Gamma(\frac{1}{\sigma^2}, \frac{1}{\sigma^2})$ is given by

$$f(z) = \frac{1}{\Gamma(\frac{1}{\sigma^2})} \left(\frac{1}{\sigma^2}\right)^{\frac{1}{\sigma^2}} z^{\frac{1}{\sigma^2}-1} \exp\left(-\frac{z}{\sigma^2}\right) \tag{3.16}$$

and is depicted in Figure 3.4.

The unconditional survival function can be derived by the Laplace transform given in (3.5):

$$S(t) = \mathbf{L}(M_0(t)) = \frac{1}{(1 + \sigma^2 M_0(t))^{\frac{1}{\sigma^2}}}. \tag{3.17}$$

This implies the unconditional probability density function

$$f(t) = \frac{\mu_0(t)}{(1 + \sigma^2 M_0(t))^{\frac{1}{\sigma^2} + 1}}$$

and the unconditional hazard function

$$\mu(t) = \frac{\mu_0(t)}{1 + \sigma^2 M_0(t)}. \tag{3.18}$$

Furthermore, it turns out that the assumption about a gamma distribution of the frailty at the start of the follow-up yields some useful mathematical results, which will be discussed in detail in the following. Mainly for reasons of convenience, frailty is assumed to be constant over time for each individual. But because of the selection process that takes place as time goes by, the distribution of the frailty in the population still at risk changes over time. In the following presentation we extend the model by including Cox type regression terms into the formulas meaning substitution of the cumulative baseline hazard $M_0(t)$ with $M_0(t)e^{\beta' \mathbf{X}}$. We will show that the frailty among survivors of a specific time point is still gamma distributed but now with new parameters depending on the original parameter σ^2 and the cumulative hazard function $M_0(t)e^{\beta' \mathbf{X}}$. Furthermore, a similar result can be obtained for individuals dying at a specific time point. These results are helpful for the development of estimation procedures especially in semiparametric gamma frailty models. Using relations (3.4), (3.8), (3.16), and (3.17), the density of the frailty distribution among the survivors (indicated by the condition $T > t$) can be written in the form

$$
\begin{aligned}
f(z | \mathbf{X}, T > t) &= \frac{S(t | \mathbf{X}, z) f(z)}{S(t | \mathbf{X})} \\
&= \frac{\exp\left(-z M_0(t)e^{\beta' \mathbf{X}}\right) z^{\frac{1}{\sigma^2} - 1} \exp\left(-\frac{z}{\sigma^2}\right)}{\Gamma(\frac{1}{\sigma^2}) \sigma^{\frac{2}{\sigma^2}} \left(1 + \sigma^2 M_0(t)e^{\beta' \mathbf{X}}\right)^{-\frac{1}{\sigma^2}}} \\
&= \frac{\left(\frac{1}{\sigma^2} + M_0(t)e^{\beta' \mathbf{X}}\right)^{\frac{1}{\sigma^2}}}{\Gamma(\frac{1}{\sigma^2})} z^{\frac{1}{\sigma^2} - 1} \exp\left(-z\left(\frac{1}{\sigma^2} + M_0(t)e^{\beta' \mathbf{X}}\right)\right),
\end{aligned}
$$

which is the density of a gamma distribution with the same value of the shape parameter $\frac{1}{\sigma^2}$ as at the begin of the follow-up. The value of the second parameter, however, is now given by $\frac{1}{\sigma^2} + M_0(t)e^{\beta' \mathbf{X}}$. In a similar way (3.9) can be used to calculate the frailty distribution of individuals who die at time point t:

$$
\begin{aligned}
f(z|\mathbf{X}, T = t) &= \frac{f(t|\mathbf{X}, z)f(z)}{f(t|\mathbf{X})} \\[2mm]
&= \frac{z\mu_0(t)\exp\left(-zM_0(t)e^{\boldsymbol{\beta}'\mathbf{X}}\right)z^{\frac{1}{\sigma^2}-1}\exp\left(-\frac{z}{\sigma^2}\right)}{\Gamma(\frac{1}{\sigma^2})\sigma^{\frac{2}{\sigma^2}}\mu_0(t)\left(1+\sigma^2 M_0(t)e^{\boldsymbol{\beta}'\mathbf{X}}\right)^{-\frac{1}{\sigma^2}-1}} \\[2mm]
&= \frac{\left(\frac{1}{\sigma^2}+M_0(t)e^{\boldsymbol{\beta}'\mathbf{X}}\right)^{\frac{1}{\sigma^2}+1}}{\Gamma(\frac{1}{\sigma^2})\frac{1}{\sigma^2}}z^{\frac{1}{\sigma^2}}\exp\left(-z(\frac{1}{\sigma^2}+M_0(t)e^{\boldsymbol{\beta}'\mathbf{X}})\right) \\[2mm]
&= \frac{\left(\frac{1}{\sigma^2}+M_0(t)e^{\boldsymbol{\beta}'\mathbf{X}}\right)^{\frac{1}{\sigma^2}+1}}{\Gamma(\frac{1}{\sigma^2}+1)}z^{\frac{1}{\sigma^2}+1-1}\exp\left(-z(\frac{1}{\sigma^2}+M_0(t)e^{\boldsymbol{\beta}'\mathbf{X}})\right).
\end{aligned}
$$

This is a gamma density with the same scale parameter $\frac{1}{\sigma^2}+M_0(t)e^{\boldsymbol{\beta}'\mathbf{X}}$ as among those surviving to t but with shape parameter $\frac{1}{\sigma^2}+1$. In particular, it follows that the mean frailty among the deaths at age t is

$$
\mathbf{E}(Z|\mathbf{X}, T = t) = \frac{1+\sigma^2}{1+\sigma^2 M_0(t)e^{\boldsymbol{\beta}'\mathbf{X}}} \tag{3.19}
$$

compared to

$$
\mathbf{E}(Z|\mathbf{X}, T > t) = \frac{1}{1+\sigma^2 M_0(t)e^{\boldsymbol{\beta}'\mathbf{X}}} \tag{3.20}
$$

among the survivors at the same age. This demonstrates the selection by early death of the high-risk individuals. The individuals dying at time t have a higher mean frailty compared to the survivors of this time point. Furthermore, it holds that the frailty variance among the individuals dying at time t is

$$
\mathbf{V}(Z|\mathbf{X}, T = t) = \frac{\sigma^2(1+\sigma^2)}{(1+\sigma^2 M_0(t)e^{\boldsymbol{\beta}'\mathbf{X}})^2} \tag{3.21}
$$

and

$$
\mathbf{V}(Z|\mathbf{X}, T > t) = \frac{\sigma^2}{(1+\sigma^2 M_0(t)e^{\boldsymbol{\beta}'\mathbf{X}})^2} \tag{3.22}
$$

among the survivors. Consequently, the variance of frailty declines also over time, so the study population becomes more homogeneous in absolute terms. However, the coefficient of variation stays constant over time, so the population does not become more homogeneous relative to the mean.

The univariate gamma frailty model (without covariates) was introduced by Vaupel et al. (1979). In an earlier paper, Beard (1959) used a two-parameter gamma frailty distribution and a Gompertz–Makeham baseline hazard.

Example 3.3

Let $\mu_0(t) = \lambda e^{\varphi t}$ be a Gompertz baseline hazard and frailty follows a gamma distribution $Z \sim \Gamma(\frac{1}{\sigma^2}, \frac{1}{\sigma^2})$. Hence, the unconditional hazard and survival function are given by the expressions

$$\mu(t) = \frac{\lambda e^{\varphi t}}{1 + \sigma^2 \frac{\lambda}{\varphi}(e^{\varphi t} - 1)}$$

$$S(t) = (1 + \sigma^2 \frac{\lambda}{\varphi}(e^{\varphi t} - 1))^{-\frac{1}{\sigma^2}}$$

as a consequence of (3.17) and (3.18).   ▯

Figures 3.5 and 3.6 deal with an important topic related to univariate frailty models, the so-called crossing-over effects in the mortality hazards of different populations. Figure 3.5 shows the logarithms of two proportional baseline hazards, where the second population has a higher mortality. Assuming a higher degree of heterogeneity in this population (the variance of the gamma-distributed frailty is larger in the second population) results in the crossing-over effect because of selection shown in Figure 3.6. Higher heterogeneity implies a higher selection pressure in the second population.

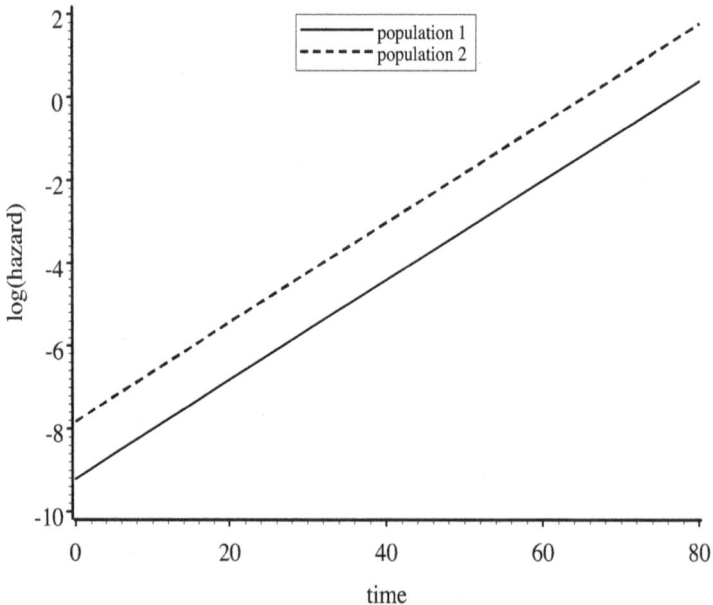

Figure 3.5: Baseline hazard functions of two populations with Gompertz hazard. The parameters are $\lambda_1 = 10^{-4}$, $\lambda_2 = 4 \times 10^{-4}$, and $\varphi_1 = \varphi_2 = 0.12$.

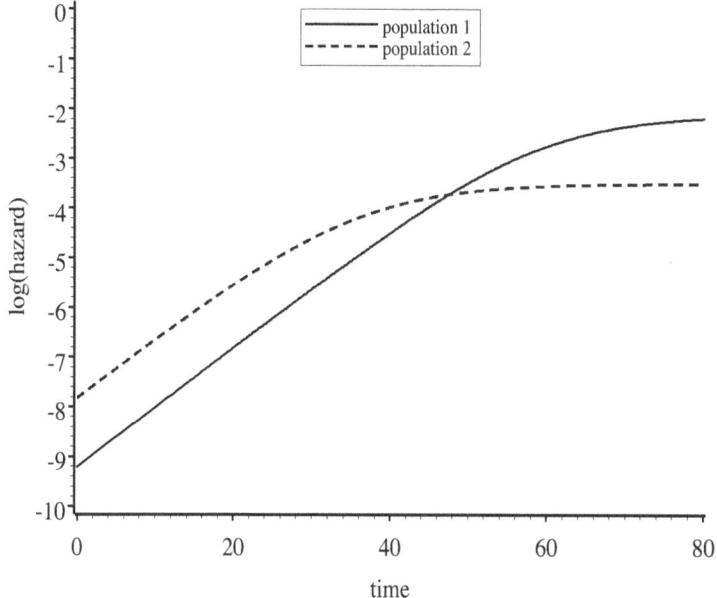

Figure 3.6: Unconditional hazards of two populations with Gompertz baseline hazard and gamma distributed frailty. The parameters of the baseline hazards are the same as in Figure 3.5. The variance of the frailty σ^2 is assumed to be one in population 1 and four in population 2.

Consequently, frailer individuals die faster in the second population than in the first. If heterogeneity is on the same level in both populations, a convergence of the hazards will be observed instead of crossing over. Such effects are described in detail by Clayton and Kaldor (1985).

These phenomena were also observed, for example, by Manton and Vaupel (1995) comparing mortality in Sweden, France, England, and Japan with that in the United States. The authors noticed that mortality was much lower in all countries except the United States up to the ages of around 65. After the age of 80, the mortality was much lower in the United States compared to the three European countries. The authors pointed out that greater heterogeneity in social and economic status and health insurance coverage in the United States may account for the higher mortality at younger ages in this country. To make this more clear, consider the form of the conditional expectation for the gamma-distributed frailty of the survivors of time t (3.20)

$$\mathbf{E}(Z|\mathbf{X}, T > t) = \frac{1}{1 + \sigma^2 M_0(t)e^{\beta'\mathbf{X}}}$$

with $M_0(t) = \int_0^t \mu_0(s)\,ds$. Clearly, the average frailty value is a decreasing function of time. The decrease is faster in situations with larger heterogeneity in the population, as measured by σ^2, a higher cumulative baseline hazard function $M_0(t)$, and larger increases due to covariates, which are modeled by the term $e^{\beta'X}$. All these factors accelerate the "frailty selection" that results from unobserved heterogeneity in individual risks.

Assume a single binary covariate X with values 0 (control group) and 1 (treatment group). Frailty selection also affects the marginal hazard ratio for treatment. Under the gamma frailty model, the marginal hazard ratio is (compare relation (3.18))

$$\frac{\mu(t|X=1)}{\mu(t|X=0)} = \frac{1+\sigma^2 M_0(t)}{1+\sigma^2 M_0(t)e^\beta}e^\beta. \tag{3.23}$$

A critical point here is that, under the proportional hazards assumption for the conditional model, the ratio of the treatment-specific population hazards is not generally timeinvariant; unless σ^2 or β is zero, the population hazard ratio (3.23) is a decreasing function. Only at time zero the population hazard ratio is equal to the conditional hazard ratio e^β. As t increases, the ratio tends to one. Under these conditions, the time-invariant hazard ratio obtained by applying a simple population model is attenuated from the conditional hazard ratio e^β. The attenuation is increased in situations with larger values of σ^2, β and $M_0(t)$, representing the three factors that accelerate frailty selection. Conversely, the attenuation is modest if any of these factors is near zero, in which case the individual- and population-averaged parameters are relatively close to each other. Formal expressions and approximations were obtained by Henderson and Oman (1999) who consider the effects of fitting a population model to conditional covariate effects. Such selection effects occur in all univariate frailty models; they are not restricted to the gamma frailty model. The advantage of the gamma frailty model is that, for all important quantities, explicit formulas can be derived in an easy way.

Example 3.4

Assume a gamma-distributed frailty model with constant baseline hazard function $\mu_0(t) = \lambda$ (exponential distribution). Consequently, using (3.17),

$$S(t) = (1+\sigma^2 M_0(t))^{-\frac{1}{\sigma^2}}$$
$$= (1+\sigma^2 \lambda t)^{-\frac{1}{\sigma^2}}$$
$$= (1+\frac{1}{\zeta}\lambda t)^{-\zeta}$$
$$= (1+\frac{1}{\omega}t)^{-\zeta}$$
$$= (\frac{\omega}{\omega+t})^\zeta,$$

with $\zeta := \frac{1}{\sigma^2}$ and $\omega := \frac{\zeta}{\lambda}$, which is a Pareto distribution with parameters ω and ζ. Clayton and Cuzick (1985a) considered this model.   ☐

3.3.1 Parametric gamma frailty model

As in the proportional hazards model in Section 2.5.1, a parametric as well as a semiparametric approach is possible. We will consider the parametric case first. Based on (3.3), the unconditional likelihood function in the frailty model is of the form

$$L(\boldsymbol{\beta}, \boldsymbol{\theta} | Z_1, \ldots, Z_n) = \prod_{i=1}^{n} \left(Z_i \mu_0(t_i; \boldsymbol{\theta}) e^{\boldsymbol{\beta}' \mathbf{X}_i} \right)^{\delta_i} e^{-Z_i M_0(t_i; \boldsymbol{\theta}) e^{\boldsymbol{\beta}' \mathbf{X}_i}}. \qquad (3.24)$$

This conditional likelihood function still depends on the unobserved frailty variables. Under the assumption of a gamma-distributed frailty, the random terms can be integrated out using relations (3.17) and (3.18), yielding the likelihood function

$$L(\boldsymbol{\beta}, \boldsymbol{\theta}, \sigma^2) = \prod_{i=1}^{n} \left(\frac{\mu_0(t; \boldsymbol{\theta}) e^{\boldsymbol{\beta}' \mathbf{X}_i}}{1 + \sigma^2 M_0(t; \boldsymbol{\theta}) e^{\boldsymbol{\beta}' \mathbf{X}_i}} \right)^{\delta_i} (1 + \sigma^2 M_0(t; \boldsymbol{\theta}) e^{\boldsymbol{\beta}' \mathbf{X}_i})^{-\frac{1}{\sigma^2}}. \qquad (3.25)$$

Example 3.5
In Table 3.3, results are given for the parametric gamma frailty model with Weibull baseline hazard function analyzing the Halluca data. For comparison, the results of the parametric proportional hazards model with Weibull baseline hazard function are given as well. The analysis was performed using PROC

Table 3.3: Parametric gamma frailty model for Halluca data

parameter	Weibull PH	gamma frailty
age (in years)	0.010 (0.003)	0.012 (0.003)
sex (females)	-0.166 (0.071)	-0.184 (0.083)
type (NSCLC)	-0.136 (0.067)	-0.114 (0.078)
ECOG (3 & 4)	0.612 (0.103)	0.861 (0.150)
stage II	0.455 (0.168)	0.516 (0.188)
stage IIIa	0.606 (0.131)	0.701 (0.148)
stage IIIb	0.970 (0.120)	1.109 (0.140)
stage IV	1.358 (0.110)	1.562 (0.136)
λ	0.029 (0.007)	0.020 (0.006)
ν	0.859 (0.019)	0.951 (0.036)
σ^2		0.254 (0.084)
log-likelihood	-4858.672	-4853.032

NLMIXED in SAS by specifying the likelihood function given in (3.25). The gamma frailty model with Weibull baseline provides a better fit compared to the Weibull proportional hazards model based on the value of the log-likelihood because of the additional parameter σ^2. The Weibull proportional hazards model is nested in the parametric gamma frailty model with Weibull baseline hazard. Consequently, the models can be compared by the likelihood ratio test, which yields a test statistic $\chi^2 = -2(-4858.672+4853.032) = 11.28$. Because the parameter value under the null hypothesis $\sigma^2 = 0$ to be tested lays on the boundary of the parameter space, standard methods cannot be applied. It turns out that the approximation of the likelihood ratio test statistic by a χ^2-distribution with one degree of freedom is too conservative (Self and Liang, 1987). Rather, a mixture of a $\frac{1}{2}\chi_0^2$ and a $\frac{1}{2}\chi_1^2$ distribution should be used (Claeskens et al. 2008). In the present example, this results in a highly significant p-value. Hence, the additional parameter in the frailty model causes a significant improvement in the fit to the data. This agrees with the small standard error of the estimate of the frailty variance, which also supports the hypothesis $\sigma^2 > 0$. In the frailty model – similar to the Weibull proportional hazards model – an increasing risk of death is seen for increasing disease stage. However, the interpretation of the hazard ratios in the frailty model is slightly different from the interpretation in the Weibull proportional hazards model. For example, the hazard ratio of patients with disease stage IV is $e^{1.562}=4.77$ times higher compared to patients in risk group I *given the same value of frailty*. Patients in group I serve as reference group. Hazard ratios have to be interpreted conditional on the frailty. In the proportional hazards model with Weibull baseline, the analogous hazard ratio for stage IV is $e^{1.358}=3.89$, meaning an increase in risk by this factor comparing patients with disease stage IV and I with similar values of all other risk factors in the model. Consequently, in the Weibull proportional hazards model (as well as in the semiparametric Cox model), comparisons are made based on (more or less hypothetical) groups where all observed covariate values are similar. In the frailty model, comparisons are made based on groups where all observed *and unobserved* covariate values are assumed to be similar.

The obtained estimates of the model parameters depend on the parametric assumption about the Weibull baseline hazard. Furthermore, in the frailty model, the parameter estimates depend additionally on the assumption of gamma distribution of frailty. In the following sections the analysis is repeated with different assumptions about frailty distribution. Typically, an absolute increase in regression parameter estimates and their standard errors can be observed. One exception here is variable type.

Different parametric gamma frailty models are applied to the Halluca data. The baseline hazard function is assumed to be exponential, Gompertz and Weibull distributed. The results are given in Table 3.4. It is easy to see that the results depend on the parametric form of the baseline hazard function. Nevertheless, in all cases, the estimated frailty variance is different from zero indicating the presence of unobserved heterogeneity. Careful considerations are necessary because the null hypothesis $\sigma^2 = 0$ is again on the boundary of the parameter space. For further details about tests for heterogeneity

Table 3.4: Parametric gamma frailty models for Halluca data

parameter	Weibull	exponential	Gompertz
age (in years)	0.012 (0.003)	0.013 (0.004)	0.012 (0.004)
sex (females)	-0.184 (0.083)	-0.192 (0.086)	-0.188 (0.085)
type (NSCLC)	-0.114 (0.078)	-0.104 (0.082)	-0.104 (0.080)
ECOG (3 & 4)	0.861 (0.150)	0.959 (0.139)	0.925 (0.160)
stage II	0.516 (0.188)	0.514 (0.195)	0.540 (0.193)
stage IIIa	0.701 (0.148)	0.726 (0.150)	0.720 (0.154)
stage IIIb	1.109 (0.140)	1.159 (0.139)	1.145 (0.151)
stage IV	1.562 (0.136)	1.630 (0.126)	1.611 (0.150)
λ	0.020 (0.006)	0.017 (0.005)	0.017 (0.005)
ν	0.951 (0.036)		
φ			-0.003 (0.007)
σ^2	0.254 (0.084)	0.344 (0.053)	0.307 (0.109)
log-likelihood	-4853.032	-4853.888	-4853.812

in the proportional hazards models see Section 7.5. The higher flexibility of the Gompertz and Weibull baseline hazard does not imply a significant improvement based on the likelihood function. If the models are not nested, then the Akaike information criteria (AIC) can be used. Consequently, the exponential model should be preferred among the three parametric models presented in Table 3.4.

This links to a general problem in the field of frailty modeling. On the one hand, parametric estimation procedures (parametric specification of the baseline hazard) are much easier to implement compared to semiparametric models. Furthermore, standard errors of the frailty variance estimate are easy to obtain. On the other hand, in many practical applications the investigator has only limited information about the form of the baseline hazard function, which makes parametric analysis difficult. Estimations in parametric frailty models can be performed with an SAS macro described by Liu and Yu (2008). This approach requires a closed-form expression of the frailty density, which is, for example, available for the gamma distribution. Otherwise, in the gamma case, the integrals in the conditional likelihood function can be integrated out explicitly without using the approximative method of Liu and Yu (2008). Here the latter method was used. □

Example 3.6

In Table 3.5 the results are given for the parametric gamma frailty model with exponential baseline hazard analyzing the EBCT data. For comparison, the results of the parametric proportional hazards model with exponential baseline hazard function are given as well. The analysis was performed using PROC NLMIXED in SAS by specifying the likelihood function given in (3.25). The gamma frailty model with exponential baseline hazard provides a better

Table 3.5: Parametric gamma frailty model for the EBCT data

parameter	gamma frailty	exponential PH
risk group II	0.23 (0.94)	0.23 (0.92)
risk group III	1.31 (0.86)	1.28 (0.83)
risk group IV	2.73 (0.82)	2.53 (0.78)
calcium (> 100)	1.60 (0.57)	1.49 (0.53)
age (55–62)	0.36 (0.51)	0.46 (0.42)
age (63–84)	0.03 (0.49)	0.15 (0.41)
λ	3.4e-4 (2.8e-4)	3.2e-4 (2.6e-4)
σ^2	0.73 (0.69)	
log-likelihood	-219.622	-220.294

fit compared to the exponential proportional hazards model based on the values of log-likelihood because of the additional parameter σ^2 in the frailty model. The exponential proportional hazards model is nested in the gamma frailty model. Consequently, the models can be compared by the likelihood ratio test, which yields a test statistic $\chi^2 = -2(-220.294 + 219.622) = 1.324$. Because of the nonstandard test situation, a mixture of a $\frac{1}{2}\chi_0^2$ and a $\frac{1}{2}\chi_1^2$ distribution should be used (Claeskens et al. 2008), which results in a p-value of p = 0.10. Hence, the additional parameter σ^2 in the frailty model does not cause a significant improvement in the fit of the data. This agrees with the large standard error of σ^2, which does not support the hypothesis $\sigma^2 > 0$. In both models we see an increasing risk for major CHD events with the higher risk group. Again, the interpretation of the hazard ratios in both models is different. For example, the hazard ratio of patients in risk group IV is $e^{2.73}$=15.3 times higher compared to patients in risk group I *given the same value of frailty* with patients in group I serving as reference group. Hazard ratios have to be interpreted conditional on unobserved frailty. However, this is in some sense similar to the traditional Cox model. In the Cox model the relative risk of a patient from risk group IV compared to a patient from risk group I is conditional on that all other risk factors (included in the model) are the same for both. In the frailty model the comparison is made under the condition that all observed, and additionally also the unobserved, factors (frailty) are equal. Furthermore, patients with calcium values higher than 100 show a $e^{1.6} = 5$ times higher risk for an event compared to patients with a calcium score less than 100 *given the same value of frailty*. Age does not play any role as a predictor. Individuals of age 23 – 54 serve as the reference group. The parameter estimates depend on the assumption about the exponential baseline hazard and, in the frailty model, on the assumption of gamma distribution of frailty. Typically, an increase in the parameter estimates away from zero as well as an increase in the standard errors can be observed. Exceptions are the estimates for the two age groups.

In Table 3.6 parametric gamma frailty models with Weibull, exponential, and Gompertz baseline hazard are compared. The gamma frailty model with

Table 3.6: Parametric gamma frailty models for the EBCT data

parameter	Weibull	exponential	Gompertz
risk group II	0.14 (1.05)	0.23 (0.94)	0.21 (0.96)
risk group III	1.62 (1.01)	1.31 (0.86)	1.36 (0.89)
risk group IV	4.29 (1.19)	2.73 (0.82)	3.06 (1.00)
calcium (> 100)	2.19 (0.73)	1.60 (0.57)	1.77 (0.65)
age (55–62)	0.16 (0.71)	0.36 (0.51)	0.27 (0.60)
age (63–84)	-0.34 (0.72)	0.03 (0.49)	-0.10 (0.59)
λ	4.9e-6 (1.0e-5)	3.4e-4 (2.8e-4)	2.2e-4 (2.4e-4)
ν	2.14 (0.50)		
φ			0.02 (0.03)
σ^2	4.45 (2.01)	0.73 (0.69)	1.60 (1.57)
log-likelihood	-215.035	-219.622	-219.402

Weibull baseline hazard function shows the best fit to the data based on the log-likelihood value. The variance of the frailty is significantly larger than zero in this model, whereas in the models with exponential and Gompertz baseline no significant unobserved heterogeneity can be detected. This makes the main drawback of parametric frailty models obvious. The interpretation of the results (here especially the question if unobserved heterogeneity is present or not) depends one the choice of the baseline hazard. Usually, the researcher has no additional prior information about the form of the baseline distribution. Consequently, the decision for the best-fitting model should be based on the likelihood ratio test if the models are nested. Here the nonstandard test situation for testing the hypothesis $\sigma^2 > 0$ versus $\sigma^2 = 0$ has been taken into account. If the models are not nested, then the Akaike information criteria (AIC) should be used. □

The unobserved frailty Z_i $(i = 1, \ldots, n)$ for each patient can be estimated based on the distribution of the frailty conditional on event time and status given in (3.19) and (3.20) by the expression

$$\hat{Z}_i = \frac{1/\hat{\sigma}^2 + \delta_i}{1/\hat{\sigma}^2 + M_0(t_i; \hat{\boldsymbol{\theta}})e^{\hat{\boldsymbol{\beta}}'\mathbf{x}_i}}. \tag{3.26}$$

Here $\hat{\sigma}^2$ denotes the estimate of the frailty variance, $\hat{\boldsymbol{\theta}}$ the vector of parameter estimates of the cumulative baseline hazard, and $\hat{\boldsymbol{\beta}}$ the vector of estimated regression coefficients. A parametric gamma frailty model with exponential baseline hazard is considered, for example, by Tomazella et al. (2008).

3.3.2   Semiparametric gamma frailty model

In the semiparametric frailty model, no assumption about the form of the baseline hazard function is made. This requires new estimation strategies compared to the parametric model. In the last section we considered the extension of the parametric proportional hazards model to the parametric gamma frailty model. In the following the extension of the semiparametric proportional hazards (Cox) model to the semiparametric gamma frailty model will be discussed. The likelihood function looks similar to the parametric model (3.25), but now the baseline hazard $\mu_0(t)$ is treated as a nuisance. In the following the EM algorithm (expectation-maximization algorithm) will be explained, which allows parameter estimation in the semiparametric gamma frailty model. This algorithm was suggested by Dempster et al. (1977) and is often used in the presence of unobserved data. It was adopted for parameter estimation in frailty models first by Nielsen et. al (1992), Klein (1992), and Guo and Rodriguez (1992). The EM algorithm iterates between two steps. In the first, one estimates the expectations of the unobserved frailties based on observed data, and current estimates are obtained. These estimates are now used in the maximization step to obtain new parameter estimates given the estimated frailties. In the gamma frailty model, closed-form expressions exist for the conditional expectations of the frailties in the expectation step. Furthermore, applying the partial likelihood approach with the estimated frailties as offset terms in the M step is easy to perform, which makes the EM algorithm useful.

First we consider the full likelihood with the frailty variables assumed to be observed random variables similar to the event times. This full likelihood results from the joint density of (t_i, δ_i, Z_i) $(i = 1, \ldots, n)$ and is of the form

$$
\begin{aligned}
L(\boldsymbol{\beta}, \sigma^2 | \mathbf{Z}) &= \prod_{i=1}^{n} f(t_i, \delta_i, Z_i; \boldsymbol{\beta}, \sigma^2) \\
&= \prod_{i=1}^{n} f(t_i, \delta_i, Z_i; \boldsymbol{\beta}) \prod_{i=1}^{n} f(Z_i; \sigma^2) \\
&= L_1(\boldsymbol{\beta} | \mathbf{Z}) L_2(\sigma^2 | \mathbf{Z})
\end{aligned}
\tag{3.27}
$$

with $\mathbf{Z} = (Z_1, \ldots, Z_n)$ and

$$
L_1(\boldsymbol{\beta} | \mathbf{Z}) = \prod_{i=1}^{n} \left(Z_i \mu_0(t_i) e^{\boldsymbol{\beta}' \mathbf{x}_i} \right)^{\delta_i} e^{-Z_i M_0(t_i) e^{\boldsymbol{\beta}' \mathbf{x}_i}}
\tag{3.28}
$$

from relation (3.25), which is the likelihood function of the observed event times conditional on the frailties.

The second term is given by the probability density of the frailty variables:

$$L_2(\sigma^2|\mathbf{Z}) = \prod_{i=1}^{n} f(Z_i; \sigma^2).$$

If the frailties Z_i were known, the regression parameters $\boldsymbol{\beta}$ could be estimated by the partial likelihood method rewriting the terms $Z_i e^{\boldsymbol{\beta}'\mathbf{X}_i}$ in (3.28) in the form $e^{\boldsymbol{\beta}'\mathbf{X}_i + \log(Z_i)}$, using the $\log(Z_i)$ as fixed offset values. Consequently, the expectation step is needed to get estimates of the frailty values. These estimates are used instead of the unknown frailties in the maximization step to obtain the estimates for the regression parameters.

Maximization-Step: Extending the partial likelihood idea in the Cox model described in Section 2.5.1, the partial likelihood for the regression parameters in the frailty model is similar to equation (2.15):

$$L(\boldsymbol{\beta}|\mathbf{Z}) = \prod_{i=1}^{n} \left(\frac{e^{\boldsymbol{\beta}'\mathbf{X}_i + \log(Z_i)}}{\sum\limits_{j \in R(t_i)} Z_j e^{\boldsymbol{\beta}'\mathbf{X}_j}} \right)^{\delta_i}. \qquad (3.29)$$

The unknown random variables Z_i and $\log(Z_i)$ are now substituted by their current expected values (at iteration step k) $\mathbf{E}_{(k)}(Z_i)$ and $\mathbf{E}_{(k)}(\log Z_i)$

$$\log L(\boldsymbol{\beta}, \sigma^2) = \sum_{i=1}^{n} \delta_i \Big[\boldsymbol{\beta}'\mathbf{X}_i + \mathbf{E}_{(k)}(\log(Z_i)) - \log \Big(\sum_{j \in R(t_i)} \mathbf{E}_{(k)}(Z_j) e^{\boldsymbol{\beta}'\mathbf{X}_j} \Big) \Big].$$

From this expression, new estimates $\boldsymbol{\beta}_{(k)}$ can be obtained using standard software. A new estimate of the frailty parameter $\sigma^2_{(k)}$ is derived by maximization of $L_2(\sigma^2|\mathbf{Z})$ also replacing the unknown variables Z_i by their current expected values at iteration step k.

Expectation-Step: Similar to the parametric gamma frailty model (3.26), the unobserved frailty Z_i $(i = 1, \ldots, n)$ of each individual can be estimated by expression

$$\mathbf{E}_{(k+1)}(Z_i) = \frac{1/\sigma^2_{(k)} + \delta_i}{1/\sigma^2_{(k)} + M_{(k)}(t_i) e^{\boldsymbol{\beta}'_{(k)}\mathbf{X}_i}}. \qquad (3.30)$$

Here $M_{(k)}(\cdot)$ is a nonparametric estimator of the cumulative baseline hazard based on the current parameter estimates at iteration step k, for example, the Nelson–Aalen estimator

$$M_{(k)}(t) = \sum_{i:t_i < t} \frac{\delta_i}{\sum\limits_{j \in R(t_i)} \mathbf{E}_{(k)}(Z_j) e^{\boldsymbol{\beta}'_{(k)}\mathbf{X}_j}}.$$

Furthermore, as the conditional distribution of Z is gamma, $\log(Z)$ has a log-gamma distribution with expectation

$$\mathbf{E}_{(k+1)}(\log(Z_i)) = \psi(1/\sigma_{(k)}^2 + \delta_i) - \log\left(1/\sigma_{(k)}^2 + M_{(k)}(t_i)e^{\beta'_{(k)}\mathbf{X}_i}\right)$$

with the digamma function $\psi(x) = \Gamma'(x)/\Gamma(x)$.

Barker and Henderson (2005) investigate the performance of the EM algorithm in the univariate gamma frailty model. In their extensive simulation study they found a large underestimation of the frailty variance similar (or even much stronger) compared to the results reported by Nielsen et al. (1992) in the shared gamma frailty model. The corresponding regression parameters are underestimated in absolute terms. To correct for this underestimation, an adaption of the EM algorithm is suggested by Barker and Henderson (2005), substituting the nonparametric Breslow estimate of the hazard function by a local likelihood formulation for the baseline hazard that allows the survival times themselves (instead of their ranks) to enter the estimation terms.

Example 3.7

To account for heterogeneity within the failure times, a semiparametric shared gamma frailty model was applied to the EBCT data. Results are given in Table 3.7. The typical inflation of the effect of the covariates is seen, combined

Table 3.7: Semiparametric gamma frailty model applied to the EBCT data

parameter	Cox model	gamma frailty
risk group II	0.23 (0.92)	0.19 (0.96)
risk group III	1.27 (0.83)	1.32 (0.89)
risk group IV	2.49 (0.78)	3.16 (1.01)
calcium (> 100)	1.48 (0.53)	1.87 (0.66)
age (55–62)	0.43 (0.42)	0.30 (0.60)
age (63–84)	0.10 (0.40)	-0.22 (0.61)
σ^2		1.95 (1.64)

with larger standard errors. One exception is the covariate risk group II, whose estimate lowers from 0.23 (0.92) in the Cox model to 0.19 (0.96) in the gamma frailty model. The variance of the frailty is large but not significantly different from zero when taking into account the size of the standard error. The simple Cox model seems to be appropriate to model the data compared to the more complex gamma frailty model. The SAS macro SPGAM written by Hien Vu (Vu and Knuiman 2002) was used for analysis. It is based on a modified version of the EM algorithm. The above-mentioned correction by Barker and Henderson (2005) is not included in this macro.   □

The second important estimation approach to the semiparametric gamma frailty model is the penalized partial likelihood (PPL) method. Introduced by McGilchrist and Aisbett (1991) for the log-normal frailty model it was described in detail by Therneau et al. (2003). It leads to the same estimates as the EM algorithm in the gamma frailty model (Therneau and Grambsch 2000, Duchateau and Janssen 2008), but this does not hold for other frailty distributions. For the following presentation it is convenient to rewrite the frailty model by

$$\mu(t|\mathbf{X}, Z) = Z\mu_0(t)e^{\boldsymbol{\beta}'\mathbf{X}} = \mu_0(t)e^{\boldsymbol{\beta}'\mathbf{X}+\ln(Z)} = \mu_0(t)e^{\boldsymbol{\beta}'\mathbf{X}+W}. \qquad (3.31)$$

We will call Z a frailty, and $W = \ln(Z)$ a random effect, to distinguish between both. In the penalized partial likelihood approach, the second part of the likelihood in (3.27) is considered to be a penalty, implying large penalties to the likelihood if the value of the random effect is far away from its expectation value. Considering the random effects as another set of parameters in the first part of the likelihood, the penalized partial likelihood can be written as the product of the partial likelihood (2.15) with $\mathbf{W} = (W_1, \ldots, W_n)$ as additional unknown parameters and the density of the random effects

$$L_{ppl}(\boldsymbol{\beta}, \sigma^2|\mathbf{W}) = \prod_{i=1}^{n} \left(\frac{e^{\boldsymbol{\beta}'\mathbf{X}_i + W_i}}{\sum\limits_{j \in R(t_i)} e^{\boldsymbol{\beta}'\mathbf{X}_j + W_j}} \right)^{\delta_i} f(W_i; \sigma^2). \qquad (3.32)$$

Consequently, the logarithm of the penalized partial likelihood can be split into two parts, where the first part does not depend on σ^2 and the second part does not depend on $\boldsymbol{\beta}$:

$$\log L_{ppl}(\boldsymbol{\beta}, \sigma^2|\mathbf{W}) = \log L_{part}(\boldsymbol{\beta}|\mathbf{W}) + \log L_{pen}(\sigma^2|\mathbf{W}) \qquad (3.33)$$

with

$$L_{pen}(\sigma^2|\mathbf{W}) = \prod_{i=1}^{n} f(W_i; \sigma^2)$$

and the density

$$f(w; \sigma^2) = \frac{(e^w)^{1/\sigma^2} e^{-e^w/\sigma^2}}{(\sigma^2)^{1/\sigma^2} \Gamma(1/\sigma^2)}.$$

This results in a penalty term of the log-likelihood

$$\log L_{pen}(\sigma^2|\mathbf{W}) = -\frac{1}{\sigma^2} \sum_{i=1}^{n} (W_i - e^{W_i}).$$

The maximization of the penalized partial likelihood consists now of an inner and an outer loop. The inner loop estimates $\boldsymbol{\beta}$ and $\mathbf{W}$ by maximization of

$\log L_{ppl}(\beta, \sigma^2 | \mathbf{W})$ based on a provisional value of σ^2. In the outer loop, σ^2 is obtained as maximization of a profiled version of the marginal likelihood. This version is obtained as follows: For a specific value of σ^2, estimates of β and $\mathbf{W}$ are obtained by maximizing the penalized partial likelihood given σ^2. Based on these estimates, other estimates for the cumulative hazard function can be found using the Nelson–Aalen estimator similar to the EM algorithm. As in the EM algorithm, this profile marginal likelihood for σ^2 is used to find an estimate for the frailty variance. The procedure is iterated until convergence. More details about the EM algorithm and the penalized partial likelihood approach in the semiparametric gamma frailty can be found in Duchateau and Janssen (2008). The interested reader is also referred to this book with respect to a detailed derivation of the fact that the estimates in both approaches coincide in the gamma frailty model. This is not true in general for other frailty distributions. In the following example the penalized partial likelihood approach is applied.

Example 3.8

We reanalyze the Halluca lung cancer data again. A semiparametric gamma frailty model is applied in Table 3.8. Results of the Cox model are given for comparisons. As expected, the effect of the covariates is smaller (the

Table 3.8: Semiparametric gamma frailty model for Halluca data

parameter	Cox model	gamma frailty
age (in years)	0.009 (0.003)	0.013 (0.004)
sex (females)	-0.162 (0.071)	-0.197 (0.091)
type (NSCLC)	-0.125 (0.067)	-0.096 (0.086)
ECOG (3 & 4)	0.610 (0.104)	1.054 (0.145)
stage II	0.455 (0.169)	0.578 (0.203)
stage IIIa	0.594 (0.131)	0.780 (0.157)
stage IIIb	0.947 (0.120)	1.232 (0.146)
stage IV	1.345 (0.110)	1.746 (0.133)
σ^2		0.460 ( )

only exception is covariate type) in the Cox model when not corrected for unobserved heterogeneity in the study population. The gamma frailty model is able to account (at least in part) for this unobserved heterogeneity. Note that the standard errors also increase in the gamma frailty model. Estimation is based on the penalized partial likelihood approach and performed by the R package coxph. This procedure (adapted from the Splus macro by Thierry Therneau) provides no standard error of the frailty variance estimate. □

The importance of the penalized partial likelihood approach stems especially from the fact that it can also be used to fit log-normal frailty models considered in the next section. Furthermore, it is much faster than the EM algorithm. The major disadvantage is that it is much more complicated to obtain a valid estimate of the standard error of the frailty variance σ^2. One solution to obtain the standard error of the frailty variance estimate are bootstrap resampling methods. Because of the speed of the penalized partial likelihood estimation procedure compared to the EM algorithm, bootstrap methods are a realistic alternative. Unfortunately, such kind of methods are not integrated in the coxph package in R, which limits its applicability.

Parner (1998) and Therneau et al. (2003) show the exact link between the gamma frailty model and penalized estimation. In the case of log-normal-distributed frailty approximation methods of more complex frailty models are given by Ripatti and Palmgren (2000).

Rondeau et al. (2003) use a different approach and penalize the hazard function, while Therneau et al. (2003) penalize the frailties. A semiparametric gamma frailty model is applied to study the effect of aluminium on the risk of dementia in a large cohort. The aim of the paper is to propose a smooth baseline hazard estimator by maximizing the penalized log-likelihood

$$\log L_{ppl}(\boldsymbol{\beta}, \sigma^2) = \log L(\boldsymbol{\beta}, \sigma^2) - \kappa \int_0^\infty \mu_0''(t)^2 \, dt, \tag{3.34}$$

where $\log L(\boldsymbol{\beta}, \sigma^2)$ is the full log-likelihood in the gamma frailty model and κ is a smoothing parameter. The integral represents a trade-off between the faithfulness to the data, as represented by the term $\log L$, and smoothness of the solution, as represented by the squared norm of the second derivative of the baseline hazard in the penalty term. For large κ, the integral will be forced toward zero, and the baseline hazard will approach a linear function. If κ is small, then the main contribution to $\log L_{ppl}$ will be $\log L$ and the curve estimate will track the data closely, but will be more irregular.

Other approaches such as the Markov Chain Monte Carlo (MCMC) method have also been suggested for estimation in the semiparametric gamma frailty model. The new PROC MCMC routine in SAS offers flexible alternatives compared to the traditional WinBugs software often used for MCMC analyses.

Another choice for estimation in frailty models is Gaussian quadrature. It approximates the integral of a parametric function with respect to a frailty density by a weighted sum over predefined abscissas for the frailties. However, all current implementations make a parametric choice of the baseline hazard function (especially exponential, piecewise constant), see Yamaguchi et al. (2002), Littell et al. (2006), Nelson et al. (2006), Liu and Huang (2008), and Liu and Yu (2008). However, a piecewise constant hazard function with raising number of pieces can be used to approximate semiparametric models. The SAS routine PROC NLMIXED provides a powerful tool for adaptive as well as nonadaptive Gaussian quadrature.

3.3.3 Gamma frailty model for current status data

The case of current status data in frailty models is considered in this section. The likelihood function for current status data is given by formula (2.8):

$$L(\boldsymbol{\theta}) = \prod_{i=1}^{n} \left(1 - S(t_i; \boldsymbol{\theta})\right)^{\delta_i} S(t_i; \boldsymbol{\theta})^{1-\delta_i}.$$

Plugging in the survival function of the gamma frailty model with Gompertz baseline from Example 3.3 and $\boldsymbol{\theta} = (\lambda, \varphi)$, the likelihood function becomes

$$L(\lambda, \varphi, \sigma^2) = \prod_{i=1}^{n} \left(1 - \left(1 + \sigma^2 \frac{\lambda}{\varphi}(e^{\varphi t_i} - 1)\right)^{-\frac{1}{\sigma^2}}\right)^{\delta_i} \left(1 + \sigma^2 \frac{\lambda}{\varphi}(e^{\varphi t_i} - 1)\right)^{-\frac{1-\delta_i}{\sigma^2}}.$$

Example 3.9

The hepatitis A and B current status data from Example 1.7 are analyzed in detail. A univariate parametric gamma frailty model with the Gompertz baseline hazard function as described earlier is fitted to the hepatitis data. Age-dependent prevalences of hepatitis A and B are shown in Figures 3.7 and 3.8, respectively. Results of the analysis are given in Table 3.9. The univariate frailty model treats time to infection by hepatitis A and B, respectively, as independent times for each individual. It turns out that the estimation of the frailty variance regarding hepatitis B is difficult, because the likelihood is very flat with respect to σ^2. This is also indicated by a large standard error of σ^2. A reason for this variability is the smaller prevalence of hepatitis B compared to hepatitis A.

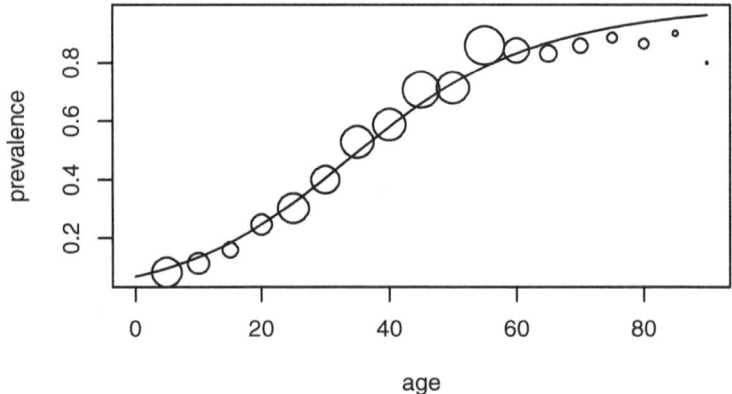

Figure 3.7: Age-specific prevalence of hepatitis A in Flanders 1994/95. The circles indicate the size of the respective age group on which the prevalence estimates are based.

Another, maybe more important reason is the irregularity in the relationship between age and prevalence of hepatitis B, which can be seen in Figure 3.8. Results depend on the choice of the baseline. Here a Gompertz model for the baseline hazard was assumed, other distributions are possible. The likelihood function was maximized by using PROC NLMIXED in SAS.

Table 3.9: Gamma frailty model for hepatitis A and B current status data

parameter	hepatitis A	hepatitis B
σ^2	2.018 (0.510)	10.037 (8.821)
λ	0.008 (0.001)	0.002 (0.001)
φ	0.085 (0.016)	0.015 (0.142)

The parameter σ^2 provides a nice interpretation as a measures of population heterogeneity in the susceptibility to hepatitis A and B, respectively. This parameter provides important implications for further programs to prevent infections as the critical vaccination coverage is higher for more heterogeneous populations. More details about this data are given in Hens et al. (2009). ▯

Another possibility to analyze interval-censored data in a frailty model is provided by the R package developed by Henschel et al. (2009).

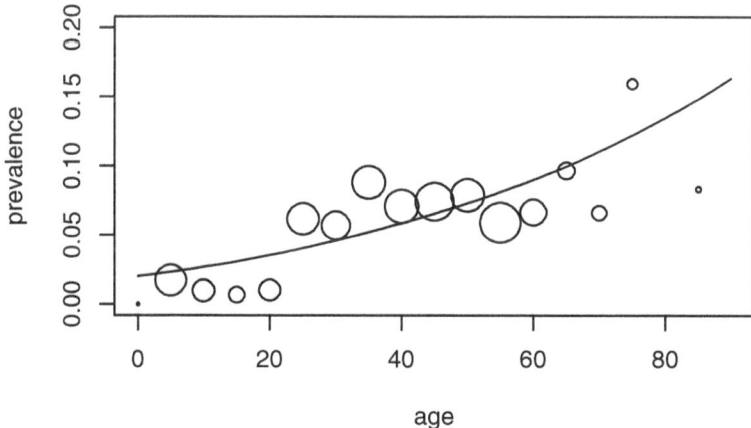

Figure 3.8: Age-specific prevalence of hepatitis B in Flanders 1994/95. The circles indicate the size of the respective age group on which the prevalence estimates are based.

3.3.4   Extensions of the gamma frailty model

An interesting extension of the univariate gamma frailty model was suggested by Semenchenko et al. (2004a,b). Consider the problem of comparing control and treatment group in animal experiments or clinical trials. The distinctive feature of the model compared to other frailty models is that it assumes that treatment influences parameters of both frailty distribution and baseline hazard function. The survival function of the control group is assumed to be

$$S_1(t) = \left(1 + \sigma^2 M_{01}(t)\right)^{-\frac{1}{\sigma^2}}$$

with cumulative baseline hazard function $M_{01}(t)$. The survival function of the treatment group can be written as

$$S_2(t) = \left(1 + r\gamma\sigma^2\left(M_{01}(t) + \frac{\lambda}{\varphi}(e^{\varphi t} - 1)\right)\right)^{-\frac{1}{\gamma\sigma^2}}.$$

One can see that the model has five unknown parameters $\lambda, \varphi, r, \gamma$, and σ^2. Parameter σ^2 indicates the presence of heterogeneity in control and treatment group. Parameters λ and φ describe changes in the baseline hazard caused by treatment. The model is based on the relation

$$M_{02}(t) = M_{01}(t) + \frac{\lambda}{\varphi}(e^{\varphi t} - 1),$$

where $M_{02}(t)$ denotes the cumulative baseline hazard of the treatment group. Frailty in the treatment group is now gamma distributed with mean r and variance $\gamma\sigma^2$. Hence, changes in the frailty distribution caused by treatment are given by parameters r and γ. Parameter $r < 1$ shows an increase in the average robustness (decrease in mean frailty), while $r > 1$ indicates an accumulation of frail individuals in the treatment group. A parameter value $\gamma \neq 1$ signalizes an increase ($\gamma > 1$) or decrease ($\gamma < 1$) in the heterogeneity by the treatment. In the above expression, $\sigma^2 M_{01}(t)$ can be substituted by $S_1(t)^{-\sigma^2} - 1$ resulting in

$$S_2(t) = \left(1 + r\gamma(S_1(t)^{-\sigma^2} - 1) + r\gamma\frac{\lambda}{\varphi}(e^{\varphi t} - 1)\right)^{-\frac{1}{\gamma\sigma^2}}.$$

The nonparametric Kaplan–Meier estimator can now be used to estimate the unknown survival function $S_1(t)$ of the control group. Consequently, the suggested model is semiparametrically in this sense.

Another extension of the gamma frailty model was recently introduced by Barker and Henderson (2004). The authors claim that it is likely that only a part of the covariates used in a Cox regression fulfill the proportional hazards assumption. To circumvent this problem they introduce a mixed model that allows for both proportional and converging hazards. Two kinds of covariates are considered, $\mathbf{X}_1$ and $\mathbf{X}_2$. The usual gamma frailty model with covariates $\mathbf{X}_2$ has a hazard of the form $\mu(t) = Z\mu_0(t)e^{\boldsymbol{\beta}_2'\mathbf{X}_2}$, but the frailty distribution is assumed to depend on covariates $\mathbf{X}_1$, namely, $Z \sim \Gamma(\frac{e^{\boldsymbol{\beta}_1'\mathbf{X}_1}}{\sigma^2}, \frac{1}{\sigma^2})$. Then the unconditional survival function is obtained as

$$S(t|\mathbf{X}_1, \mathbf{X}_2) = \int_0^\infty e^{-zM_0(t)e^{\boldsymbol{\beta}_2'\mathbf{X}_2}} f(z|\mathbf{X}_1)\, dz$$

$$= \left(1 + \sigma^2 M_0(t)e^{\boldsymbol{\beta}_2'\mathbf{X}_2}\right)^{-\frac{e^{\boldsymbol{\beta}_1'\mathbf{X}_1}}{\sigma^2}}. \tag{3.35}$$

When the frailty variance σ^2 is zero, the model reduces to the standard Cox proportional hazards model with covariates $\{\mathbf{X}_1, \mathbf{X}_2\}$. If $\boldsymbol{\beta}_2 = 0$, the model reduces to the proportional hazards model with covariates $\mathbf{X}_1$, whereas if $\boldsymbol{\beta}_1 = 0$ holds, it is clear from equation (3.35) that the suggested mixed model reduces to the univariate gamma frailty model with covariates $\mathbf{X}_2$. The baseline hazard function in this model is left unspecified.

In the following we a nontypical extension of the univariate gamma frailty model is presented to demonstrate the strengths of this approach. Consider a bivariate outcome (T, L) in the following analysis, where the first component T is an event time, but the second one L is a nonnegative integer number. For example, T could be the lifetime of a woman, and L the number of their children. The aim of such an approach is to analyze both outcomes in parallel, assuming a dependence between lifetime and number of children caused by unobserved underlying factors influencing lifetime as well as fecundability. The difference to a Cox regression model with number of children as covariate is the causal relationship. If number of children is modeled as an independent variable, and lifetime as a dependent variable, a causal relationship between number of children and lifetime is assumed. The model presented in this paragraph assumes an association between both variables, but no assumption about the direction of a causal relationship is made. Let the expression

$$S(t|Z) = e^{-ZM_0(t)}$$

denote the conditional survival function of lifetime T, conditional on the frailty (random effect) Z. Furthermore, let $p > 0$, and the integer number L be conditional Poisson distributed, conditional on the random effect Z with parameter pZ:

$$\mathbf{P}(L = l|Z) = \frac{(pZ)^l}{l!}e^{-pZ}.$$

The dependence between T and L is based on the unobserved random effect Z. Let Z be gamma distributed with expectation one and variance σ^2. Then the model can be derived in the following way:

$$\mathbf{P}(T > t, L = l) = \mathbf{E}\mathbf{P}(T > t, L = l|Z)$$

$$= \mathbf{E}S(t|Z)\mathbf{P}(L = l|Z)$$

$$= \mathbf{E}e^{-ZM_0(t)}\frac{(pZ)^l}{l!}e^{-pZ}$$

$$= \frac{1}{\Gamma(k)l!}\int e^{zM_0(t)}e^{-pz}(pz)^l \lambda^k z^{k-1}e^{-\lambda z}\, dz.$$

Consequently,

$$
\begin{aligned}
\mathbf{P}(T > t, L = l) &= \frac{\lambda^k \Gamma(k+l) p^l \int (\lambda + M_0(t) + p)^{k+l} z^{k+l-1} e^{-(\lambda + M_0(t)+p)z} \, dz}{\Gamma(k) l! (\lambda + M(t) + 1)^{k+l} \Gamma(k+l)} \\
&= \frac{\lambda^k \Gamma(k+l) p^l}{\Gamma(k) l! (\lambda + M_0(t) + p)^{k+l}} \\
&= \binom{l+k-1}{k-1} \left(\frac{\lambda}{\lambda + M_0(t) + p}\right)^k \left(\frac{p}{\lambda + M_0(t) + p}\right)^l
\end{aligned}
$$

Now we consider the two marginal distributions in more detail. The event time distribution is obtained by

$$
\begin{aligned}
S(t) &= \sum_{l=0}^{\infty} \mathbf{P}(T > t, L = l) \\
&= \sum_{l=0}^{\infty} \binom{l+k-1}{k-1} \left(\frac{\lambda}{\lambda + M_0(t) + p}\right)^k \left(\frac{p}{\lambda + M_0(t) + p}\right)^l \\
&= (1 + \frac{1}{\lambda} M_0(t))^{-k} \sum_{l=0}^{\infty} \binom{l+k-1}{k-1} \left(\frac{\lambda + M_0(t)}{\lambda + M_0(t) + p}\right)^k \left(\frac{p}{\lambda + M_0(t) + p}\right)^l \\
&= (1 + \frac{1}{\lambda} M_0(t))^{-k},
\end{aligned}
$$

which results because the infinite sum is the probability function of a negative binomial distribution with parameters k and $\frac{\lambda + M_0(t)}{\lambda + M_0(t) + p}$. If now the restriction $k = \lambda = \frac{1}{\sigma^2}$ is used, we obtain the unconditional survival function with gamma frailty in (3.17).

The count data distribution can be derived from the joint distribution by

$$
\mathbf{P}(L = l) = \mathbf{P}(T > 0, L = l) = \binom{l+k-1}{k-1} \left(\frac{\lambda}{\lambda + p}\right)^k \left(\frac{p}{\lambda + p}\right)^l,
$$

which is a negative binomial distribution with parameters k and $\frac{\lambda}{\lambda + p}$. Using again parameterization $k = \lambda = \frac{1}{\sigma^2}$ results in

$$
\mathbf{P}(L = l) = \binom{l + \frac{1}{\sigma^2} - 1}{\frac{1}{\sigma^2} - 1} \left(\frac{1}{1 + p\sigma^2}\right)^{\frac{1}{\sigma^2}} \left(\frac{p\sigma^2}{1 + p\sigma^2}\right)^l,
$$

a negative binomial distribution with parameters $\frac{1}{\sigma^2}$ and $\frac{1}{1+p\sigma^2}$, implying expectation p and variance $p(1+p\sigma^2)$. The parameters p and σ^2 give the model enough flexibility to fit the marginal distribution of the number of children in the population. Furthermore, σ^2 can be interpreted in some sense as an association parameter. Large values speak in favor of a strong association between lifetime and number of children, whereas small values do not.

The negative binomial distribution has been widely used to model count data. One of the first applications was used by Greenwood and Yule (1920) to model the number of accidents of women working in munition shell production during World War I in England. Up to this time the Poisson distribution was considered as a universal count data distribution based on the book by von Bortkiewicz (1898). Greenwood and his colleagues observed discrepancies between the observed and expected numbers of accidents and suggested an extension of the Poisson distribution to the negative binomial distribution by assuming the Poisson parameter to be a random mixture variable that follows a gamma distribution. Consequently, heterogeneity was assumed in the population. This was the starting point for a series of accident studies based on the theory of accident proneness. The idea was that it should be able to reduce the number of accidents by identifying the most accident-prone individuals with the help of such heterogeneity models.

There are many applications of the univariate gamma frailty model in the literature. For the first time the model was used by Beard (1959). Lancaster (1979) suggested this model for the duration of unemployment spells, and Vaupel et al. (1979) used it to calculate individual hazard functions and to adjust life tables in the case of heterogeneous populations. Manton et al. (1981) compared the mortality experience of heterogeneous populations, and Manton and Stallard (1981) explained the black/white mortality crossing-over effects observed in the United States. Manton et al. (1986) compared the inverse normal and the gamma models, together with Gompertz and Weibull baseline hazards, in a study of survival at advanced ages, based on data from U.S. Medicare insurance. Aalen (1987) studied the expulsion of intrauterine contraceptive devices. Ellermann et al. (1992) used a parametric model to analyze recidivism among criminals. Andersen et al. (1993) applied the model to the malignant melanoma data from Example 1.2. Jones (1998) used a gamma–Gompertz model for analyzing the impact of selective lapsation on mortality in life insurance. Jeong et al. (2003) used a gamma frailty to model long-term follow-up survival data from breast cancer clinical trials when the treatment effect diminishes over time as an alternative to the proportional hazards model. Solid cancer incidence data from atomic bomb survivors in Japan were used by Izumi and Ohtaki (2004) to check two different hypotheses about individual hazard functions. Balakrishnan and Peng (2006) consider an extension of the gamma frailty model which also includes the log-normal frailty model considered in the following section. The use of gamma-distributed frailty in univariate models is supported by the results of Abbring and van den Berg (2007), who showed that, under some regularity assumptions, frailty among survivors converges against a gamma distribution even if the original frailty distribution is not a gamma distribution.

Parametric gamma frailty models are implemented in STATA and in the SAS macro PGAM by Vu. Furthermore, NLMIXED in SAS can be used based on Liu and Yu (2008). Semiparametric versions are included in R/S plus (Therneau) and SAS macros by Vu (SPGAM) and Klein (GAMFRAIL).

3.4   Log-normal Frailty Model

The log-normal distribution together with the gamma distribution is the most important and often-used frailty distribution. Increasing computer power helps to overcome the restrictions of this model, which needs the solution of numerical integrals because of the lack of closed-form expressions for the marginal survival function and the resulting terms in the likelihood. The strong link to random effects/mixed models makes this model very attractive. As it will be shown in the subsequent chapters, log-normal frailty models are especially useful in modeling dependence structures in multivariate problems. Their main advantage is the large flexibility in the dependence structures by means of multivariate normal distribution. However, log-normal distribution has also been applied in univariate cases, for example, by Flinn and Heckman (1982). Log-normal distribution is in fact very close to inverse Gaussian distribution.

Two variants of the log-normal frailty model exist. We assume a normally distributed random variable $W \sim N(m, s^2)$ to generate frailty as $Z = e^W$, with N denoting the normal distribution. The parameters of this normal distribution are some functions of the frailty parameters μ and σ^2 (see, for example, Hutchinson and Lai 1991)

$$\mu = \mathbf{E}Z = e^{m + \frac{s^2}{2}} \tag{3.36}$$

$$\sigma^2 = \mathbf{V}(Z) = e^{2m + s^2}(e^{s^2} - 1). \tag{3.37}$$

Simple calculations show that under the constraint $\mu = 1$ this results in

$$m = \mathbf{E}\ln(Z) = -\frac{1}{2}s^2$$
$$s^2 = \mathbf{V}(\ln(Z)) = \ln(1 + \sigma^2).$$

First, following the historical definition of frailty originally introduced in the field of demography (Vaupel et al. 1979), one can use the restriction $\mu = 1$. Second, one can use the restriction $m = 0$. This means that the logarithm of the frailty has a mean of zero. In this case, a "standard" individual has the logarithm of the hazard rate, which is equal to $\ln\left(\mu_0(t)\right)$. Any individual in a population has the logarithm of the hazard rate distorted by some random variable $W = \ln(Z)$. This value is added to the "true" logarithm of the hazard rate $\ln\left(\mu_0(t)\right)$ to provide the logarithm of hazard rate of the individual. In this interpretation, it is natural to assume that the distortions W have a normal distribution with an expectation of zero.

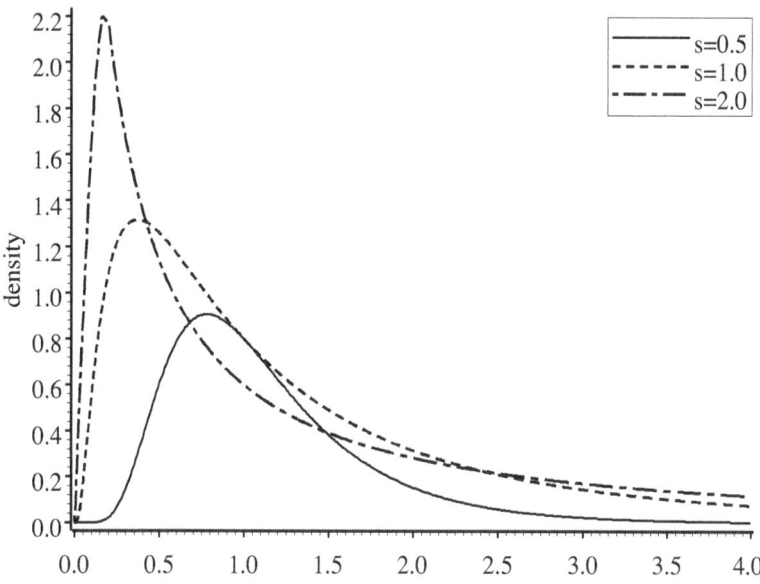

Figure 3.9: Probability density functions of log-normal distributions with parameter values $m = 0$ and $s^2 = 0.25$, 1, and 4.

The density of the frailty distribution based on the parameters m and s^2 is given by the expression

$$f(z) = \frac{1}{\sqrt{2\pi}sz}e^{-\frac{(\ln(z))^2}{2s^2}},$$

where the form of the density for different parameters is shown in Figure 3.9. In this model, a "standard" individual has the hazard rate $\mu_0(t)$. Individual i has the hazard rate of a "standard" individual multiplied by the frailty Z_i. This restriction on μ means that the average frailty in a population equals 1 (at the beginning of the follow-up). This makes the model comparable with other frailty models considered in the preceding sections. Despite this advantage of comparability of frailty variances in different models, the parameterization based on $\mathbf{E}W = m = 0$ is much more common in the literature and standard in statistical packages. The reason is that the normally distributed random effect acts on the linear predictor, which suits nicely generalized linear models and the assumption of normality of the linear predictor. To take advantage of the theoretical research results and software solutions provided in the fast-growing field of mixed models, we will use this approach in the following as well. Furthermore, interpretation of the log-normal frailty model as a random effects model with normally distributed random effects makes this model class more convenient for application by researchers not especially trained in the field of survival analysis/frailty models.

3.4.1 Parametric log-normal frailty model

Unfortunately, no explicit form of unconditional likelihood exists because of the intractable Laplace transform. The likelihood of the data $(t_i, \delta_i, \mathbf{X}_i)$ $(i = 1, \ldots, n)$ is of the form

$$L(\boldsymbol{\beta}, \boldsymbol{\theta}, s^2) = \prod_{i=1}^{n} \int \left(\mu_0(t_i; \boldsymbol{\theta})e^{\boldsymbol{\beta}'\mathbf{X}_i + w_i}\right)^{\delta_i} e^{-M_0(t_i;\boldsymbol{\theta})e^{\boldsymbol{\beta}'\mathbf{X}_i + w_i}} \, d\Phi(w_i) \quad (3.38)$$

with Φ as cumulative distribution function of the normal distribution with mean zero and variance s^2. Consequently, more sophisticated estimation strategies are required, for example, numerical integration in the maximum likelihood approach or MCMC methods. In the parametric case, numerical integration of the normally distributed random effects based on the Laplace approximation or (adaptive/nonadaptive) Gaussian quadrature can be used. We follow this approach here by making three different assumptions about the baseline hazard in the Halluca study. The results are given in Table 3.10.

Table 3.10: Parametric log-normal frailty models for Halluca lung cancer data

parameter	Weibull	exponential	Gompertz
age (in years)	0.013 (0.004)	0.013 (0.004)	0.013 (0.004)
sex (females)	-0.192 (0.089)	-0.198 (0.088)	-0.203 (0.091)
type (NSCLC)	-0.126 (0.084)	-0.120 (0.083)	-0.132 (0.086)
ECOG (3 & 4)	0.938 (0.149)	0.900 (0.136)	0.958 (0.146)
stage II	0.545 (0.203)	0.533 (0.200)	0.562 (0.207)
stage IIIa	0.738 (0.159)	0.742 (0.155)	0.769 (0.163)
stage IIIb	1.197 (0.152)	1.181 (0.143)	1.229 (0.156)
stage IV	1.669 (0.147)	1.654 (0.130)	1.713 (0.149)
s^2	0.516 (0.134)	0.475 (0.073)	0.578 (0.134)
λ	0.013 (0.005)	0.014 (0.004)	0.012 (0.004)
ν	1.013 (0.041)		
φ			0.006 (0.006)
log-likelihood	-4848.24049	-4848.26798	-4847.85248

The estimates of the regression parameters are very similar to each other, indicating robustness of the analysis with respect to the choice of the baseline hazard. Small differences occur between the estimates of the random effects variance. The likelihood ratio test indicates that the simple exponential model is significantly better compared to the more complex Gompertz or Weibull model. Analysis was performed by SAS procedure NLMIXED. The variance s^2 of the random effect differs significantly from zero in all three models. It cannot be directly compared with frailty variance σ^2 from the gamma model.

3.4.2 Semiparametric log-normal frailty model

If the form of the underlying baseline hazard function is known, the parametric approach is efficient. However, in most practical applications, this information is not available, and semiparametric models are preferred. If no assumptions about the form of the baseline hazard function are made, parameter estimation becomes much more difficult. One way to solve the estimation problem is the penalized partial likelihood approach, already considered in the case of the gamma frailty model. Similar to the gamma case, the random effects are considered as another set of parameters in the first part of the likelihood. Note that, due to (3.31), the relation $\mathbf{E}W = 0$ is used to keep the model identifiable instead of $\mathbf{E}Z = 1$. Furthermore, the model is parameterized in terms of the variance of the random effects $\mathbf{V}(W) = s^2$, which is different from the gamma model. Based on (3.32), the logarithm of the penalized partial likelihood can be split in a partial likelihood L_{part} and a penalty term L_{pen} and written in the form

$$\log L_{ppl}(\boldsymbol{\beta}, s^2|\mathbf{W}) = \log L_{part}(\boldsymbol{\beta}|\mathbf{W}) + \log L_{pen}(s^2|\mathbf{W})$$

with $\mathbf{W} = (W_1, \ldots, W_n)$,

$$L_{pen}(s^2|\mathbf{W}) = \prod_{i=1}^{n} f(W_i; s^2)$$

and the density of a normal distribution with mean zero and variance s^2

$$f(w; s^2) = \frac{1}{\sqrt{2\pi s^2}} e^{-\frac{w^2}{2s^2}}.$$

This results in a penalty term of the log-likelihood

$$\log L_{pen}(s^2|\mathbf{W}) = -\frac{1}{2} \sum_{i=1}^{n} \left(\frac{W_i^2}{s^2} + \ln(2\pi s^2)\right).$$

The maximization of the penalized partial likelihood consists again of an inner and an outer loop. The inner loop is similar to the gamma frailty model and estimates $\boldsymbol{\beta}$ and $\mathbf{W}$ by a Newton–Raphson procedure to maximize $\log L_{ppl}(\boldsymbol{\beta}, s^2|\mathbf{W})$ based on a provisional value of s^2 (best linear unbiased predictor – BLUB). The outer loop is different from the gamma model. The restricted maximum likelihood estimator for s^2 is based on the BLUBs. Then the procedure is iterated until convergence occurs. The asymptotic variance for the estimates of the regression parameters can be found in McGilchrist and Aisbett (1991). Asymptotic variance of the random effects variance estimate is given in McGilchrist (1993). The more technical details of the algorithm can be found elsewhere (Therneau and Grambsch 2000, Duchateau and Janssen 2008) and are therefore omitted here.

Example 3.10

The penalized partial likelihood approach is illustrated with an application to the Halluca data. In Table 3.11 the results of a semiparametric log-normal frailty model are given with the Cox model for comparison. We see the typical pattern of stronger covariate effects (estimates of the regression parameters are further away from zero) with variable type as an exception. Furthermore, standard errors for the regression coefficients are larger in the frailty model. Estimation was performed by means of the R procedure COXPH based on a penalized partial likelihood approach. This procedure does not provide a standard error for the frailty variance estimate. Comparing the results

Table 3.11: Cox and semiparametric log-normal frailty model for Halluca lung cancer data

parameter	Cox model	log-normal frailty
age (in years)	0.009 (0.003)	0.012 (0.003)
sex (females)	-0.162 (0.071)	-0.194 (0.088)
type (NSCLC)	-0.125 (0.067)	-0.112 (0.083)
ECOG (3 & 4)	0.610 (0.104)	0.924 (0.134)
stage II	0.455 (0.169)	0.552 (0.198)
stage IIIa	0.594 (0.131)	0.742 (0.154)
stage IIIb	0.947 (0.120)	1.177 (0.142)
stage IV	1.345 (0.110)	1.667 (0.130)
s^2		0.498 ( )

of the log-normal frailty model and the gamma frailty model in Table 3.8, one has to note that frailty in the log-normal model with a parameterization based on $\mathbf{E}W = m = 0$ is not standardized to $\mathbf{E}Z = \mu = 1$. Despite this fact the estimates for the regression coefficients are similar in both models. Further caution is needed when variances in the two models are compared. The parameter σ^2 describes the variance of the frailty term Z in the gamma model, whereas s^2 denotes the variance of the random effect $W = \ln(Z)$ in the log-normal frailty model. Both quantities cannot be directly compared. However, both estimates are similar ($\sigma^2 = 0.46$ compared to $s^2 = 0.498$).

In general, the variance of the random effect W in a log-normal frailty model is larger than the variance of the respective frailty $Z = e^W$ (in the same model), and the difference becomes more pronounced the larger the frailty variance is. In situations with reasonable small frailty variance, there is no big difference between σ^2 and s^2 (Duchateau and Janssen 2008). The results show robustness regarding the frailty distribution. Similar to the gamma model, the results from parametric and semiparametric models support the robustness of parametric frailty analysis regarding the baseline hazard. ⬚

3.5 Inverse Gaussian Frailty Model

The inverse Gaussian (inverse normal) distribution was introduced as a frailty distribution alternative to the gamma distribution by Hougaard (1984) and was used, for example, by Manton et al. (1986), Klein et al. (1992), Keiding et al. (1997), Price and Manatunga (2001), Economou and Caroni (2005), Kheiri et al. (2007), and Duchateau and Janssen (2008). Similar to the gamma frailty model, simple closed-form expressions exist for the unconditional survival and hazard functions, which makes the model attractive. The probability density function of an inverse Gaussian distributed random variable with parameters $\mu > 0$ and $\lambda > 0$ is given by

$$f(z) = \frac{\sqrt{\lambda}}{\sqrt{2\pi z^3}} \exp\left(-\frac{\lambda}{2\mu^2 z}(z - \mu)^2\right).$$

The form of the density function for different parameter values is depicted in Figure 3.10.

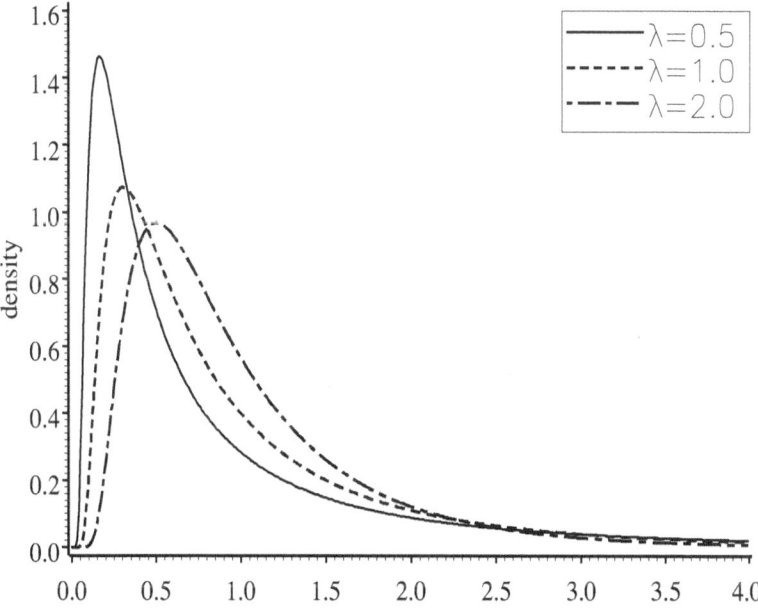

Figure 3.10: Probability density functions of inverse Gauss distributions with expectation 1 and variances 0.5, 1, and 2.

The density given above is the starting point to derive the Laplace transform of the inverse Gaussian distribution:

$$\mathbf{L}(u) = \mathbf{E}e^{-uZ}$$

$$= \int \frac{\sqrt{\lambda}}{\sqrt{2\pi z^3}} e^{-uz} \exp\left(-\frac{\lambda}{2\mu^2 z}(z-\mu)^2\right) dz$$

$$= \int \frac{\sqrt{\lambda}}{\sqrt{2\pi z^3}} \exp\left(-\frac{(\lambda + 2\mu^2 u)z^2 - 2\mu\lambda z + \lambda\mu^2}{2\mu^2 z}\right) dz$$

$$= \int \frac{\sqrt{\lambda}}{\sqrt{2\pi z^3}} \exp\left(-\frac{z}{2}\frac{\lambda + 2\mu^2 u}{\mu^2} + \frac{\lambda}{\mu} - \frac{\lambda}{2z}\right) dz$$

$$= \exp\left(-\frac{\lambda\sqrt{1 + \frac{2\mu^2 u}{\lambda}}}{\mu} + \frac{\lambda}{\mu}\right)$$

$$\times \int \frac{\sqrt{\lambda}}{\sqrt{2\pi z^3}} \exp\left(-\frac{\lambda z}{2}\frac{1 + \frac{2\mu^2 u}{\lambda}}{\mu^2} + \frac{\lambda\sqrt{1 + \frac{2\mu^2 u}{\lambda}}}{\mu} - \frac{\lambda}{2z}\right) dz \qquad (3.39)$$

Because of the relation

$$-\frac{\lambda z}{2}\frac{1 + \frac{2\mu^2 u}{\lambda}}{\mu^2} + \frac{\lambda\sqrt{1 + \frac{2\mu^2 u}{\lambda}}}{\mu} - \frac{\lambda}{2z} = -\frac{\lambda}{2\frac{\mu^2}{1 + \frac{2\mu^2 u}{\lambda}} z}\left(z - \frac{\mu}{\sqrt{1 + \frac{2\mu^2 u}{\lambda}}}\right)^2,$$

the expression

$$\frac{\sqrt{\lambda}}{\sqrt{2\pi z^3}} \exp\left(-\frac{\lambda z}{2}\frac{1 + \frac{2\mu^2 u}{\lambda}}{\mu^2} + \frac{\lambda\sqrt{1 + \frac{2\mu^2 u}{\lambda}}}{\mu} - \frac{\lambda}{2z}\right) =$$

$$\frac{\sqrt{\lambda}}{\sqrt{2\pi z^3}} \exp\left(-\frac{\lambda}{2\frac{\mu^2}{1 + \frac{2\mu^2 u}{\lambda}} z}\left(z - \frac{\mu}{1 + \frac{2\mu^2 u}{\lambda}}\right)^2\right)$$

in (3.39) is the density of an inverse Gaussian distribution with parameters $\frac{\mu}{\sqrt{1 + \frac{2\mu^2 u}{\lambda}}}$ and λ. Thus, the integral equals one. As a consequence, the Laplace transform of an inverse Gaussian distributed random variable simplifies to the expression

$$\mathbf{L}(u) = \exp\left(-\frac{\lambda\sqrt{1 + \frac{2\mu^2 u}{\lambda}}}{\mu} + \frac{\lambda}{\mu}\right) = \exp\left(\frac{\lambda}{\mu}\left(1 - \sqrt{1 + \frac{2\mu^2 u}{\lambda}}\right)\right). \qquad (3.40)$$

The first and second derivatives of the Laplace transform are given by

$$\mathbf{L}'(u) = -\frac{\mu}{\sqrt{1 + \frac{2\mu^2 u}{\lambda}}} \exp\left(\frac{\lambda}{\mu}\left(1 - \sqrt{1 + \frac{2\mu^2 u}{\lambda}}\right)\right)$$

and

$$\mathbf{L}''(u) = \frac{\mu^3}{\lambda(1 + \frac{2\mu^2 u}{\lambda})^{3/2}} \exp\left(\frac{\lambda}{\mu}\left(1 - \sqrt{1 + \frac{2\mu^2 u}{\lambda}}\right)\right)$$

$$+ \frac{\mu^2}{1 + \frac{2\mu^2 u}{\lambda}} \exp\left(\frac{\lambda}{\mu}\left(1 - \sqrt{1 + \frac{2\mu^2 u}{\lambda}}\right)\right).$$

Expectation and variance of the frailty distribution can now be calculated by evaluating the derivatives at $u = 0$:

$$\mathbf{E}Z = -\mathbf{L}'(0) = \mu$$

$$\mathbf{V}(Z) = \mathbf{L}''(0) - (\mathbf{L}'(0))^2 = \frac{\mu^3}{\lambda}.$$

Taking $\mathbf{E}Z = \mu = 1$ and $\mathbf{V}(Z) = \sigma^2 = 1/\lambda$ results in the following simplified Laplace transform:

$$\mathbf{L}(u) = e^{\frac{1}{\sigma^2}(1 - \sqrt{1 + 2\sigma^2 u})}.$$

Hence, the unconditional survival and hazard function can be written in the form

$$S(t) = e^{\frac{1}{\sigma^2}(1 - \sqrt{1 + 2\sigma^2 M_0(t)})}$$

and

$$\mu(t) = \frac{\mu_0(t)}{(1 + 2\sigma^2 M_0(t))^{1/2}}.$$

In the following we include regression terms $e^{\beta' X}$ into the model. The aim is to evaluate the effect of unobserved heterogeneity on the regression parameters in the inverse Gaussian frailty model. We consider the marginal hazards of two individuals with only one binary covariate in the model. The hazard ratio for two individuals with covariate values one (meaning, for example, experimental treatment) and zero (for example, placebo treatment) is of the form

$$\frac{\mu(t|X = 1)}{\mu(t|X = 0)} = \frac{(1 + 2\sigma^2 M_0(t))^{1/2}}{(1 + 2\sigma^2 M_0(t)e^\beta)^{1/2}} e^\beta.$$

This hazard ratio is e^β at time point $t = 0$ and converges towards $e^{\beta/2}$ for $t \to \infty$. Similar to the gamma frailty model, this marginal model is no longer a proportional hazards model. The effect of the covariate weakens over time. The time-independent hazard ratio obtained from the conditional model is attenuated from the conditional hazard ratio e^β. The influence of unobserved heterogeneity is stronger in situations with larger values of σ^2, β, or $M_0(t)$, representing the three factors that accelerate selection.

The density of the frailty distribution among the survivors at time point t can be written in the form

$$
\begin{aligned}
f(z|\mathbf{X}, T > t) &= \frac{S(t|\mathbf{X}, z)f(z)}{S(t|\mathbf{X})} \\
&= \frac{\exp\left(-zM_0(t)e^{\boldsymbol{\beta}'\mathbf{X}}\right)\exp\left(-\frac{(z-1)^2}{2\sigma^2 z}\right)}{\sqrt{2\pi^2 z^3}\exp\left(\frac{1}{\sigma^2}(1 - \sqrt{1 + 2\sigma^2 M_0(t)e^{\boldsymbol{\beta}'\mathbf{X}}})\right)} \\
&= \frac{\exp\left(-\frac{z^2(1+2\sigma^2 M_0(t)e^{\boldsymbol{\beta}'\mathbf{X}})-2z+1}{2\sigma^2 z}\right)}{\sqrt{2\pi^2 z^3}\exp\left(\frac{1}{\sigma^2}(1 - \sqrt{1 + 2\sigma^2 M_0(t)e^{\boldsymbol{\beta}'\mathbf{X}}})\right)} \\
&= \frac{1}{\sqrt{2\pi^2 z^3}}\exp\left(-\frac{\left(z - (1 + 2\sigma^2 M_0(t)e^{\boldsymbol{\beta}'\mathbf{X}})^{-1/2}\right)^2}{\frac{2\sigma^2 z}{1+2\sigma^2 M_0(t)e^{\boldsymbol{\beta}'\mathbf{X}}}}\right).
\end{aligned}
$$

This is the density of an inverse Gaussian-distributed frailty variable with expectation

$$
\mathbf{E}(Z|\mathbf{X}, T > t) = \frac{1}{\sqrt{1 + \sigma^2 M_0(t)e^{\boldsymbol{\beta}'\mathbf{X}}}}
$$

among the survivors at time t. This demonstrates selection by early death of the high-risk individuals, for example, individuals with high values of frailty Z and high values of observed risk factors. The variance of frailty among the survivors at time point t is given by

$$
\mathbf{V}(Z|\mathbf{X}, T > t) = \frac{\sigma^2}{(1 + \sigma^2 M_0(t)e^{\boldsymbol{\beta}'\mathbf{X}})^2}.
$$

The frailty distribution of those who die at time t is a "generalized" inverse Gaussian one, which is a much more complicated distribution, and is not considered in detail here. Parametric versions of the inverse Gaussian frailty model are available in the STATA package. Possible choices for the baseline hazard in STATA are exponential, Weibull, Gompertz, log-logistic, log-normal, and gamma distributions.

3.6   Positive Stable Frailty Model

A distribution is called stable if the normalized sum of n independent random variables from this distribution has the same distribution as a scale factor multiplied by a single random variable. The normalization is given by $n^{\frac{1}{\gamma}}$, where the parameter γ is from the interval $(0, 2]$ and called a *characteristic exponent*. To ensure a distribution on the positive numbers, we restrict here to the case of positive stable distributions, characterized by $\gamma \in (0, 1]$. The probability density function of such a one-parameter positive stable random distribution is given by (Feller 1971)

$$f(z) = \frac{1}{\pi} \sum_{\kappa=1}^{\infty} (-1)^{\kappa+1} \frac{\Gamma(\kappa\gamma + 1)}{\kappa!} z^{-\kappa\gamma-1} \sin(\kappa\gamma\pi)$$

with $z \geq 0$ and $0 < \gamma \leq 1$. This expression is a power series, converging fast for large values of z, and slow for small values of z. In the special case of $\gamma = 1$, the frailty distribution becomes degenerated at the point mass $Z = 1$. Although the probability density function of a random variable with positive stable distribution can only be represented by infinite series, the Laplace transform has a very simple form. This makes the distribution especially attractive as a frailty distribution because many characteristics of the unconditional survival distribution of the event times follow from the Laplace transform and can easily be deduced:

$$\mathbf{L}(u) = e^{-u^{\gamma}}. \tag{3.41}$$

All moments of this distribution are infinite. Consequently, the expectation of the frailty is infinite, and variance does not exists. In the first view this seems to be a disadvantage because an infinite expectation is more difficult to work with. However, infinite expectation was one of the main reasons why this frailty distribution was introduced. The first derivative of the Laplace transform is used to show this fact for the expectation (Duchateau and Janssen 2008)

$$\lim_{u \to +0} \mathbf{L}'(u) = -\gamma \lim_{u \to +0} \frac{e^{-u^{\gamma}}}{u^{1-\gamma}} = -\infty,$$

where $\lim_{u \to +0}$ denotes the right limit. Here the comparison of the population hazard function with the conditional hazard function for a subject with frailty value one makes no sense because the expectation of the frailty variable does not exist. Consequently, an individual with frailty equal to one cannot serve as a standard individual as in other frailty models with finite expectation of the frailty. This infinite expectation result is also important with respect to identifiability issues treated by Elbers and Ridder (1982). They found that a finite mean of the frailty distribution is one condition (among others) for the identifiability of univariate frailty models. This was the main reason why the positive stable distribution was introduced as a frailty distribution. Especially in bivariate/multivariate applications, much attention is given to overcoming confounding problems in shared (gamma) frailty models, considered later in this book (for more details see Section 4.9). Using the Laplace transform of a positive stable frailty variable given earlier, the unconditional survival and density functions are

$$S(t) = e^{-M_0(t)^\gamma} \qquad (3.42)$$

and

$$f(t) = \gamma\mu_0(t)M_0(t)^{\gamma-1}e^{-M_0(t)^\gamma},$$

respectively, resulting in the unconditional hazard function

$$\mu(t) = \gamma\mu_0(t)M_0(t)^{\gamma-1}. \qquad (3.43)$$

The positive stable model implies some interesting features, which are given in the following examples. The most important one is that the positive stable distribution is the only frailty distribution that preserves the proportional hazards condition in unconditional hazards after integrating out the frailty. In the following we introduce observed covariates to the model. In the case of only one binary 0-1 covariate, the ratio of two hazards with different individual covariate values is

$$\frac{\mu(t|X=1)}{\mu(t|X=0)} = e^{\gamma\beta}.$$

The two marginal hazards are still proportional but with proportionality factor $e^{\gamma\beta}$ instead of e^β. This shows that parameter estimates are biased in a proportional hazards model if relevant covariates are not included. Since $0 < \gamma < 1$, the population hazard ratio will typically be closer to one. The more the parameter γ deviates from one, the more the population hazard ratio will deviate from the conditional hazard ratio.

Example 3.11
Let $M_0(t) = \lambda t^\nu$ (Weibull) and assume that the frailty variable is positive stable distributed with parameter γ. Then the resulting survival function is given by

$$S(t) = e^{-M_0(t)^\gamma} = e^{-\lambda^\gamma t^{\gamma\nu}}.$$

This is again a Weibull distribution but with parameters λ^γ and $\gamma\nu$. □

Example 3.12

In the following, the positive stable frailty model is applied to the Halluca data. The survival and hazard function, respectively, are given by (3.42) and (3.43) for a parametric analysis. Results can be found in Table 3.12. The

Table 3.12: Parametric positive stable frailty models for Halluca lung cancer data with different baseline hazard functions

parameter	Weibull	exponential	Gompertz
age (in years)	0.011 (0.001)	0.011 (0.001)	0.010 (0.003)
sex (females)	-0.192 (0.085)	-0.193 (0.083)	-0.176 (0.078)
type (NSCLC)	-0.162 (0.078)	-0.161 (0.077)	-0.139 (0.073)
ECOG (3 & 4)	0.708 (0.121)	0.705 (0.121)	0.663 (0.114)
stage II	0.535 (0.193)	0.532 (0.196)	0.489 (0.184)
stage IIIa	0.702 (0.155)	0.707 (0.152)	0.649 (0.144)
stage IIIb	1.134 (0.146)	1.131 (0.140)	1.038 (0.135)
stage IV	1.576 (0.124)	1.584 (0.128)	1.457 (0.129)
γ	0.863 (0.018)	0.859 (0.019)	0.919 (0.031)
λ	0.017 (0.004)	0.016 (0.004)	0.020 (0.005)
ν	0.999 (0.042)		
φ			-0.013 (0.005)
log-likelihood	-4858.66462	-4858.66470	-4855.45463

estimates of the regression parameters are very similar, indicating robustness of the analysis with respect to the choice of the baseline hazard function. The values of the log-likelihood function indicate that the Weibull and exponential models provide a similar fit to the data. The Gompertz model fits the data significantly better than the two other models. In the positive stable model no moments of frailty exist. Consequently, the model parameter $\gamma \in (0, 1]$ has no interpretation as frailty variance. Despite this fact, γ can be used as a measure of heterogeneity in the population. For $\gamma = 1$, there is no heterogeneity in the population. The smaller the values of γ, the larger the heterogeneity. In all three models the parameter estimates for γ are significantly different from one. The foregoing analysis was performed by maximizing the parametric log-likelihood function using the SAS procedure NLMIXED. □

The positive stable frailty distribution was introduced as a frailty distribution by Hougaard (1986b) and applied by Wang et al. (1995), Lam and Kuk (1997), Qiou et al. (1999), and Manatunga and Oakes (1999). Fine et al. (2003) and Martinussen and Pipper (2005) recently suggested new estimation procedures in the shared positive stable frailty model. It was further extended by Hougaard's power variance function distribution (Hougaard, 1986a) and Aalen's compound Poisson distribution (Aalen 1988, 1992).

3.7   PVF Frailty Model

A generalized family of frailty distributions that includes gamma, inverse Gaussian, and positive stable distributions is the family of power variance function distributions suggested by Tweedy (1984) and derived independently by Hougaard (1986a). This is a three-parameter family with parameters $\mu > 0, \lambda > 0$ and $0 < \gamma \le 1$. The probability density function is given by

$$f(z) = e^{-\lambda(1-\gamma)(\frac{z}{\mu} - \frac{1}{\gamma})}$$

$$\times \frac{1}{\pi} \sum_{\kappa=1}^{\infty} (-1)^{k+1} \frac{(\lambda(1-\gamma))^{\kappa(1-\gamma)} \mu^{\kappa\gamma}}{\gamma^\kappa} \frac{\Gamma(\kappa\gamma+1)}{\kappa!} z^{-\kappa\gamma-1} \sin(\kappa\gamma\pi)$$

The derivation of the Laplace transform from this density function is difficult and therefore omitted here. The interested reader is referred to Aalen (1992). The Laplace transform is

$$\mathbf{L}(u) = e^{\frac{\lambda(1-\gamma)}{\gamma}\left(1-(1+\frac{\mu u}{\lambda(1-\gamma)})^\gamma\right)}. \tag{3.44}$$

The first and second derivatives are given by

$$\mathbf{L}'(u) = -\mu(1 + \frac{\mu u}{\lambda(1-\gamma)})^{\gamma-1} e^{-\frac{\lambda(1-\gamma)}{\gamma}\left(1-(1+\frac{\mu u}{\lambda(1-\gamma)})^\gamma\right)}$$

and

$$\mathbf{L}''(u) = \frac{\mu^2}{\lambda}(1 + \frac{\mu u}{\lambda(1-\gamma)})^{\gamma-2} e^{-\frac{\lambda(1-\gamma)}{\gamma}\left(1-(1+\frac{\mu u}{\lambda(1-\gamma)})^\gamma\right)}$$

$$+ \mu^2(1 + \frac{\mu u}{\lambda(1-\gamma)})^{2\gamma-2} e^{-\frac{\lambda(1-\gamma)}{\gamma}\left(1-(1+\frac{\mu u}{\lambda(1-\gamma)})^\gamma\right)}$$

Similar to the gamma model, expectation and variance of a PVF-distributed random variable Z are derived with the help of the first and second derivatives of the Laplace transform:

$$\mathbf{E}Z = -\mathbf{L}'(0) = \mu \tag{3.45}$$

$$\mathbf{V}(Z) = \mathbf{L}''(0) - (\mathbf{L}'(0))^2 = \frac{\mu^2}{\lambda}. \tag{3.46}$$

The positive stable distribution can be obtained as a special case of the PVF distribution. To show this fact, some asymptotic considerations are necessary. Following the presentation in the book by Duchateau and Janssen (2008), we rewrite the logarithm of the Laplace transform of a PVF-distributed random variable in the following way:

$$
\log \mathbf{L}(u) = \frac{\lambda(1-\gamma)}{\gamma}\left(1 - \left(1 + \frac{\mu u}{\lambda(1-\gamma)}\right)^{\gamma}\right)
$$

$$
= \frac{\lambda(1-\gamma)}{\gamma}\left(1 - \left(\frac{\mu}{\lambda(1-\gamma)}\right)^{\gamma}\left(\frac{\lambda(1-\gamma)}{\mu} + u\right)^{\gamma}\right)
$$

$$
= \frac{\lambda(1-\gamma)}{\gamma}\left(\frac{\mu}{\lambda(1-\gamma)}\right)^{\gamma}\left(\left(\frac{\lambda(1-\gamma)}{\mu}\right)^{\gamma} - \left(\frac{\lambda(1-\gamma)}{\mu} + u\right)^{\gamma}\right) \quad (3.47)
$$

Now it is necessary that $\frac{\lambda}{\mu}$ converges to zero in an appropriate way by μ converging toward infinity and λ converging toward zero. Assuming the convergence

$$
\frac{\mu^{\gamma}}{\lambda^{\gamma-1}} \xrightarrow[\mu\to\infty,\lambda\to 0]{} \frac{\gamma}{(1-\gamma)^{1-\gamma}},
$$

the first factor in the expression (3.47) converges against one, and the second one goes to $-u^{\gamma}$. This is the logarithm of the Laplace transform of a positive stable-distributed random variable.

Using the standard assumption in frailty models that $\mathbf{E}Z = \mu = 1$, and introducing the frailty variance as a model parameter by the relationship $\mathbf{V}(Z) = \frac{1}{\lambda} := \sigma^2$, the Laplace transform (3.44) of a PVF random variable becomes

$$
\mathbf{L}(u) = e^{\frac{1-\gamma}{\gamma\sigma^2}\left(1-(1+\frac{\sigma^2 u}{1-\gamma})^{\gamma}\right)}.
$$

This implies the unconditional survival and hazard function in the PVF frailty model

$$
S(t) = e^{\frac{1-\gamma}{\gamma\sigma^2}\left(1-(1+\frac{\sigma^2 M_0(t)}{1-\gamma})^{\gamma}\right)}
$$

and

$$
\mu(t) = \frac{\mu_0(t)}{(1 + \frac{\sigma^2}{1-\gamma}M_0(t))^{1-\gamma}}.
$$

If $\gamma = 0$, the gamma frailty model with frailty distribution $\Gamma(1/\sigma^2, 1/\sigma^2)$ is easily obtained from the foregoing hazard function by comparison with (3.18). When comparing the Laplace transforms, the gamma distribution is derived as a limiting case after application of the rule by L'Hospital. For $\gamma = 0.5$, the inverse Gaussian distribution is obtained.

To quantify the effect of unobserved heterogeneity in the PVF frailty model, observed covariates are introduced into the model. Similar to the other frailty models, we assume again for ease of presentation that there exists only one single binary covariate with possible individual values zero and one in the model. Then the ratio of the marginal hazards becomes

$$\frac{\mu(t|X=1)}{\mu(t|X=0)} = \frac{(1 + \frac{\sigma^2}{1-\gamma} M_0(t))^{1-\gamma}}{(1 + \frac{\sigma^2}{1-\gamma} M_0(t)e^\beta)^{1-\gamma}} e^\beta,$$

which is e^β at the beginning of the follow-up $t=0$ and converges towards $e^{\gamma\beta}$ as time goes to infinity. This is the same value as the ratio of the marginal hazards in the positive stable frailty model. However, in contrast to the positive stable frailty model, the marginal hazards are not parallel in the PVF frailty model.

To calculate the frailty distribution among the survivors at a specific time point, we restrict again to the case $\mu=1$ and drop the observed covariates to keep the formulas simple:

$$f(z|T>t) = \frac{S(t|z)f(z)}{S(t)}$$

$$= \frac{\exp\left(-zM_0(t)\right)}{\exp\left(\frac{1-\gamma}{\gamma\sigma^2}\left(1 - (1 + \frac{\sigma^2 M_0(t)}{1-\gamma})^\gamma\right)\right)} e^{-\frac{1-\gamma}{\sigma^2}(z-\frac{1}{\gamma})}$$

$$\times \frac{1}{\pi} \sum_{\kappa=1}^{\infty} (-1)^{\kappa+1} \frac{(1-\gamma)^{\kappa(1-\gamma)}}{\sigma^{2\kappa(1-\gamma)}\gamma^\kappa} \frac{\Gamma(\kappa\gamma+1)}{\kappa!} z^{-\kappa\gamma-1} \sin(\kappa\gamma\pi)$$

$$= e^{\frac{-(1-\gamma)}{\sigma^2 A^{-\gamma}}\left(\frac{z}{A^{\gamma-1}}-\frac{1}{\gamma}\right)}$$

$$\times \frac{1}{\pi} \sum_{\kappa=1}^{\infty} (-1)^{\kappa+1} \frac{(1-\gamma)^{\kappa(1-\gamma)} A^{\kappa\gamma(\gamma-1)}}{(\sigma^2 A^{-\gamma})^{\kappa(1-\gamma)}\gamma^\kappa} \frac{\Gamma(\kappa\gamma+1)}{\kappa!} z^{-\kappa\gamma-1} \sin(\kappa\gamma\pi)$$

This is the density of a PVF-distributed random variable with parameters $A = 1 + \frac{\sigma^2 M_0(t)}{1-\gamma}$ (instead of μ), $\sigma^2 A^{-\gamma}$ (instead of σ^2) and γ.

On the one hand, the PVF frailty model is easily tractable because of closed-form expressions for the marginal survival function. On the other hand, the model is flexible in the sense that it contains many other interesting frailty models as special cases. That makes the model attractive for applications, and it is often used. Crowder (1989) studied the PVF frailty model to generate a multivariate distribution with Weibull marginals and one parameter governing association, which may be positive or negative. Hougaard et al. (1992) applied the model to lifetimes of Danish twins. Mallick and Ravishanker (2004) used a PVF frailty distribution and a Weibull baseline hazard. Inference was carried out in the Bayesian framework using Markov Chain Monte Carlo techniques. The model was extended regarding the baseline hazard function by Mallick and Ravishanker (2006).

3.8 Compound Poisson Frailty Model

The compound Poisson distribution was introduced by Aalen (1988, 1992) as a frailty distribution. The probability density function is similar to the density of the PVF distribution

$$f(z) = e^{-\lambda(1-\gamma)(\frac{z}{\mu} - \frac{1}{\gamma})} \tag{3.48}$$

$$\times \frac{1}{\pi} \sum_{\kappa=1}^{\infty} \frac{(\lambda(1-\gamma))^{\kappa(1-\gamma)}\mu^{\kappa\gamma}}{\gamma^{\kappa}} \frac{\Gamma(\kappa\gamma+1)}{\kappa!} (-z)^{-\kappa\gamma-1} \sin(\kappa\gamma\pi),$$

with parameters $\mu > 0, \lambda > 0$ and (different from the PVF distribution) $\gamma < 0$. An interesting property of the model is that it allows for a subgroup of zero frailty, which never experiences the event of interest. In the case of total mortality, this is impossible because nobody is immortal. But this model is relevant to medicine and demography, for example, when considering cause-specific mortality or the occurrence of a disease. Despite the fact that the density of the continuous part is only given as an infinite series that has to be calculated numerically, the distribution is mathematically convenient. It may also be seen as a natural choice. The distribution can be constructed as the sum of a Poisson-distributed number of independent and identically gamma-distributed random variables. This can be viewed as a hit model where each individual experiences a random number of hits, each of random size. More formally, the frailty Z of individuals in the study population is

$$Z = \begin{cases} V_1 + V_2 + \ldots + V_N & : \text{ if } N > 0, \\ 0 & : \text{ if } N = 0, \end{cases} \tag{3.49}$$

where N is Poisson distributed with expectation ρ. The variables $V_1, V_2, \ldots$ are independent and gamma distributed with $V_i \sim \Gamma(k, \lambda)$. Furthermore, N is assumed to be independent of $V_1, V_2, \ldots$ Laplace transforms of gamma and Poisson distributions are given by $\mathbf{L}_V(u) = (1 + \frac{u}{\lambda})^{-k}$ and $\mathbf{L}_N(u) = e^{-\rho + \rho e^{-u}}$, respectively. The Laplace transform of the frailty can now be derived by

$$\mathbf{L}(u) = \mathbf{E}e^{-uZ}$$

$$= \mathbf{P}(N=0) + \sum_{\kappa=1}^{\infty} \mathbf{E}(e^{-u(V_1+\ldots+V_N)}|N=\kappa)\mathbf{P}(N=\kappa)$$

$$= e^{-\rho} + \sum_{\kappa=1}^{\infty} \prod_{i=1}^{\kappa} (1 + \frac{u}{\lambda})^{-k} \frac{\rho^{\kappa}}{\kappa!} e^{-\rho}$$

$$= e^{-\rho} \sum_{\kappa=0}^{\infty} \frac{(\rho(1+\frac{u}{\lambda})^{-k})^{\kappa}}{\kappa!}$$

$$= e^{-\rho(1-(1+\frac{u}{\lambda})^{-k})}. \tag{3.50}$$

In the following we will switch to another, more convenient parameterization, given by

$$\rho = -\frac{k\lambda^\gamma}{\gamma}, \qquad \lambda = \lambda, \qquad k = -\gamma.$$

The Laplace transform of a compound Poisson-distributed random variable then becomes

$$\mathbf{L}(u) = \exp\Big[\frac{k\lambda^\gamma}{\gamma}\{1 - (1 + \frac{u}{\lambda})^\gamma\}\Big].$$

The first and second derivatives of the Laplace transform are

$$\mathbf{L}'(u) = -k\lambda^{\gamma-1}(1 + \frac{u}{\lambda})^{\gamma-1}\exp[\frac{k\lambda^\gamma}{\gamma}\{1 - (1 + \frac{u}{\lambda})^\gamma\}]$$

$$\mathbf{L}''(u) = -k\lambda^{\gamma-2}(\gamma - 1)(1 + \frac{u}{\lambda})^{\gamma-2}\exp[\frac{k\lambda^\gamma}{\gamma}\{1 - (1 + \frac{u}{\lambda})^\gamma\}]$$

$$+ k^2\lambda^{2\gamma-2}(1 + \frac{u}{\lambda})^{2\gamma-2}\exp[\frac{k\lambda^\gamma}{\gamma}\{1 - (1 + \frac{u}{\lambda})^\gamma\}].$$

Expectation and variance of frailty distribution can now be calculated by evaluating the derivatives at $u = 0$

$$\mathbf{E}Z = k\lambda^{\gamma-1} \tag{3.51}$$

$$\mathbf{V}(Z) = k(1 - \gamma)\lambda^{\gamma-2}. \tag{3.52}$$

Using the standard relation $\mathbf{E}Z = 1$ and $\sigma^2 = \frac{1-\gamma}{\lambda}$, the Laplace transform becomes

$$\mathbf{L}(u) = \exp\Big[\frac{1-\gamma}{\gamma\sigma^2}\Big(1 - (1 + \frac{\sigma^2 u}{1-\gamma})^\gamma\Big)\Big]. \tag{3.53}$$

This Laplace transform implies the marginal survival and hazard function in the case of a compound Poisson frailty model given by

$$S(t) = e^{\frac{1-\gamma}{\gamma\sigma^2}\left(1 - (1 + \frac{\sigma^2 M_0(t)}{1-\gamma})^\gamma\right)} \tag{3.54}$$

and

$$\mu(t) = \frac{\mu_0(t)}{(1 + \frac{\sigma^2}{1-\gamma}M_0(t))^{1-\gamma}}.$$

Because the Laplace transforms of the PVF distribution and the compound Poisson distribution are equal (except for the range of parameter γ, which can be negative in the compound Poisson model), the properties obtained from the Laplace transform are the same. Consequently, the population survival and hazard functions of the compound Poisson frailty model coincides with the respective functions in the PVF frailty model. Also, the ratio of the marginal hazards is similar to the PVF model when introducing a single binary observed covariate into the model

$$\frac{\mu(t|X=1)}{\mu(t|X=0)} = \frac{\left(1 + \frac{\sigma^2}{1-\gamma}M_0(t)\right)^{1-\gamma}}{\left(1 + \frac{\sigma^2}{1-\gamma}M_0(t)e^\beta\right)^{1-\gamma}}e^\beta,$$

which is e^β at $t=0$ and converges toward $e^{\gamma\beta}$ for $t \to \infty$.

Using the frailty representation (3.49), it is easy to derive the density of the continuous part of the distribution following the presentation in Duchateau and Janssen (2008). Denote by $f(z|N=\kappa)$ the probability density function of the sum $V_1 + \ldots + V_\kappa$. Because $V_1, \ldots, V_\kappa$ are i.i.d. random variables with gamma distribution $\Gamma(k, \lambda)$,

$$\mathbf{E}e^{-(V_1+\ldots+V_\kappa)s} = \left(1 + \frac{s}{\lambda}\right)^{-\kappa k},$$

meaning $V_1 + \ldots + V_\kappa \sim \Gamma(\kappa k, \lambda)$. Hence, the density can be written as

$$f(z) = \sum_{\kappa=1}^\infty f(z|N=\kappa)\mathbf{P}(N=\kappa)$$

$$= \sum_{\kappa=1}^\infty \frac{\lambda^{\kappa k} z^{\kappa k-1}e^{-\lambda z}}{\Gamma(\kappa k)}\frac{\rho^\kappa}{\kappa!}e^{-\rho}$$

$$= e^{-\rho-\lambda z}\sum_{\kappa=1}^\infty \frac{\lambda^{\kappa k}\rho^\kappa}{\Gamma(\kappa k)\kappa!}z^{\kappa k-1}$$

$$= e^{\frac{1-\gamma}{\gamma\sigma^2} - \frac{1-\gamma}{\mu\sigma^2}z}\sum_{\kappa=1}^\infty \frac{\left(\frac{1-\gamma}{\mu\sigma^2}\right)^{-\kappa\gamma}\left(-\frac{1-\gamma}{\gamma\sigma^2}\right)^\kappa}{\Gamma(-\kappa\gamma)\kappa!}z^{-\kappa\gamma-1}$$

$$= e^{-\frac{1-\gamma}{\sigma^2}\left(\frac{z}{\mu}-\frac{1}{\gamma}\right)}\sum_{\kappa=1}^\infty \frac{\left(\frac{1-\gamma}{\sigma^2}\right)^{\kappa(1-\gamma)}\mu^{\kappa\gamma}}{\gamma^\kappa\Gamma(-\kappa\gamma)\kappa!}(-z)^{-\kappa\gamma-1}$$

$$= e^{-\frac{1-\gamma}{\sigma^2}\left(\frac{z}{\mu}-\frac{1}{\gamma}\right)}\frac{1}{\pi}\sum_{\kappa=1}^\infty \frac{\left(\frac{1-\gamma}{\sigma^2}\right)^{\kappa(1-\gamma)}\mu^{\kappa\gamma}}{\gamma^\kappa}\frac{\Gamma(\kappa\gamma+1)}{\kappa!}(-z)^{-\kappa\gamma-1}\sin(\kappa\gamma\pi),$$

where the last equation holds because of the relation

$$\frac{1}{\Gamma(-\kappa\gamma)} = \frac{1}{\pi}\Gamma(\kappa\gamma+1)\sin(\kappa\gamma\pi).$$

This is the density given in (3.48) with $\lambda = \frac{1}{\sigma^2}$. It should be noted that the integral of $\mu(t)$ over $[0, \infty)$ is finite if $\gamma < 0$. Consequently, the survival function is incomplete because a fraction of individuals has zero frailty and will never experience the event under study. The size of the nonsusceptible fraction is given by

$$S(t) = e^{\frac{1-\gamma}{\gamma\sigma^2}\left(1-(1+\frac{\sigma^2}{1-\gamma}M_0(t))^\gamma\right)} \xrightarrow[t\to\infty]{} e^{\frac{1-\gamma}{\gamma\sigma^2}}.$$

The parameter γ divides the class of distributions in two major subfamilies: For $\gamma \geq 0$, the distribution is a PVF distribution. The extension to $\gamma < 0$ was suggested by Aalen (1988) and yields the compound Poisson distribution. The two subclasses are separated by the gamma distribution ($\gamma = 0$). Note that a different parameterization was applied by Aalen. The notation $cP(\gamma, k, \lambda)$ is used for a compound Poisson distribution.

It is necessary to mention that a connection exists between the probability of susceptibility and the frailty distribution in the compound Poisson frailty model. A model relaxing this assumption is considered in Section 3.12.

The model was used by Aalen (1992) to model the incidence of marriage of women born in Denmark. Marriage is an example of an event that not everybody experiences. A certain percentage of individuals never marry, and models of marriage incidence have to account for this. The fact that the observed incidence peaks around age 23 and becomes rather low after age 30 is therefore interpreted to be a selection phenomenon due to heterogeneity. This means that those who are most prone to marriage will marry quite early, and the reminder will have a lower tendency to marry.

A second interesting application of Aalen (1992) deals with fertility data in Norwegian women. It is a well-known fact that around 5% to 10% of all couples are unable to conceive children. Naturally, $\mathbf{P}(Z = 0)$ (where Z denotes the frailty to conceive a child) will be the probability of infertility, and the variation of Z expresses the varying fecundabilities among fertile couples.

Hougaard et al. (1994) applied the model to diabetic nephropathy onset data, a serious complication for insulin-dependent diabetic patients. Data are interval-censored because measurement of protein takes place only at selected time points. Less than 50% of diabetics with long-term survival develop nephropathy, suggesting that only some but not all patients are susceptible.

Aalen and Tretli (1999) applied the compound Poisson model to testicular cancer. Testicular cancer has two striking epidemiological features. First, its incidence has increased rapidly over the past few decades. Second, the incidence is greatest among younger men, and then declines from a certain age. The idea of the model is that a subgroup of men is particularly susceptible to testicular cancer, which results in selection over time. The model is fit to incidence data from the Norwegian Cancer Registry collected between 1953 and 1993. This work is being continued by Moger et al. (2004a).

Haukka et al. (2003) applied the model to schizophrenia data from the Finnish population born between 1950 and 1968. They concluded that only a small part of the population is susceptible to schizophrenia and found increasing individual risk with higher age among the susceptible part of the study population.

Example 3.13

To illustrate the many interesting features of the compound Poisson frailty model, the malignant melanoma data from Example 1.2 is considered. Here we apply three parametric models with Gompertz baseline to this data: the proportional hazards model, the gamma frailty model, and the compound Poisson/PVF frailty model. The results are given in Table 3.13.

Table 3.13: PH, gamma frailty, and compound Poisson frailty model applied to the malignant melanoma data

parameter	Gompertz model	gamma frailty	cP/PVF frailty
age	0.014 (0.009)	0.011 (0.011)	-0.001 (0.015)
gender	-0.528 (0.266)	-0.729 (0.388)	-0.886 (0.509)
thickness	0.144 (0.033)	0.241 (0.114)	0.286 (0.150)
λ	5.5e-5 (3.2e-5)	4.6e-5 (3.6e-5)	4.0e-5 (4.7e-5)
φ	-1.9e-5 (1.4e-4)	3.7e-7 (4.2e-7)	1.4e-6 (1.1e-6)
σ^2		2.064 (2.029)	3.823 (3.151)
γ			-0.822 (1.153)
log-likelihood	-554.638	-554.153	-553.666

The proportional hazards model with Gompertz baseline hazard suggests that women face a lower risk of death caused by malignant melanoma compared to men. Increasing age and tumor size result in higher mortality. The gamma frailty model implies an increase in the effect of the covariates gender and thickness, whereas the effect of age is decreased. Standard errors are also increased. The heterogeneity estimate σ^2 is not significantly greater than zero. The compound Poisson/PVF frailty model extends the gamma frailty model. Estimates of the regression parameters are different from the estimates in the gamma frailty model. The compound Poisson model shows only a nonsignificant improvement in the fit compared to the gamma frailty model ($\gamma = 0$), which is also supported by the large standard error of the estimate of parameter γ. Comparing all three models, the proportional hazards model with Gompertz baseline shows the best fit with respect to the likelihood ratio test. The estimate of γ is negative, implying that this is a compound Poisson frailty model. Consequently, some patients will never die from this disease. This is possible because only death by malignant melanoma was studied and not total mortality. That means a part of the population seems to be protected against mortality from malignant melanoma. The estimated proportion with zero risk is around $e^{\frac{1-\gamma}{\gamma\sigma^2}} = 56\%$. A possible conclusion would be that this is a cure or nonsusceptible fraction. But caution is necessary, especially in the present case where the compound Poisson frailty model does not show a significant better fit compared to the gamma frailty model. ☐

3.9 Quadratic Hazard Frailty Model

Making appropriate distributional assumptions about frailty, it is often possible to find a complete analytical form of the likelihood function. One disadvantage of the log-normal frailty model considered in Section 3.4 the absence of explicit expressions for the survival and hazard functions. To avoid this problem and to combine the flexibility of the normal distribution with advantages of frailty models that provide an analytic survival function, Aalen (1987) and Yashin and Iachine (1996) suggested the quadratic hazard frailty model. Their model is based on the idea of quadratic conditional hazard and normal distribution of the random effects. Assume $Z = W^2$ and let W be a normally distributed random variable with $W \sim N(m, s^2)$. The model is given in terms of the conditional hazard function (without covariates):

$$\mu(t|Z) = Z\mu_0(t) = W^2\mu_0(t).$$

The Laplace transform can be calculated in the following way:

$$\mathbf{L}(u) = \mathbf{E}\exp(-uW^2)$$

$$= \frac{1}{\sqrt{2\pi}s} \int_{-\infty}^{\infty} \exp(-w^2u)\exp\left(-\frac{(w-m)^2}{2s^2}\right) dw$$

$$= \frac{1}{\sqrt{2\pi}s} \int_{-\infty}^{\infty} \exp\left(-\frac{2s^2w^2u + w^2 - 2mw + m^2}{2s^2}\right) dw$$

$$= \frac{1}{\sqrt{2\pi}s} \int_{-\infty}^{\infty} \exp\left(-\frac{w^2 - \frac{2mw}{1+2s^2u} + \frac{m^2}{(1+2s^2u)^2} + \frac{m^2}{1+2s^2u} - \frac{m^2}{(1+2s^2u)^2}}{2\frac{s^2}{1+2s^2u}}\right) dw$$

$$= \frac{1}{\sqrt{1+2s^2u}} \exp\left(-\frac{\frac{m^2}{1+2s^2u} - \frac{m^2}{(1+2s^2u)^2}}{2\frac{s^2}{1+2s^2u}}\right)$$

$$\times \frac{1}{\sqrt{2\pi}\frac{s}{\sqrt{1+2s^2u}}} \int_{-\infty}^{\infty} \exp\left(-\frac{(w - \frac{m}{1+2s^2u})^2}{2\frac{s^2}{1+2s^2u}}\right) dw$$

$$= \frac{1}{\sqrt{1+2s^2u}} \exp\left(-\frac{m^2u}{1+2s^2u}\right), \qquad (3.55)$$

where the last equation holds because the integral equals to one as it is over the density of a normal distribution. It is easy to see that, in case of $m = 0$, the frailty $Z = W^2$ is gamma distributed with shape parameter $k = 1/2$ and form parameter $\lambda = 1/2s^2$.

The first and second derivatives need some algebra.

$$\mathbf{L}'(u) = -s^2(1+2s^2u)^{-\frac{3}{2}} e^{-\frac{m^2u}{1+2s^2u}} - m^2(1+2s^2u)^{-\frac{5}{2}} e^{-\frac{m^2u}{1+2s^2u}}$$

$$\begin{aligned}
\mathbf{L}''(u) &= 2m^2s^2(1+2s^2u)^{-\frac{7}{2}} e^{-\frac{m^2u}{1+2s^2u}} + 3s^4(1+2s^2u)^{-\frac{5}{2}} e^{-\frac{m^2u}{1+2s^2u}} \\
&= 3m^2s^2(1+2s^2u)^{-\frac{7}{2}} e^{-\frac{m^2u}{1+2s^2u}} + m^2s^2(1+2s^2u)^{-\frac{7}{2}} e^{-\frac{m^2u}{1+2s^2u}} \\
&= m^4(1+2s^2u)^{-\frac{11}{2}} e^{-\frac{m^2u}{1+2s^2u}}
\end{aligned}$$

Expectation and variance of the frailty $Z = W^2$ are then given by

$$\mathbf{E}Z = -\mathbf{L}'(0) = m^2 + s^2$$

and

$$\begin{aligned}
\mathbf{V}(Z) &= \mathbf{L}''(0) - (\mathbf{L}'(0))^2 \\
&= 3s^4 + 6m^2s^2 + m^4 - (s^2 + m^2)^2 \\
&= 2s^4 + 4m^2s^2.
\end{aligned}$$

The unconditional survival function is

$$S(t) = \frac{1}{\sqrt{1+2s^2 M_0(t)}} \exp\left(-\frac{m^2 M_0(t)}{1+2s^2 M_0(t)} \right),$$

resulting in the unconditional hazard function

$$m(t) = m_0(t)\left(\frac{m^2}{(1+2s^2 M_0(t))^2} + \frac{s^2}{1+2s^2 M_0(t)} \right).$$

One nice feature of this model is the Gaussian property of the conditional distribution $\mathbf{P}(W \le w | T > t)$:

$$\begin{aligned}
\mathbf{P}(W \le w | T > t) &= \frac{\mathbf{P}(T > t, W \le w)}{S(t)} \\
&= \frac{1}{S(t)} \int_{-\infty}^{w} \mathbf{P}(T > t|s) f_W(s)\, ds \\
&= \frac{1}{S(t)} \frac{1}{\sqrt{2\pi}s} \int_{-\infty}^{w} \exp(-s^2 M_0(t)) \exp\left(-\frac{(s-m)^2}{2s^2} \right) ds \\
&= \frac{1}{S(t)} \frac{1}{\sqrt{2\pi}s} \int_{-\infty}^{w} \exp\left(-\frac{s^2 - \frac{2ms}{1+2s^2 M_0(t)} + \frac{m^2}{(1+2s^2 M_0(t))^2}}{2\frac{s^2}{1+2s^2 M_0(t)}} \right) ds \\
&= \frac{1}{\sqrt{2\pi}\frac{s}{\sqrt{1+2s^2 M_0(t)}}} \int_{-\infty}^{w} \exp\left(-\frac{(s - \frac{m}{1+2s^2 M_0(t)})^2}{2\frac{s^2}{1+2s^2 M_0(t)}} \right) ds.
\end{aligned}$$

Consequently, W (square root of frailty) among survivors of age t is normally distributed with parameters

$$W|(T > t) \sim N\left(\frac{m}{1 + 2s^2 M_0(t)}, \frac{s^2}{1 + 2s^2 M_0(t)}\right).$$

The common constraint $\mathbf{E}Z = \mathbf{E}W^2 = 1$ implies the relation $s^2 + m^2 = 1$, which restricts possible values of m and s^2 and limits the applicability of the model to real-life problems. Substituting m^2 by the expression $1 - s^2$ (and keeping in mind $s^2 \leq 1$) results in the following unconditional survival and hazard functions:

$$S(t) = \frac{1}{\sqrt{1 + 2s^2 M_0(t)}} e^{-\frac{(1-s^2) M_0(t)}{1 + 2s^2 M_0(t)}} \tag{3.56}$$

and

$$\mu(t) = \mu_0(t) \frac{1 + 2s^4 M_0(t)}{(1 + 2s^2 M_0(t))^2}. \tag{3.57}$$

To quantify the effect of unobserved heterogeneity in the quadratic hazard frailty model, observed covariates are introduced into the model. Considering only one single binary 0-1 covariate in the model, the ratio of the marginal hazards becomes

$$\frac{\mu(t|X = 1)}{\mu(t|X = 0)} = \frac{1 + 2s^4 M_0(t)e^{\beta}}{(1 + 2s^2 M_0(t)e^{\beta})^2} \frac{(1 + 2s^2 M_0(t))^2}{1 + 2s^4 M_0(t)} e^{\beta},$$

which is e^{β} at $t = 0$ and converges towards e^{β} as time goes to infinity. Hence, the marginal hazards are not time independent as in the positive stable frailty model, but the ratio of the marginal hazards converges against the ratio of the conditional hazards. This means that the marginal and conditional hazard ratios coincide at time point zero, are becoming more and more different during the first part of the follow-up and finally converge again as time goes to infinity.

It is necessary to keep in mind that s^2 is the variance of the random effect W but not the variance of the frailty term $Z = W^2$. To underline this difference, s^2 is used as the variance parameter for the random effect, whereas σ^2 is used as the variance parameter for the frailty term. Frailty variance can easily be calculated by using the 4th moments of normal distributed random variables and the restriction $m^2 = 1 - s^2$ introduced above for identifiability reasons

$$\begin{aligned} \mathbf{V}(Z) &= \mathbf{E}W^4 - (\mathbf{E}W^2)^2 \\ &= 2s^4 + 4m^2 s^2 \\ &= 2s^2(2 - s^2). \end{aligned} \tag{3.58}$$

As a consequence, it holds that $0 \leq V(Z) \leq 2$. This means that the amount of unobserved heterogeneity is restricted in this model by an upper bound. Furthermore, it is easy to see that, in the limiting case $s^2 \to 0$, the original Cox proportional hazards model without unobserved heterogeneity is obtained.

Example 3.14

The quadratic hazard frailty model is applied to the Halluca lung cancer data from Example 1.3. The hazard and survival functions have an explicit form in this model (see (3.56) and (3.57)) and can be used in the likelihood function for parametric analysis. Similar to other frailty models considered before a Weibull, exponential, and Gompertz baseline hazard function is used, and the results of the analysis are given in Table 3.14.

Table 3.14: Parametric quadratic hazard frailty models with different baseline hazard functions applied to the Halluca lung cancer data

parameter	Weibull	exponential	Gompertz
age (in years)	0.012 (0.002)	0.013 (0.004)	0.013 (0.004)
sex (females)	-0.183 (0.084)	-0.188 (0.086)	-0.188 (0.086)
type (NSCLC)	-0.104 (0.080)	-0.101 (0.082)	-0.098 (0.082)
ECOG (3 & 4)	0.943 (0.160)	1.007 (0.145)	1.012 (0.145)
stage II	0.522 (0.190)	0.540 (0.194)	0.541 (0.194)
stage IIIa	0.707 (0.149)	0.738 (0.150)	0.738 (0.150)
stage IIIb	1.119 (0.140)	1.159 (0.138)	1.159 (0.138)
stage IV	1.584 (0.134)	1.642 (0.126)	1.643 (0.126)
s^2	0.065 (0.017)	0.078 (0.011)	0.078 (0.011)
λ	0.018 (0.006)	0.016 (0.004)	0.016 (0.004)
ν	0.964 (0.035)		
φ			1e-8 (0.001)
log-likelihood	-4851.86641	-4852.41278	-4852.41104

Estimates of the regression parameters are very similar in the three models, indicating robustness of the analysis with respect to the choice of the baseline hazard function. The values of the log-likelihood function indicate that the Weibull and Gompertz models do not fit the data significantly better than the exponential model. Only small differences occur between the estimates of the random effects variance. In general, the variance of the random effects is small (but significantly away from zero in all three models). Using formula (3.58), the variance of the frailty term σ^2 is around 0.3. Analysis was performed by maximizing the parametric log-likelihood function using the SAS procedure NLMIXED. □

3.10 Lévy Frailty Models

A common problem is statistics is the comparison of groups with respect to their event time outcome. When applying a frailty model one usually assumes the same frailty distribution for all groups and that the individuals in one group have a proportionally higher conditional hazard than in the other groups. Integrating out the frailty and calculating the unconditional hazards, one finds that these hazards are no longer proportional (with one exception – the positive stable distribution). Aalen and Hjort (2002) suggest the use of different frailty distributions in the groups. One way of constructing this is to think of a damage process that has generated frailty in the groups. This process is assumed to have run its course before the current observations start. In high-risk groups, this process has been running for a longer time, or at a higher rate, thereby yielding greater frailty than in low-risk groups. The use of frailty distributions based on Lévy processes implies proportionality of the population hazards, which is of course a very convenient feature of this approach.

Aalen and Hjort (2002) and Aalen et al. (2008) consider frailty distributions which are generated by a nonnegative Lévy process $D = \{D(s), s \geq 0\}$, that is a random process with nonnegative, independent, time-homogeneous increments. The Laplace transform of such a damage process is given by the Lévy–Chinchin formula

$$\mathbf{L}(u; s) = e^{-s\psi(u)}.$$

This is a valid Laplace transform for all nonnegative s when function ψ is a characteristic exponent of the Lévy process. Here s denotes the time which the frailty generating Lévy process has been running prior to the follow-up. Larger values of s indicate higher risks because of a longer running damage process. More details about Laplace exponents and Lévy processes can be found in Bertoin (1996). The family of Lévy processes contains a number of interesting special cases such as compound Poisson processes, PVF processes, gamma processes, stable processes, etc. The survival function in this model is given by

$$S(t) = e^{-s\psi(M_0(t))}$$

and the unconditional hazard function is

$$\mu(t) = s\mu_0(t)\psi'\big(M_0(t)\big).$$

One can see that s is a proportionality parameter and there is a natural link to the proportional hazards model. Of course, the special Laplace transform of a Lévy process produces this result. Aalen and Hjort (2002) present a number of examples of frailty models based on Lévy processes. The majority of the frailty distributions applied in practice follow from them. The connection to the compound Poisson frailty model in the parameterization (3.50) used by Aalen and Hjort (2002) is obtained by $\psi(u) = \rho\big(1 - (1 + \frac{u}{\lambda})^{-k}\big)$, resulting in the Laplace transform

$$\mathbf{L}(u; s) = e^{-s\rho\big(1-(1+\frac{u}{\lambda})^{-k}\big)}.$$

Here it is clearly to see that the additional parameter s influences only ρ from the original model which is the parameter of the Poisson distribution of the number of damaging hits. The parameters k and λ describing the gamma distribution of the hits are not influenced by s. It is necessary to note that the compound Poisson frailty distribution in this model depends on s and is therefore no longer restricted to expectation one. In the gamma frailty model as another example the characteristic exponent is of the form

$$\psi(u) = k \ln(1 + \frac{u}{\lambda}) \tag{3.59}$$

which gives

$$\mathbf{L}(u; s) = (1 + \frac{u}{\lambda})^{-sk}.$$

This is the Laplace transform of a gamma distribution $\Gamma(sk, \lambda)$. Consequently, s influences only the shape parameter of the gamma distribution, but not the form parameter. Again, the restriction of zero expectation does no longer hold for different values of s if the other two parameters are fixed. For different values of s proportional hazards are obtained, which is clearly a nice and interesting feature of this approach, especially when event times of different groups need to be compared.

3.11   Log-t Frailty Model

The logarithm of a t-distribution is used as a frailty distribution in very few cases in the literature. Matsuyama et al. (1998) used this approach in a multi-center cancer clinical trial to compare the effect of institutions. Sahu and Dey (2004) applied the model to the kidney infection data by McGilchrist and Aisbett (1991) and rat litter tumor data by Mantel, Bohidar, and Ciminera (1977). Sargent (1998) applied the model also to rat tumor data. All papers used a Bayesian approach, which is rather complex and does not allow fitting analytic methods. Consequently, MCMC methods were used to estimate the model parameters. The R package COXPH as alternative includes the log-t distribution as an option for frailty (beside gamma and log-normal frailty distribution). But the author does not have good experience with this model because several example data could not be fitted due to numerical problems in the R package.

3.12   Univariate Frailty Cure Models

The Cox model is commonly used in the analysis of survival time data. An often unstated assumption of this model (and of frailty models with frailty distributions without mass point zero) is that all individuals are susceptible to experiencing the event of interest. Consequently, if follow-up is long enough, all individuals will experience the event. However, in some situations it makes sense to assume the existence of a fraction of individuals who are not expected to experience the event. These individuals are nonsusceptible or cured, for example, by a genetic predisposition or a vaccination. For instance, researchers may be interested in analyzing the recurrence of a disease. Many individuals may never experience a recurrence of that disease; therefore, a fraction in the study population exists that has recovered from disease and is now protected. Historically, cure models were first presented by Boag (1949) and Berkson and Gage (1952), and have been utilized to estimate the cured (or nonsusceptible) fraction. Cure models are survival models that allow for a cured fraction of individuals. These models extend the understanding of time-to-event data by allowing for the formulation of more accurate and informative conclusions than previously made. These conclusions would otherwise be unobtainable from an analysis that fails to account for a cured fraction in the population. If a cured fraction component is not present, the analysis is reduced to standard approaches of survival analysis. A key characteristic of data modeled by cure models is that there needs to be sufficient follow-up time to determine that a cure fraction is present in the study population. For the proportion of individuals in the population experiencing the event under study, there exist many ways to model the distribution of their event times. For example, Peng et al. (1998) used the generalized F distribution, whereas Kuk and Chen (1992) and Sy and Taylor (2000) applied a proportional hazards approach to model event times.

Cure models assume that individuals prone to experience the event are homogeneous in risk. This section deals with extensions of cure models in order to allow for heterogeneity among the fraction under risk by using frailty models. Or, depending on the point of view, it deals with extensions of frailty models to allow for a cured fraction in the study population. In this case, the distribution of frailty is a combination of discrete and continuous distributions. Spilerman (1972) considered the "spiked-gamma" as an example of such a distribution.

In cure models, the population is divided into two subpopulations. An individual is either cured with probability $1 - \phi$, or has a proper survival function $S(t)$, with probability ϕ. Individuals regarded as cured will never experience the event of interest, and their survival time will be defined as infinity. Therefore, hazard and survival functions of cured individuals are set to zero and one, respectively, for all finite values of t. A model of survival times that incorporates a cured fraction is given by Berkson and Gage (1952):

$$S^*(t) = (1 - \phi) + \phi S(t).$$

Longini and Halloran (1996) have proposed frailty cure (cure-mixture) models that extends a model by Farewell (1977). In their model the frailty variable has point mass at zero with probability $1 - \phi$ while heterogeneity among those experiencing the event of interest is modeled via a continuous distribution with probability ϕ. In the gamma frailty cure model, the survival function S of the susceptible individuals is substituted by the marginal survival function in the gamma frailty model (3.17):

$$S^*(t) = (1 - \phi) + \phi(1 + \sigma^2 M_0(t))^{-1/\sigma^2}. \tag{3.60}$$

The idea behind this model is similar but not equivalent to the compound Poisson frailty model suggested by Aalen (1988, 1992). In the model by Longini and Halloran (1996), the shape of the frailty distribution is assumed to be independent of the size of the cure fraction, while in the compound Poisson frailty model there exists a connection between the shape of the frailty density and the probability of susceptibility.

An interesting work about cure models is that of Maller and Zhou (1996). Price and Manatunga (2001) give a comprehensive introduction to the area and apply different cure, frailty, and frailty cure models to leukemia remission data. They conclude that frailty models are useful in modeling data with a cured fraction and found that the gamma frailty cure model provides a better fit to their remission data compared to the standard cure model.

The next example provides an extension of the foregoing model to include censored observations. Consider two types of expressions for a disease: the incidence and the age of disease onset. Risk models for overall susceptibility (lifetime risk) that consider only the first expression by treating the disease as a binary trait of being affected or not can give wrong results. The reason is, that for individuals without the disease, due to censoring, it is often not known whether they will eventually develop the disease. On the other hand, models from survival analysis typically assume that everyone has the same susceptibility to the disease and will eventually be effected if followed up for a sufficiently long period of time. It is possible that these models do not accurately describe the disease risk factors. In models dealing with both types of expressions, the effect of a covariate can act on either the overall susceptibility or the age at onset or both. Such a model is considered later in (3.63). The following model is a special case of the binary frailty model. Here, one of the two point masses is located at zero, resulting in a cure fraction with hazard zero with respect to the event of interest.

The application of mixture models for joint modeling of the overall risk of a disease and the age-at-onset distribution of the individuals at risk is popular (Farewell 1977, Kuk and Chen 1992, Lam et al. 2005). We define an individual to be susceptible if she or he will eventually develop the disease after being followed for a sufficiently long time. Define

$$Y = \begin{cases} 1 & : \quad \text{if the individual is susceptible} \\ 0 & : \quad \text{if not} \end{cases} \tag{3.61}$$

and let T denote the age at onset when $Y = 1$. With the foregoing concept, let $\phi = \mathbf{P}(Y = 1)$ and $S(t) = \mathbf{P}(T > t | Y = 1)$ describe the distribution of Y and of the failure time T. It is impossible to observe Y, but it is possible to observe whether or not a subject has experienced the event during the period of its follow-up time.

- For those individuals that experience the event, it holds that $\Delta = 1$. Obviously, if $Y = 1$, then the survival function for the uncensored observations is of the form $\mathbf{P}(Y = 1)\mathbf{P}(T \leq C | Y = 1) = \phi(1 - S(C))$, where C denotes the censoring time.

- For the other observations, a failure is not observed ($\Delta = 0$). This may occur either because $Y = 0$ or because the observation is really censored. Therefore, $\mathbf{P}(Y = 0) + \mathbf{P}(Y = 1)\mathbf{P}(T > C | Y = 1) = (1 - \phi) + \phi S(C)$.

Combining these results, the likelihood function takes the form

$$L(\boldsymbol{\theta}, \phi) = \prod_{i=1}^{n} \left(\phi f(t_i; \boldsymbol{\theta}) \right)^{\delta_i} \left(1 - \phi + \phi S(t_i; \boldsymbol{\theta}) \right)^{1 - \delta_i}. \tag{3.62}$$

This is a generalization of (2.6) and (2.7) because these relations are easily obtained with $\phi = 1$.

Example 3.15
Three different frailty models are applied to age at onset of breast cancer in 11,714 Swedish female twins described in Example 1.6. The results are given in Table 3.15.

Table 3.15: Frailty and frailty cure models for the breast cancer data of Swedish twins

parameter	gamma	gamma cure	compound Poisson
σ^2	59.060 (7.677)	9.182 (11.14)	45.079 (15.42)
γ	0		-0.089 (0.133)
ϕ	1.000	0.221 (0.174)	0.237 ( )
λ	2.4e-7 (1.6e-7)	1.8e-6 (2.6e-6)	3.9e-7 (3.1e-7)
φ	0.162 (0.013)	0.150 (0.017)	0.150 (0.017)
log-likelihood	-5236.5914	-5236.2517	-5236.2751

In the first column of Table 3.15, the gamma frailty model is applied to account for heterogeneity in the study population. This model is described in detail in Section 3.3. The model ignores the existence of a cure fraction, and the parameter $\phi = 1$ indicates that all individuals are (more or less) susceptible. This model is extended to the gamma frailty cure model (second column, see (3.60)), which allows for a fraction of nonsusceptible individuals, for example, patients who are not at risk of suffering from breast cancer. The third model is the compound Poisson frailty model (Section 3.8). The size of the susceptible fraction is calculated by $\phi = 1 - \exp(\frac{1-\gamma}{\gamma\sigma^2})$. That is why no standard error is given for this quantity. All models are parametric models using a Gompertz baseline hazard function with parameters λ and φ.

In the gamma frailty model, the size of the susceptible fraction is 100% per definition as in classical survival analysis. The gamma frailty cure model gives an estimate of 22.1% of the size of the susceptible fraction, for example, only 22.1% of all women are at risk for breast cancer. The respective number calculated from the compound Poisson frailty model is similar, with 23.7%. The gamma frailty model is a special case of the gamma frailty cure model (when $\phi = 1$) and the compound Poisson frailty model (when $\gamma = 0$). These estimates are in good agreement with results found by Chatterjee and Shih (2001) and Wienke et al. (2003a) in bivariate analyses and estimates of a lifetime risk of breast cancer of around 8–12% (Feuer et al. 1993, Rosenthal and Puck 1999, Ries et al. 1999) in current Western populations. The latter numbers give a lower boundary for the size of the susceptible fraction. A huge estimate of σ^2 in the gamma model indicates the existence of large heterogeneity in the study population, which is at least partially accounted for by the introduction of a nonsusceptible fraction in the gamma frailty cure model, where the heterogeneity is smaller, but still large. In the compound Poisson frailty model, the estimate of γ is negative, indicating the existence of a nonsusceptible fraction. However, differences between the three models are not significant in terms of the log-likelihood function. This speaks in favor of the most simple gamma frailty model. To compare the nested gamma model ($\gamma = 0$) with the compound Poisson model standard test theory can be applied because the value $\gamma = 0$ is no longer on the boundary of the parameter space. The fit of the compound Poisson frailty model to the Swedish breast cancer data is demonstrated in Figure 3.11.

It is necessary to mention that the correlation between the ages at onset of breast cancer in the twin pairs is neglected in these univariate models. We will reanalyze the data using a bivariate model later on to account for the correlated observation times. ▯

Model (3.60) was extended to the mixture cure frailty model with gamma frailty by Peng and Zhang (2008a):

$$S^*(t|\mathbf{X}_1, \mathbf{X}_2) = (1 - \phi(\mathbf{X}_2)) + \phi(\mathbf{X}_2)(1 + \sigma^2 M_0(t)e^{\boldsymbol{\beta}_1'\mathbf{X}_1})^{-1/\sigma^2}. \qquad (3.63)$$

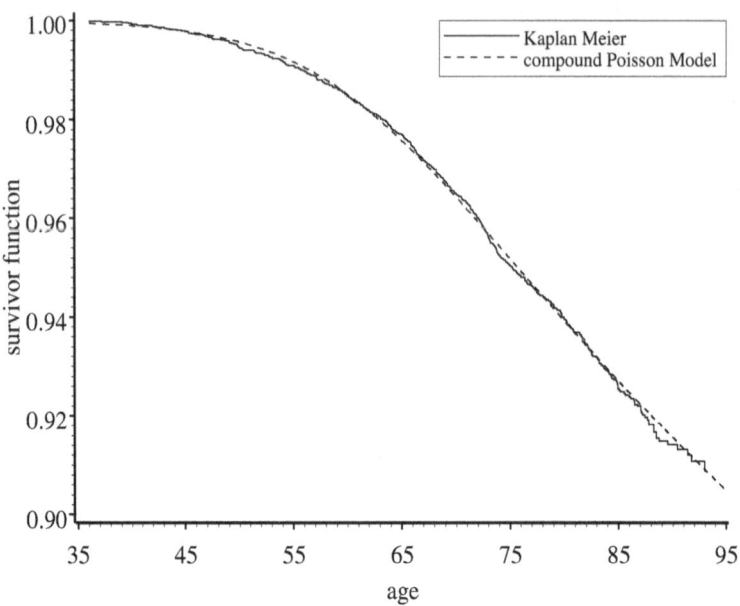

Figure 3.11: Kaplan–Meier estimator and compound Poisson model for Swedish breast cancer data.

Here $\mathbf{X}_2$ denotes the vector of covariates that may have effects on the cure rate. The vector $\mathbf{X}_1$ represents the covariates that influence the event times of those individuals who are susceptible to the event. Without frailty, the model reduces to the proportional hazards model with cure fraction. Without cure fraction, the model becomes the gamma frailty model considered earlier. Without both cure fraction and the frailty the common proportional hazards model is obtained. If the probability of cure depends on observable covariates, a common way to introduce this into the model is logistic regression (Farewell 1982)

$$\phi(\mathbf{X}_2) = \frac{e^{\boldsymbol{\beta}_2' \mathbf{X}_2}}{1 + e^{\boldsymbol{\beta}_2' \mathbf{X}_2}}$$

with $\boldsymbol{\beta}_2$ as the vector of regression parameters to be estimated. Other link functions such as the probit link and the log–log link can also be used.

Cure models suffer from an inherent identifiability problem due to right-censored observations. The event under study has not occurred at the end of the follow-up either because the person is nonsusceptible or because the person is susceptible, but follow-up was not long enough to observe the event. A key component of identifiability is the presence of covariates in both components of the mixture model. In fact, Li et al. (2001) show that, if the baseline hazard is nonparametric and independent of covariates, and if the cure fraction is taken to be constant (independent of covariates), the mixture cure survival model is not identifiable. The situation becomes less restricted in models with parametric baseline hazard functions. There exists a series of results regarding identifiability in competing risk models, which are analogous to identifiability in mixture cure models (Heckman and Honoré 1989, Abbring and van den Berg 2003, Peng and Zhang 2008b). All of these results are based on the presence of observed covariates in the models.

As a consequence of these identifiability results, estimating the proportion of nonsusceptibles is not easy. However, it is tempting to try it, especially when the Kaplan–Meier curves appear to level off above zero. For a detailed discussion of pros and cons of univariate frailty models as cure models, see Schumacher (1989). The identifiability problem grows with increasing amount of censoring but is reduced by the parametric modeling of the baseline hazard. In cure models with fixed censoring times (caused by end of study), censoring is no longer noninformative. The proportion of censored observations contains important information about the model parameters; for example, in the case of no censoring, it holds that $\phi = 1$.

Further interesting examples of cure models based on a frailty approach are considered in Price and Manatunga (2001). An application of the model to the analysis of colorectal cancer incidence data in Norway can be found in Svensson et al. (2006).

3.13 Missing Covariates in PH Models

In most practical situations it is impossible to include all relevant covariates into the model. Sometimes researchers are not able to measure an important prognostic factor because of time or financial restrictions. In other situations there might exist important prognostic factors that are unknown yet. For example, these could be genetic factors as researcher usually do not know all genes having a relevant influence on the event time. In other cases, maybe the information about covariates is lost or incomplete. This consideration is true for all regression models. The standard approach is to ignore such kind of variables, which means that the unobserved heterogeneity is absorbed by the error term. The consequence of omitted covariates in linear regression models is known: parameter estimates are unbiased unless the omitted risk factors are correlated with the included observed covariates. In hazard regression models, even this result does not hold. The omission of influential covariates implies biased parameter estimates. The main goal of univariate frailty models is therefore to reduce this bias. We will consider a proportional hazards model with vectors of observed and unobserved covariates $\mathbf{X}_1$ and $\mathbf{X}_2$, respectively:

$$\mu(t|\mathbf{X}_1, \mathbf{X}_2) = \mu_0(t)e^{\boldsymbol{\beta}_1'\mathbf{X}_1 + \boldsymbol{\beta}_2'\mathbf{X}_2}. \tag{3.64}$$

Here β_2 denotes the vector of regression parameters of unobserved covariates. Because the vector $\mathbf{X}_2$ is unknown, the model cannot be used in practice. That is why it is assumed that the expression $Z = e^{\beta_2' \mathbf{X}_2}$ is a random unobservable variable, combining the effect of all unobserved covariates in the frailty Z. For convenience it is assumed that the distribution of Z is independent of $\mathbf{X}_1$ and time t. Both assumptions are reasonable because, in the classical proportional hazards models with observed covariates, it is also assumed that there is no interaction between the covariates and that the covariates are time independent. Now all that matters is the distribution of frailty, discussed throughout the previous sections. As shown there, for some frailty distributions, the (unconditional) hazard function can be given in an explicit form.

Many biostatistical studies dealing with univariate survival have focused on evaluating the effect of omitted covariates on the estimates of the regression parameters β, see, for example, Gail et al. (1984), Hougaard et al. (1986a), Schumacher et al. (1987), Schumacher (1989), Bretagnolle and Huber-Carol (1988), Chamberlain (1992), Schmoor and Schumacher (1997), Keiding et al. (1997), and Oakes and Jeong (1998). The present section deals with the problem of unobserved covariates. Modeling of this unobserved heterogeneity was the main reason for the introduction of univariate frailty models by Vaupel et al. (1979) and Lancaster (1979) to the scientific community. The main aim is to reduce the bias caused by unobserved covariates in the proportional hazards model.

We will consider the analytical result by Gail et al. (1984) a little bit more in detail. If the baseline hazard is assumed to be known (parametric model), if frailty is erroneously ignored in the model, and if there is no censoring, then the parameter estimates β are consistently estimated by the classical maximum likelihood method. Unfortunately, this nice result does not generalize to more realistic settings. In general, hazard models (including censored observations) neglecting a subset of the important covariates leads to biased estimates of both regression coefficients and the hazard rate. The reason for such bias is the time-dependent hazard function, a unique element in survival analysis. To understand this result, we consider the example of a population initially consisting of two subpopulations, a high-risk group and a low-risk group, each subject to a constant risk binary frailty model. If this heterogeneity is not accounted for and a common hazard is assumed for the whole population, the estimated hazard will not be a simple average of the hazards of the two groups as depicted in Figure 3.2. It will increase less fast over time (or even level off or decrease) compared to the hazards of the two subpopulations because of the selection effect, which drops out high-risk individuals early.

Consequently, in a proportional hazards model with observed covariates, an omitted covariate may result in biased parameter estimates for the remaining factors. This even holds when the distribution of the omitted characteristics is initially the same in all categories of included covariates. The problem is that the distribution of characteristics cannot remain the same across categories over time. This results because high-risk individuals with certain values of the omitted covariate will die earlier, and so the distribution of omitted characteristics within each category of an included covariate must also change over time. As a consequence, all parameter estimates must be contaminated by the effect of the omitted risk factor. This is quite disturbing since one can never know the true model.

Bretagnolle and Huber-Carol (1988) predict the sign of the bias in the two following cases: first, when there is only one covariate left in the model, whatever the number of omitted covariates is. Then the effect on the survival of the covariate under study is always underestimated. Second, in case of several covariates remaining in the analyzed model, the authors prove that the same result of underestimation holds for each of them at least up to some fixed time, which, in practical cases, is reasonably long. The asymptotic bias resulting from such omissions is not negligible, as shown by simulations. In the case of left-truncated and right-censored data, it may even happen that the estimates cross zero. That means a beneficial covariate ($\beta < 0$) results through the biased estimate in an unfavorable one ($\beta > 0$). Nevertheless, this crossing zero phenomenon does not happen with only right censoring if one assumes that censoring is independent of the included covariates.

Univariate frailty models are one (but not the only) way to account for the effect of omitted covariates in a proportional hazards model. For reasons of convenience, analysts frequently choose parametric representations of the frailty distribution that are mathematically tractable. We follow this line throughout the book. With such parametric assumptions about heterogeneity, the hazard function can be represented parametrically or nonparametrically. There could be the problem of misspecifying the frailty distribution. Heckman and Singer (1982b) demonstrate, however, that for a given parametric baseline hazard, results can be very sensitive to the choice of the parametric form of the frailty distribution even when a flexible form is chosen (see also Heckman and Singer 1984a, and Keiding et al. 1997). For this purpose, Heckman and Singer (1982b) use simple parametric distribution families (log-normal, normal, and gamma distribution) for the random effects to investigate this sensitivity. The authors propose a discrete nonparametric frailty distribution and show through simulations that the regression parameters can be estimated with great precision. The frailty distribution is approximated by a discrete mixture with a finite number of mass points where the number, location, and probability mass associated with each point are to be estimated (Section 3.2). The results of Heckman and Singer (1982b) indicate that the distribution of heterogeneity cannot be approximated well. Thus their procedure corrects for heterogeneity without clearly identifying its exact distribution.

It should be noted that Heckman and Singer's (1982b) arguments against parametric assumptions about the frailty distribution are points of discussion and controversies by authors who claim that Heckman and Singer (1982b) misspecified the duration dependence in the example data used to demonstrate the potentials of their nonparametric approach. Newer studies conclude that parameter estimates are not that sensitive with respect to the choice of frailty distribution (see Manton et al. 1986, Klein et al. 1992, Guo and Rodriguez 1992, Guo 1993).

To get any results at all with a nonparametric frailty distribution, one must impose a parametric form on the baseline hazard function like the Weibull or Gompertz distribution. What is not mentioned in Heckman and Singer (1982b) but is demonstrated, though not emphasized, by Manton et al. (1981) is that results can also be sensitive to the functional form of the assumed baseline hazard. Trussell and Richards (1985) show that parameter estimates could be very sensitive with respect to the assumed parametric form of the baseline hazard function when using the nonparametric frailty distribution suggested by Heckman and Singer (1982b).

Henderson and Oman (1999) intend to quantify the bias that may occur in estimated covariate effects. They fit marginal distributions when frailty is present in the survival data but ignored in a wrongly specified proportional hazards analysis. The authors investigate this problem for positive stable frailty models. In general, however, no explicit solution was found. Henderson and Oman (1999) used first-order approximations to estimate the bias in different situations. It turns out that the amount of bias depends on the form of frailty distribution, but to the first-order approximation the bias is independent of the covariate distribution. Censoring in the Koziol–Green model (Koziol and Green 1976), where the censoring survival is a power of the baseline survival function, and type I censoring show that the asymptotic bias is reduced by censoring, particularly with log-normal frailty. For the very specific situation of noncensored survival times and gamma-distributed frailty with variance parameter σ^2, the following approximation was derived by Henderson and Oman (1999)

$$\beta = (1 + \sigma^2)\beta^*, \tag{3.65}$$

where β, β^* denote the unbiased and biased parameters, respectively, in the Cox model, assuming that the covariates are centered. Consequently, the bias due to omitted covariates becomes greater with increasing heterogeneity (frailty variance), and relation (3.65) could be used to compensate for the frailty effect.

Congdon (1995) investigates the influence of different frailty distributions (gamma, inverse Gaussian, stable, and binary) on the analysis of cause-specific and total mortality data from the London area during the years 1988 – 1990 by using Weibull and Gompertz baseline hazard functions.

Chapter 4

Shared Frailty Models

So far we have focused on the frailty model as a way of dealing with possible heterogeneity due to unobserved covariates. This is the main interpretation of frailty in the application to univariate time-to-event data. As discussed in the last chapter, this results in selection over time; for example, this is shown as leveling-off or crossing-over effects in population hazards. The concept of frailty introduced by Vaupel et al. (1979) to biostatistics and by Lancaster (1979) to the econometric literature originates from this kind of models.

Another, completely different, aspect of this approach is to use the frailty term to model associations between event times, which goes back to the work of Clayton (1978). Implicitly, most of the statistical models and methods for failure time data, and here especially the Cox proportional hazards model, were developed under the assumption that the observations from different subjects are statistically independent of each other. While this is sensible in many applications, it has become obvious that this assumption does not hold in certain situations that are more common as originally thought.

In the following section the two main approaches in multivariate survival analysis – marginal and frailty models – are outlined and compared, followed by a description and discussion of the shared frailty model in the subsequent sections. The shared frailty model is a mixture model because the common risk in each cluster (the frailty Z) is assumed to be random. The model assumes that all event times in a cluster are independent given the frailty variables. In other words, it is a conditional independence model where the frailty is common to all individuals in a cluster and therefore responsible for creating dependence between event times. This is the reason for the concept of *shared frailty*. A shared frailty model can be considered as a mixed (random effects) model in survival analysis with group variation (frailty) and individual variation described by the hazard function. In contrast, mixed models show a more symmetric handling of these two sources of variation. Because of the censored observations the Cox model and the frailty models do not belong to the class of generalized linear mixed models. It is assumed that there is independence between the observations from different clusters. If the variation of the frailty variable is zero, this implies independence between event times in the clusters; otherwise, there is positive dependence between event times. A more detailed presentation of shared frailty models can be found in the excellent book by Duchateau and Janssen (2008).

4.1   Marginal versus Frailty Model

Multivariate survival analysis may provide an effective tool for analyzing information from multiple/recurrent events in situations where independence between event times cannot be assumed. The following three examples given in Liang et al. (1995) may serve to illustrate different problems in multivariate event-time data analysis.

- Diabetic retinopathy is one of the most important causes of visual loss and blindness. Given the relatively high prevalence of this disease, new treatments to delay the onset of severe visual loss are critical. In 1971, the Diabetic Retinopathy Study was initiated to study the effectiveness of laser photocoagulation. This randomized, controlled clinical trial involved more than 1700 patients enrolled at 15 medical centers in the United States. Patients with diabetic retinopathy and visual acuity of 20/100 or higher in both eyes were eligible to participate in the study. The design protocol randomly selected one of each participant's eyes that was treated, and the other eye was observed without having received treatment. The event was the occurrence of visual acuity less than 5/200 at two consecutively completed follow-ups of four months. This design differs from conventional trials in that each patient served as his own control. Consequently, each patient contributed two correlated observations to the analysis, one from each eye.

- Family studies are critical in assessing the role which genetics play in the disease process. Statistical methods such as variance component models and path analysis have been developed and adopted to analyze family data with quantitative traits such as cholesterol. Variance component models aim to measure the extent to which the total variation in the quantitative trait is due to a correlation between relatives, as well as the degree of correlation among full siblings and other relatives. When the considered trait is onset age of a disease, conventional methods are not appropriate. This is mainly due to censoring/truncation of this variable but also to the need for a measure of within-family correlation that incorporates time, a feature not shared by conventional measures such as the correlation coefficient.

- The trial on gamma interferon as described in Fleming and Harrington (1991) is a typical example of recurrent events. In their study, patients with chronic granulomatous disease (CGD) were randomly assigned to either gamma interferon or placebo, with the event of interest being the diagnosis of a serious infection. It is clear that infections can reoccur. Thus both the time and the number of infection occurrences may be informative about the effectiveness of the treatment.

These three examples share an important feature, namely, that the failure times for observations from the same cluster correlate with one another. In Examples one and three the cluster is an individual, in Example two it is a family. In these examples, the cluster sizes are small relative to the number of clusters. These three examples, however, differ from one another in terms of their scientific objectives. The main objective of examples one and three is to examine the effectiveness of a new treatment, which presumably can be characterized through regression modeling. The within-cluster correlation in these examples is usually of secondary interest, although ignoring it could lead to erroneous conclusions. The within-family association, for example, two is of primary interest, although regression adjustment for each related subject is critical in order to minimize the potential that the observed association is mainly due to environmental factors shared by family members. Furthermore, the mechanisms behind within-cluster associations may vary so that different statistical models to describe the associations may be needed. It is clear that the mechanism leading to the correlation between two fellow eyes is different from that attributed to the correlation of observations measured over time from the same eye.

Another typical example with clustered event times are multicenter clinical trials with event-time outcome. Here the treatment centers are the clusters. Event times of patients in a cluster are assumed to be correlated because of center-specific differences in treatment, care, and diagnosis of the patients, or in the composition of the center-specific study populations. The lung cancer data from the Halluca study provide such an example. Dependent on the prevalence of the disorder of interest, there are sometimes many centers with only a few patients (rare diseases) or a few centers with a large number of patients each (common diseases).

Available statistical models fall into two broad classes – marginal and frailty models (Wei and Glidden 1997). Marginal methods specify models for the effect of covariates on the hazards of the individuals (the margins) under the working independent assumption. That means, for the point estimates of the parameters, independence between the event times in a cluster is assumed. To take into account the fact that observed event times are correlated, the variance estimates need to be adjusted but without the need for explicitly modeling the correlation (Wei et al. 1989, Lee et al. 1992, Cai and Prentice 1995). The association between the events is considered a nuisance parameter. The marginal baseline hazards can be modeled differently (Wei et al. 1989) or with a common functional form (Lee et al. 1992). As with the analysis of longitudinal data, regression parameters are estimated from generalized estimating equations, and the corresponding variance–covariance estimators are corrected properly to account for the dependence structure. Yu and Peng (2008) suggested a marginal model with cure fraction where both the margins as well as the cure fraction may depend on observed covariates. An excellent and detailed review of the robust and well-developed marginal approach is given in Lin (1994).

The other commonly used and general approach to the problem of modeling multivariate data is the specification of independence among observed data items conditional on a set of unobserved or latent variables (random effects). A multivariate model for the observed data is then induced by averaging over an assumed distribution for the latent variables. The dependence structure in the multivariate model arises when dependent latent variables enter into the conditional models for multiple observed data items, and the dependence parameters may often be interpreted as variance components. Frailty models for multivariate survival data are derived under a conditional independence assumption by specifying latent variables that act multiplicatively on the baseline hazard function. Different assumptions about the distribution of the random effects can create different dependence structures in the cluster as discussed in detail for the shared frailty model in the book by Duchateau and Janssen (2008). This popular approach with its strong link to the field of generalized linear mixed models is one of the building blocks for the present monograph.

Two main differences between the two approaches should be kept in mind. First, the interpretation of regression parameters in both models is different. In the marginal model, the parameters describe the population level relative risk, whereas in the frailty model, the parameters have a cluster-level relative risk interpretation. That is, in the latter approach, the hazard ratio refers to comparisons within clusters where individuals share the same frailty. In the marginal approach, the hazard ratio refers to comparisons between individuals randomly drawn from the total study population, independent of which cluster the individuals belong to. As such, the estimates are not expected to be the same in marginal and frailty models since they estimate different quantities, unless the within-cluster correlation is zero (meaning that clustering does not play any role) and both models comply with the Cox model for independent data.

Second, the marginal approach, although effective, can predict only marginal survival probabilities of single individuals. In contrast, in the frailty approach it is possible to perform joint prediction of survival for individuals from the same cluster. Frailty models also allow the prediction of survival based on the current status of the other individuals in the cluster. Such kind of analysis is of special interest in small clusters, for example, in event times of sibships. Practical comparisons of both methods show that the confidence intervals for regression parameter estimates are smaller in frailty models compared to that in the marginal approach (Chuang and Cai 2006). This is based on the fact that the frailty approach makes stronger model assumptions by specifying the correlation structure.

An interesting approach occupying an intermediate position between the two aforementioned models to allow estimation both regression coefficients with traditional interpretation as well as correlations between event times is described by Mahé and Chevret (1999).

4.2   The Concept of Shared Frailty

In this section we would like to focus on multivariate event-time models with dependent hazards as described earlier. This concept provides multivariate extensions of the traditional univariate frailty model (Vaupel et al. 1979, Lancaster 1979), and it allows mutual dependence of clustered event times to be taken into account in the analysis of event-time data. Survival models for dependent event times are especially useful because they allow more sophisticated questions about the nature of aging, disease, disability, and the mortality processes to be addressed. Such dependence occurs, for example, in event times of related individuals (e.g., family members) or in duration times of recurrent events (e.g., asthma attacks).

One important and mostly used approach in this field is the shared frailty concept. The hazard model for each individual in this approach, however, looks exactly the same as in the standard univariate frailty model considered in the last chapter. The only, but important, difference is that, in a shared frailty model, frailty is defined as a measure of the relative risk that individuals in a group share. Thus the frailty variable is associated with groups of individuals rather than individuals as such.

The shared frailty approach assumes that all failure times in a cluster are conditionally independent given the frailties. The value of the frailty term is constant over time and common to all individuals in the cluster, and thus it is responsible for creating dependence between event times in a cluster. This dependence is always positive in shared frailty models. Originally, the model was introduced to the literature by David Clayton and was considered in the bivariate case without using the notion of frailty (Clayton 1978), modeling the event times of sons and their fathers. The shared frailty model dominates the literature on multivariate frailty models and was extensively studied in the monographs by Hougaard (2000), Therneau and Grambsch (2000), and Duchateau and Janssen (2008). That is the reason why we will treat this model only in brief to develop the main ideas of multivariate frailty models, but without going into much details here. This lays the basis for extensions of the shared frailty model in different directions. These extensions are one of the main tasks of the present monograph and will be considered in the next chapter.

In the special case of degenerated frailty Z (meaning the variable Z is a nonrandom constant), no dependence exists between the lifetimes within a group. In this situation, the shared frailty model reduces to the case of independent event times without unobserved heterogeneity, and that means the proportional hazards model. The univariate frailty model considered in the last chapter is a special case of the shared frailty model with cluster size one. In this case the interpretation of the model is different from that of the multivariate frailty model. In the univariate case, modeling of unobserved heterogeneity caused by unobserved covariates is the main goal of the analysis. In the multivariate approach, modeling of or adjusting for the correlation in the regression models is the main focus. This conceptional difference is the main reason for treating the univariate and the shared frailty model in separate chapters in the present monograph.

Event times from different clusters are considered to be independent. The number of observations in a cluster is assumed to be known. Twin studies provide typical examples of bivariate event data. Another example are the times to failure for several similar human organs, like time to blindness of the right and the left eye as in studies on diabetic retinopathy. In family studies one is often faced with small and unequal cluster sizes. Event time data from multi-center clinical trials are an example for moderate to large and unequal cluster sizes.

In all cases, a probability distribution is assigned to the frailty variable for practical reasons. Some results exist, especially in the econometric literature, on mixed proportional hazards (frailty) models deriving specific conditions that make models identifiable even in case of a nonspecified frailty distribution. For a comprehensive overview in this field, see van den Berg (2001). We will not consider this situation here. Frailty distributions were discussed in detail in Chapter 3. Assuming a random frailty means that we have to integrate the frailty out of the likelihood expression or use more sophisticated estimation approaches to obtain parameter estimates. In the first case, almost all calculations can be made based on the Laplace transform of the respective frailty distribution, and in the second case, MCMC or numerical integration techniques are applied. In the examples in the following sections we will (similar to the last chapter) focus on parameter estimation strategies that are included in easily accessible statistical packages (R, S plus, SAS, STATA) to allow also nonspecialists in this field to apply the discussed models without extensive programming. Despite the fact described earlier that univariate and multivariate frailty models differ widely, software routines analyzing data wit frailty models can usually deal with both types, the univariate and the shared frailty models. The routine only needs different cluster variables in the data sets, indicating individuals (cluster size one) or groups of individuals as cluster.

In the following paragraph the basic definition of the model is given. A shared frailty model in survival analysis is defined as follows. Suppose there are n clusters and that cluster i has n_i observations and associates with the unobserved frailty Z_i $(1 \leq i \leq n)$. The vector $\mathbf{X}_{ij}$ $(1 \leq i \leq n, 1 \leq j \leq n_i)$ contains the covariate information of the event time T_{ij} of the jth observation in the ith cluster. Conditional on the frailty term Z_i, the survival times in cluster i $(1 \leq i \leq n)$ are assumed to be independent and their hazard functions to be of the form

$$\mu(t|\mathbf{X}_{ij}, Z_i) = Z_i \mu_0(t) e^{\boldsymbol{\beta}' \mathbf{X}_{ij}},$$

where $\mu_0(t)$ denotes the baseline hazard function, and $\boldsymbol{\beta}$ is a vector of fixed-effect parameters to be estimated. The frailties Z_i $(i = 1, \ldots, n)$ are assumed to be independently and identically distributed random variables with density function $f(z)$. The frailty density depends on unknown parameters to be estimated. Similar to the univariate case a semiparametric shared frailty model is one with a nonparametric baseline hazard $\mu_0(t)$. Furthermore, please note that, with the foregoing notation, the case of event times from clustered individuals as well as the case of recurrent event times in individuals is covered. However, in the analysis of recurrent event-time data, there may be specific information about the ordering of the events, and the time scale used needs careful consideration. For specific aspects with shared frailty models in recurrent event times, see Chapter 9 of Hougaard (2000) and Duchateau et al. (2003).

The main assumption of a shared frailty model is that all individuals in cluster i share the same value of frailty Z_i $(i = 1, \ldots, n)$, and this is why the model is called the shared frailty model. The lifetimes are assumed to be conditionally independent with respect to the shared (common) frailty. This shared frailty is the cause of dependence between lifetimes within the clusters. We derive in the following paragraphs the quantities based on this conditional formulation. Independence of the lifetimes within the clusters corresponds to a degenerate frailty distribution (no variability in Z_i). In all other cases, the dependence is positive. It is assumed that there is independence between event times from different clusters. If condition $\mathbf{P}(Z_i > 0) = 1$ holds, the shared frailty model leads to absolute continuous distributions and thus cannot model dependence due to common events. Consequently, it is not appropriate for event-related dependence (shock models) because an event in one individual is not relevant to the partner; it only changes the information available on the frailty. One exception to this general assumption is the shared compound Poisson frailty model, which does not fulfill the condition $\mathbf{P}(Z_i > 0) = 1$. In this specific model, it is possible that all individuals in a cluster share the frailty value zero (with positive probability) and are nonsusceptible to the event of interest (cure model).

Using an argument similar to that in equation (3.5), we can derive the joint conditional multivariate survival function for the individuals in the ith cluster. Conditional on frailty Z_i which is shared by all individuals in cluster i, it holds that

$$S(t_{i1}, \ldots, t_{in_i} | \mathbf{X}_i, Z_i) = S(t_{i1} | \mathbf{X}_{i1}, Z_i) \ldots S(t_{in_i} | \mathbf{X}_{in_i}, Z_i)$$

$$= \exp\left(-Z_i \sum_{j=1}^{n_i} M_0(t_{ij}) e^{\boldsymbol{\beta}' \mathbf{X}_{ij}}\right) \tag{4.1}$$

where $M_0(t) = \int_0^t \mu_0(s)\, ds$ denotes the cumulative baseline hazard function and $\mathbf{X}_i = (\mathbf{X}_{i1}, \ldots, \mathbf{X}_{in_i})$ is the covariate matrix of the individuals in the ith cluster. This is the starting point to derive the unconditional joint survival function. Averaging expression (4.1) with respect to the frailty Z_i gives the marginal survival function:

$$S(t_{i1}, \ldots, t_{in_i} | \mathbf{X}_i) = \mathbf{E} S(t_{i1}, \ldots, t_{in_i} | \mathbf{X}_i, Z_i)$$

$$= \mathbf{E} \exp \left(- Z_i \sum_{j=1}^{n_i} M_0(t_{ij}) e^{\boldsymbol{\beta}' \mathbf{X}_{ij}} \right)$$

$$= \mathbf{L} \left(\sum_{j=1}^{n_i} M_0(t_{ij}) e^{\boldsymbol{\beta}' \mathbf{X}_{ij}} \right),$$

where $\mathbf{L}$ denotes the Laplace transform of the frailty variable. Thus, the multivariate survival function is expressed as the Laplace transform of the frailty distribution, evaluated at the cumulative baseline hazard. The joint survival function for all event-time data is now the product of the survival functions of all the clusters because of the assumption about independence between clusters

$$S(t_{11}, \ldots, t_{nn_n} | \mathbf{X}_1, \ldots, \mathbf{X}_n) = \prod_{i=1}^{n} \mathbf{L} \left(\sum_{j=1}^{n_i} M_0(t_{ij}) e^{\boldsymbol{\beta}' \mathbf{X}_{ij}} \right).$$

The univariate unconditional survival functions can be expressed by means of the Laplace transform

$$S(t_{ij} | \mathbf{X}_{ij}) = \mathbf{E} S(t_{ij} | \mathbf{X}_{ij}, Z_i)$$

$$= \mathbf{E} \exp \left(- Z_i M_0(t_{ij}) e^{\boldsymbol{\beta}' \mathbf{X}_{ij}} \right)$$

$$= \mathbf{L} \left(M_0(t_{ij}) e^{\boldsymbol{\beta}' \mathbf{X}_{ij}} \right).$$

Denote by $\mathbf{L}^{-1}$ the inverse function of the Laplace transform $\mathbf{L}$. Consequently, $M_0(t_{ij}) e^{\boldsymbol{\beta}' \mathbf{X}_{ij}} = \mathbf{L}^{-1}(S(t_{ij} | \mathbf{X}_{ij}))$, and the unconditional survival function of the ith cluster is given by

$$S(t_{i1}, \ldots, t_{in_i} | \mathbf{X}_i) = \mathbf{L} \left(\mathbf{L}^{-1} \left(S(t_{i1} | \mathbf{X}_{i1}) \right) + \ldots + \mathbf{L}^{-1} \left(S(t_{in_i} | \mathbf{X}_{in_i}) \right) \right),$$

the Archimedian copula family of Genest and MacKay (1986). There is a strong link between frailty models and copula models. For an illustrative discussion in this field we refer to Goethals et al. (2008), Duchateau and Janssen (2008), and Chapter 6 of this monograph.

4.3 Shared Gamma Frailty Model

Similar to the univariate case in the last chapter, the standard assumption about frailty in shared frailty models is that it follows a gamma distribution. The main reason for the popularity of the gamma distribution is their nice mathematical properties, especially the simple form of the Laplace transform. In the shared frailty model, another aspect has to be considered additionally with respect to frailty distribution. Each frailty distribution implies a specific form of dependence between event times in clusters. For example, the gamma distribution models late dependence in shared frailty models (Duchateau and Janssen 2008). Assuming for frailty a gamma distribution with expectation one and variance σ^2, averaging equation (4.1) with respect to the cluster-specific random variable Z_i produces the multivariate survival function for the ith cluster

$$
\begin{aligned}
S(t_{i1}, \ldots, t_{in_i} | \mathbf{X}_i) &= \mathbf{L}\Big(\sum_{j=1}^{n_i} M_0(t_{ij}) e^{\boldsymbol{\beta}' \mathbf{X}_{ij}} \Big) \\
&= \Big(1 + \sigma^2 \sum_{j=1}^{n_i} M_0(t_{ij}) e^{\boldsymbol{\beta}' \mathbf{X}_{ij}} \Big)^{-\frac{1}{\sigma^2}} \\
&= \Big(\sum_{j=1}^{n_i} S(t_{ij} | \mathbf{X}_{ij})^{-\sigma^2} - (n_i - 1) \Big)^{-\frac{1}{\sigma^2}},
\end{aligned} \tag{4.2}
$$

where the last relation is a consequence of equation (3.17). It should be noted that the concept of shared frailty is different from that of individual frailty introduced by Vaupel et al. (1979) and Lancaster (1979) in their analysis of univariate duration data. This difference has gone largely unrecognized, perhaps because of the superficial similarity of the individual hazards in the two approaches. Frailty in the shared frailty model is only a part of individual frailty, capturing only the components of frailty shared by all individuals in a cluster. Noncommon unobserved risk factors are not included in the shared frailty model and require extensions of the shared gamma frailty model considered in the next chapter.

In some situations we will pay special attention to the case of bivariate frailty models ($n_i = 2$, $i = 1, \ldots, n$). Examples of bivariate data, based on event times from Danish and Swedish twins, are analyzed and discussed in detail in the present and the following chapters. In the bivariate case, the survival function (4.2) simplifies to

$$
S(t_1, t_2) = \big(S_1(t_1)^{-\sigma^2} + S_2(t_2)^{-\sigma^2} - 1 \big)^{-\frac{1}{\sigma^2}}, \tag{4.3}
$$

where we drop the cluster index i in the following for ease of presentation but assume a single binary covariate X representing two strata under the assumption of strata-specific baseline hazard functions. This results in two different marginal survival functions for the partners in each pair. In this situation it holds that $S(t|X) = S_1(t)$ if $X = 1$ (strata 1) and $S(t|X) = S_2(t)$ if $X = 2$ (strata 2).

The correlations between lifetimes of randomly selected pairs are always the same in the shared frailty model, implying a symmetric situation. This symmetry (which is equivalent to the compound symmetry assumption in linear mixed models) makes the model less useful for modeling correlations in family studies with groups of different relatives (mother–father, mother–daughter, grandfather–son, brother–brother, etc.), which are, for example, of special interest in genetic studies. In the following we will distinguish between the parametric and the semiparametric shared gamma frailty models.

4.3.1   Parametric shared gamma frailty model

Different parametric forms can be assumed for the baseline hazard function. In most examples, a Gompertz or Weibull baseline hazard is assumed, but the theory is developed in general. In the parametric shared gamma frailty model, the unconditional likelihood function can be easily derived. Similar to the univariate case, the regression parameters $\boldsymbol{\beta}$, the parameter vector $\boldsymbol{\theta}$ of the baseline hazard function μ_0, and the variance of the frailty σ^2 are the parameters to be estimated. Consider first the conditional likelihood in the case of n clusters of size n_i $(i = 1, \ldots, n)$:

$$L(\boldsymbol{\beta}, \boldsymbol{\theta}, \sigma^2) = \prod_{i=1}^{n} \int_0^\infty \prod_{j=1}^{n_i} \left(z_i \mu_0(t_{ij}; \boldsymbol{\theta}) e^{\boldsymbol{\beta}' \mathbf{X}_{ij}} \right)^{\delta_{ij}} e^{-z_i M_0(t_{ij}; \boldsymbol{\theta}) e^{\boldsymbol{\beta}' \mathbf{X}_{ij}}} f(z_i; \sigma^2) dz_i$$

with

$$f(z_i; \sigma^2) = \frac{z_i^{1/\sigma^2 - 1} e^{-\frac{z_i}{\sigma^2}}}{\sigma^{2/\sigma^2} \Gamma(1/\sigma^2)}$$

denoting the density function of a gamma distribution with expectation one and variance σ^2. A closed form solution to this integral exists. Using the simplification

$$y_i = 1/\sigma^2 + \sum_{j=1}^{n_i} M_0(t_{ij}; \boldsymbol{\theta}) e^{\boldsymbol{\beta}' \mathbf{X}_{ij}}$$

the foregoing likelihood can be written in the form

$$L(\boldsymbol{\beta}, \boldsymbol{\theta}, \sigma^2) = \prod_{i=1}^{n} \frac{\prod_{j=1}^{n_i} \left(\mu_0(t_{ij}; \boldsymbol{\theta}) e^{\boldsymbol{\beta}' \mathbf{X}_{ij}} \right)^{\delta_{ij}}}{y_i^{1/\sigma^2 + d_i} \sigma^{2/\sigma^2} \Gamma(1/\sigma^2)} \int_0^\infty (y_i z_i)^{1/\sigma^2 + d_i - 1} e^{-y_i z_i} y_i d(z_i),$$

where the expression $d_i = \sum_{j=1}^{n_i} \delta_{ij}$ denotes the number of observed events in cluster i $(i = 1, \ldots, n)$. Now the integral can be solved giving

$$L(\boldsymbol{\beta}, \boldsymbol{\theta}, \sigma^2) = \prod_{i=1}^{n} \frac{\Gamma(1/\sigma^2 + d_i) \prod_{j=1}^{n_i} \left(\mu_0(t_{ij}; \boldsymbol{\theta}) e^{\boldsymbol{\beta}' \mathbf{X}_{ij}}\right)^{\delta_{ij}}}{\left(1/\sigma^2 + \sum_{j=1}^{n_i} M_0(t_{ij}; \boldsymbol{\theta}) e^{\boldsymbol{\beta}' \mathbf{X}_{ij}}\right)^{1/\sigma^2 + d_i} \sigma^{2/\sigma^2} \Gamma(1/\sigma^2)}.$$

By taking the natural logarithm of this expression we obtain the well-known unconditional log-likelihood function of the shared gamma frailty model (Klein 1992, Duchateau and Janssen 2008):

$$\log L(\boldsymbol{\beta}, \boldsymbol{\theta}, \sigma^2) = \sum_{i=1}^{n} \Big[d_i \log \sigma^2 + \log \Gamma(1/\sigma^2 + d_i) - \log \Gamma(1/\sigma^2)$$

$$- (1/\sigma^2 + d_i) \log(1 + \sigma^2 \sum_{j=1}^{n_i} M_0(t_{ij}; \boldsymbol{\theta}) e^{\boldsymbol{\beta}' \mathbf{X}_{ij}})$$

$$+ \sum_{j=1}^{n_i} \delta_{ij} (\boldsymbol{\beta}' \mathbf{X}_{ij} + \log \mu_0(t_{ij}; \boldsymbol{\theta})) \Big]. \qquad (4.4)$$

In the parametric shared gamma frailty model with observed covariates, the unobserved frailty Z_i $(i = 1, \ldots, n)$ in each cluster can be estimated (Nielsen et al. 1992) by the expression

$$\hat{Z}_i = \frac{1/\hat{\sigma}^2 + \sum_{j=1}^{n_i} \delta_{ij}}{1/\hat{\sigma}^2 + \sum_{j=1}^{n_i} M_0(t_{ij}; \hat{\boldsymbol{\theta}}) e^{\hat{\boldsymbol{\beta}}' \mathbf{X}_{ij}}}. \qquad (4.5)$$

Here $\hat{\sigma}^2$ is the estimate of the frailty variance, $\hat{\boldsymbol{\theta}}$ the vector of the estimated parameters of the cumulative baseline hazard function, and $\hat{\boldsymbol{\beta}}$ the vector of estimated regression coefficients. This is a natural extension of formula (3.26) in the univariate case.

Example 4.1

We consider the Halluca study from Example 1.3 and apply three different parametric shared gamma frailty models with exponential, Gompertz, and Weibull baseline hazards (Table 4.1). It turns out that the exponential hazard function is not flexible enough, the Gompertz and Weibull model show a significant better fit to the data with respect to the likelihood ratio test (the exponential model is nested in the Gompertz as well as the Weibull model). The Weibull model shows a slightly better fit compared to the Gompertz model, but parameter estimates and standard errors are similar in both models and also closed to the values obtained in the semiparametric shared gamma frailty model (Table 4.2) considered in the next section.

Table 4.1: Parametric shared gamma frailty models of the Halluca lung cancer data

parameter	Weibull	exponential	Gompertz
age (in years)	0.009 (0.003)	0.009 (0.003)	0.009 (0.003)
sex (females)	-0.162 (0.073)	-0.172 (0.073)	-0.160 (0.073)
type (NSCLC)	-0.107 (0.068)	-0.119 (0.068)	-0.098 (0.068)
ECOG (3 & 4)	0.595 (0.108)	0.627 (0.108)	0.610 (0.108)
stage II	0.450 (0.170)	0.476 (0.170)	0.449 (0.170)
stage IIIa	0.613 (0.133)	0.651 (0.133)	0.606 (0.133)
stage IIIb	0.978 (0.123)	1.043 (0.123)	0.961 (0.123)
stage IV	1.324 (0.113)	1.413 (0.112)	1.312 (0.113)
λ	0.033 (0.009)	0.023 (0.006)	0.029 (0.008)
ν	0.878 (0.020)		
φ			-0.018 (0.003)
σ^2	0.318 (0.116)	0.403 (0.134)	0.305 (0.113)
log-likelihood	-4891.1150	-4908.4594	-4891.8328

In all three models we see an increase in risk with higher age, ECOG status 3 or 4 (compared to ECOG status $0 - 2$), and higher stage of the disease (reference group is stage I). Females and patients with a non-small cell lung carcinoma experience a lower risk. The estimates of the regression and frailty parameters depend on the parametric assumption regarding the baseline hazard. This limits the applicability of the parametric shared gamma frailty model because more detailed investigations about the shape of the baseline hazard function are necessary. In most practical cases, there is no additional information about the form of the baseline hazard function, which makes the parametric approach questionable. Analysis is performed using SAS PROC NLMIXED based on the suggestion by Liu and Yu (2008). ☐

An interesting application of the shared gamma frailty model with piecewise constant baseline hazard function to the lifetimes of Danish adoptees and their biological and adoption parents is presented in Petersen et al. (2010).

4.3.2 Semiparametric shared gamma frailty model

In the last section the parametric shared gamma frailty model was discussed in detail. Here we consider the semiparametric shared gamma frailty model. This model is a standard tool to analyze multivariate survival data. As already discussed, in many practical situations there is little or no information about the form of the baseline hazard function. Consequently, if the sample size is large enough, a semiparametric approach is often preferred because it does not rely on assumptions that are difficult to verify. The log-likelihood in the semiparametric shared gamma frailty model looks similar to (4.4), but the vector of model parameters to be estimated contains only the regression and frailty parameters, and the baseline hazard function is treated as an infinite dimensional nuisance parameter. For such a model, direct maximization of the marginal likelihood is no longer possible, and more sophisticated estimation procedures are necessary.

Semiparametric proportional hazards models without frailty are analyzed by means of the partial likelihood method (Cox 1972, 1975). To adapt this approach to proportional hazard models with frailty, the EM algorithm (Expectation-Maximization algorithm) can be used.

The algorithm was suggested by Dempster et al. (1977) and is typically used in the presence of unobserved data. The EM algorithm iterates between two steps. In the first one, an estimate (the expectation) of the unobserved frailties based on observed data and current parameter estimates is obtained. These estimates are used in the maximization step to obtain new parameter estimates given the estimated frailties. In the gamma frailty model, closed-form expressions exists for the conditional expectations of the frailties in the E step, which is very convenient for the estimation procedure. Furthermore, applying the partial likelihood concept with the estimated frailties as off-set terms in the M step is easy to perform, which makes the EM algorithm useful. The EM algorithm is described in more detail for the univariate gamma frailty model in Section 3.3.2, and for the shared gamma frailty in the book by Duchateau and Janssen (2008). Therefore we omit further details of the algorithm here.

Similar to the parametric shared gamma frailty model, the unobserved frailty Z_i, $(i = 1, \ldots, n)$ in each cluster can be estimated (Nielsen et al. 1992) by the expression

$$\hat{Z}_i = \frac{1/\hat{\sigma}^2 + \sum_{j=1}^{n_i} \delta_{ij}}{1/\hat{\sigma}^2 + \sum_{j=1}^{n_i} \hat{M}_0(t_{ij})e^{\hat{\beta}' \mathbf{x}_{ij}}}. \tag{4.6}$$

Here the difference from relation (4.5) lies in the expression $\hat{M}_0$, which is now a nonparametric estimator of the cumulative baseline hazard (for example, the Nelson–Aalen estimator). This approach was used by Carvalho et al. (2003) to investigate the quality of dialysis centers in Brazil represented by the unobserved frailty values assigned to each center. This underlines the possibility of using frailty models to rank treatment centers or other institutions with respect to their estimated frailties.

Example 4.2

We consider the Halluca data again and apply the semiparametric shared gamma frailty model. Patients in the study are clustered by the center where the lung carcinoma was diagnosed. Altogether, there were 53 diagnosing centers representing the clusters. A univariate and a shared gamma frailty model is applied to the data in Table 4.2, where in the univariate approach the clustering of the data is not taken into account.

Table 4.2: Univariate and shared gamma frailty
model of the Halluca lung cancer data

parameter	univariate frailty	shared frailty
age (in years)	0.013 (0.004)	0.009 (0.003)
sex (females)	-0.197 (0.091)	-0.158 (0.073)
type (NSCLC)	-0.096 (0.086)	-0.097 (0.068)
ECOG (3 & 4)	1.054 (0.145)	0.600 (0.108)
stage ll	0.578 (0.203)	0.450 (0.170)
stage IIIa	0.780 (0.157)	0.600 (0.133)
stage IIIb	1.232 (0.146)	0.957 (0.123)
stage IV	1.746 (0.133)	1.314 (0.113)
σ^2	0.460 ( )	0.311 ( )

In general, the effect of the covariates is weakened (an exception from this general rule is the covariate type) when applying the shared gamma frailty model instead of the univariate gamma frailty model. Please note that the interpretation of the parameter estimates is different in both models. In the univariate model the estimates of the regression parameters are adjusted for the unobserved heterogeneity in the population and only conditional given the same frailty. Frailty variance is interpreted as a measure of unobserved heterogeneity in the study population. In the shared gamma frailty model the parameters are adjusted for the correlation in the clusters, and the frailty variance is interpreted as a measure of the correlation between the lifetimes in the clusters. Again, the parameter estimates are conditional given the same frailty (or, which is equivalent in the shared frailty model, conditional on being from the same cluster). It is important to note these subtle differences between the models. Unfortunately, in the literature about frailty models, sometimes this difference is overlooked and a clear distinction between these two classes of models is missed, leading to wrong interpretations of the results.

In both models, estimates are obtained by means of the COXPH function of the statistical package R, which does not provide estimates for the standard error of frailty variance.   ⧠

The asymptotic properties of the maximum likelihood estimates in the non-parametric shared gamma frailty model are well established. Murphy shows consistency (Murphy 1994) and asymptotic normality (Murphy 1995) in the model without observed covariates. These results were generalized to the correlated gamma frailty model (which includes the shared gamma frailty as a special case and will be considered in detail in the next chapter) with covariates by Parner (1998). Gorfine et al. (2006) suggest new estimates and provide large sample theory for the general semiparametric shared frailty model with covariates. Their method needs only a finite first moment of the frailty distribution, but also makes use of the specific frailty distribution.

Regarding goodness-of-fit, Shih and Louis (1995b) introduced a graphical method for assessing the assumption about the gamma distribution of the frailty when the baseline hazard function is parametric and in the absence of covariates. This work was continued by Shih (1998), introducing a simple test statistic for a goodness-of-fit test in the shared gamma frailty model, allowing for censored observations, but in the absence of observed covariates. Fine and Jiang (2000) suggest a goodness-of-fit test that allows for observed covariates, which are included via semiparametric accelerated failure time regression models. Glidden (1999) suggests a test for the semiparametric gamma frailty model without covariates. A graphical as well as numerical method for checking the adequacy of the gamma distribution in a shared frailty model is suggested by Cui and Sun (2004). Their test is based on the posterior expectation of frailties given the observable data over time, extending the work by Glidden (1999). Viswanathan and Manatunga (2001) use kernel regression smoothing in order to distinguish between gamma and positive stable frailty distribution. Papers by Chen and Bandeen-Roche (2005), Glidden (2007), and Economou and Caroni (2008) contain additional material about graphical procedures checking the dependence structure in shared frailty models. These are important results that can be used for the decision about the frailty distribution to be applied to the data in specific situations.

The choice of the gamma distribution as a frailty distribution is supported in addition by asymptotic results obtained by Abbring and van den Berg (2007). Their main results focus on univariate models but are also proven in a specific bivariate model.

4.3.3 Shared gamma frailty model for current status data

In this section the parametric shared gamma frailty model will be applied to current status data. The parametric univariate gamma frailty model for current status data was already considered in Section 3.3.3. In the bivariate case with unconditional survival function $S(t_1, t_2; \boldsymbol{\theta})$, the likelihood function contains four components, depending on the censoring status of the observed data:

$$
\begin{aligned}
L_i(\boldsymbol{\theta}) = {} & \delta_1 \delta_2 \big(1 - S_1(t_1; \boldsymbol{\theta}) - S_2(t_2; \boldsymbol{\theta}) + S(t_1, t_2; \boldsymbol{\theta})\big) \\
& + \delta_1 (1 - \delta_2) \big(S_2(t_2; \boldsymbol{\theta}) - S(t_1, t_2; \boldsymbol{\theta})\big) \\
& + (1 - \delta_1) \delta_2 \big(S_1(t_1; \boldsymbol{\theta}) - S(t_1, t_2; \boldsymbol{\theta})\big) \\
& + (1 - \delta_1)(1 - \delta_2) S(t_1, t_2; \boldsymbol{\theta})
\end{aligned}
$$

with $S_1(t_1; \boldsymbol{\theta}) = S(t_1, 0; \boldsymbol{\theta})$ and $S_2(t_2; \boldsymbol{\theta}) = S(0, t_2; \boldsymbol{\theta})$ as marginal survival functions. One interesting research problem deals with the question how much information is lost when current status data are observed instead of (right-censored) lifetimes in the usual way. To answer this question, simulations are performed based on the bivariate shared gamma frailty model under different censoring assumptions.

Data are generated following the bivariate shared gamma frailty model with frailty variance $\mathbf{V}(Z) = \sigma^2 = 1$, expectation $\mathbf{E}Z = 1$, and Gompertz baseline. One thousand samples of sample size 1000 are generated. We consider two scenarios as follows. In the first scenario, the censoring/monitoring times are assumed to be independent. Consequently, current status data contain information about the two-dimensional distribution of the event times. In the second scenario, both censoring/monitoring times are assumed to be equal. This is a typical situation in current status data, where blood samples are used to test for the presence of different infections.

Scenario 1: Both censoring/monitoring times are independent.

Table 4.3: Simulation (Scenario 1) of the shared gamma frailty model with current status data

parameter	true	current status	right censored
σ^2	1.000	1.003 (0.076)	1.002 (0.054)
λ_1	0.100	0.101 (0.015)	0.100 (0.007)
φ_1	0.120	0.121 (0.026)	0.121 (0.015)
λ_2	0.100	0.100 (0.014)	0.100 (0.008)
φ_2	0.120	0.121 (0.025)	0.121 (0.015)

Each data set is analyzed under two different censoring mechanisms. In the case of right censoring (last column in Table 4.3), $(T_1, T_2, \Delta_1, \Delta_2)$ are assumed to represent common right-censored lifetimes. The second analysis (third column in Table 4.3) assumes that the data represent current status data, which means monitoring times are observed instead of event times. The estimates based on right-censored data are very similar to those based on current status data (and very close to the true values). The standard errors are larger than in the case of the current status data, but in general the information loss when switching from right-censored event time data to current status data is moderate in this scenario.

Scenario 2: Both censoring/monitoring times are equal.
Again, each data set is analyzed under two different censoring mechanisms, once in the case of right-censored lifetimes and once data are assumed to represent current status data. The parameter estimates based on the right-censored data are very similar to the estimates based on current status data (and very close to the true parameter values). The standard errors are larger with the current status data, but in general the information loss when

Table 4.4: Simulation (Scenario 2) of the shared gamma frailty model with current status data

parameter	true	current status	right censored
σ^2	1.000	0.996 (0.072)	0.998 (0.052)
λ_1	0.100	0.101 (0.015)	0.100 (0.008)
φ_1	0.120	0.120 (0.026)	0.120 (0.015)
λ_2	0.100	0.100 (0.015)	0.100 (0.008)
φ_2	0.120	0.121 (0.026)	0.121 (0.014)

switching from right-censored event times to current status data is similarly compared to Scenario 1. These simulations are undertaken to mimic the data considered in the following example.

Example 4.3
The hepatitis A and B current status data from Example 1.7 are analyzed in a bivariate model. In the second column of Table 4.5, the results from a shared gamma frailty model, and in the third column from the univariate frailty model (compare Table 3.9), are presented. The univariate frailty models treat

Table 4.5: Hepatitis A and B current status data analyzed with the shared gamma frailty model

parameter	shared frailty	univariate frailty
σ_1^2	0.522 (0.028)	2.018 (0.510)
λ_1	0.012 (0.001)	0.008 (0.001)
φ_1	0.037 (0.002)	0.085 (0.016)
σ_2^2	0.522 (0.028)	10.037 (8.821)
λ_2	0.002 (0.001)	0.002 (0.001)
φ_2	-0.001 (0.007)	0.015 (0.142)
log-likelihood	-2843.5100	-2841.4151

time to infection by hepatitis A and B, respectively, as independent times. It allows for different variances. The shared gamma frailty model is restricted to similar variances. Because of this constraint, the bivariate frailty model provides no better fit compared to the univariate model. This is based on the comparison of the loglikelihoods keeping in mind that the shared frailty model contains one parameter less. More details including the SAS code can be found in Hens et al. (2009). □

4.4 Shared Log-normal Frailty Model

Together with the gamma distribution, the log-normal distribution is the most important frailty distribution. The gamma distribution has a long tradition as a frailty distribution for the last 30 years since the introduction of the frailty model by Vaupel et al. (1979) and Lancaster (1979). The reason for the popularity of the gamma distribution is its mathematical convenience, especially due to the explicit representation of the survival function based on the simple Laplace transform. This yields simple expressions of the likelihood function, which are important for ML parameter estimation.

However, normally distributed random effects allow much more flexibility, especially in modeling multivariate correlation structures. This point of view becomes more pronounced in the next chapter. The development of new user-friendly parameter estimation procedures, for example, in SAS (MCMC, adaptive Gaussian quadrature techniques) in connection with a huge increase in computational power, this flexibility of normal distributed random effects outweighs its disadvantage of no explicit solution to the marginal survival function including the normal integral.

Example 4.4

Analogous to the last section with gamma-distributed frailty, the Halluca data set is analyzed, starting with parametric frailty models based on three different baseline hazard functions.

Table 4.6: Parametric shared log-normal frailty model of the Halluca lung cancer data

parameter	Weibull	exponential	Gompertz
age (in years)	0.009 (0.003)	0.009 (0.003)	0.009 (0.003)
sex (females)	-0.163 (0.073)	-0.173 (0.073)	-0.160 (0.073)
type (NSCLC)	-0.106 (0.068)	-0.119 (0.068)	-0.097 (0.068)
ECOG (3 & 4)	0.601 (0.108)	0.633 (0.108)	0.613 (0.108)
stage II	0.448 (0.170)	0.475 (0.170)	0.440 (0.170)
stage IIIa	0.612 (0.133)	0.648 (0.133)	0.604 (0.133)
stage IIIb	0.977 (0.123)	1.040 (0.123)	0.964 (0.123)
stage IV	1.324 (0.113)	1.412 (0.112)	1.314 (0.113)
λ	0.029 (0.008)	0.019 (0.005)	0.025 (0.007)
ν	0.880 (0.020)		
φ			0.025 (0.007)
σ^2	0.305 (0.105)	0.376 (0.125)	0.297 (0.103)
log-likelihood	-4836.43904	-4853.51499	-4837.138

Analysis is performed using SAS PROC NLMIXED, which allows writing down of the conditional likelihood function, including the random effects. By means of adaptive Gaussian quadrature techniques, the likelihood function is integrated out and maximized. This is a very user-friendly approach that allows for flexible modeling, especially in more complex models. It is easy to see that the one-parameter exponential baseline hazard is not flexible enough to model the mortality pattern accurately. The two-parameter Weibull and Gompertz models show a much better fit based on the likelihood function with slight advantage for the Weibull model. Parameter estimates in the Weibull and Gompertz model are more similar to each other compared to the exponential model. The exponential model seems to overestimate the frailty variance, resulting in stronger fixed effects estimates. □

Example 4.5

We perform a semiparametric analysis similar to Example 4.2 but with log-normal-distributed frailty. The results given in Table 4.7 are very close to the estimates obtained in the semiparametric shared gamma frailty model. This underlines the robustness of the method against misspecification of the

Table 4.7: Univariate and shared log-normal frailty model of the Halluca lung cancer data

parameter	univariate frailty	shared frailty
age (in years)	0.012 (0.003)	0.008 (0.003)
sex (females)	-0.194 (0.088)	-0.160 (0.072)
type (NSCLC)	-0.112 (0.083)	-0.097 (0.068)
ECOG (3 & 4)	0.924 (0.134)	0.605 (0.108)
stage II	0.552 (0.198)	0.450 (0.170)
stage IIIa	0.742 (0.154)	0.599 (0.133)
stage IIIb	1.177 (0.142)	0.956 (0.123)
stage IV	1.667 (0.130)	1.314 (0.113)
σ^2	0.498 ( )	0.283 ( )

frailty distribution. Parameter estimates are obtained by using the routine COXPH in the R package which does not provide standard errors for the frailty variance estimates. □

The shared log-normal model was applied by McGilchrist and Aisbett (1991), McGilchrist (1993), Gustafson (1997), and Bellamy et al. (2004). In the latter paper, the case of interval-censored data is considered with underlying Weibull baseline hazard function. The shared log-normal frailty model was extended to allow for heterogeneity in the frailty distribution (dispersed frailty) by Lee and Lee (2003).

4.5 Shared Positive Stable Frailty Model

The shared positive stable frailty model is of special interest for two reasons. First, similar to the gamma frailty model, the simple form of the Laplace transform allows simple maximum likelihood estimation in the parametric model. Second, there exists no moments of this distribution. This was the reason why Hougaard (1986a) introduced this distribution in the shared frailty approach. Because of the infinite mean, the univariate positive stable frailty model is not identifiable. This makes sense because, in shared frailty models, the frailty parameter is interpreted as an association parameter, that should not be identifiable from univariate observations. The shared positive stable frailty model was discussed in detail by Hougaard (2000) and Duchateau and Janssen (2008). The Laplace transform of a positive stable random variable with parameter γ is given in (3.41) by $\mathbf{L}(u) = e^{-u^{\gamma}}$. Starting from this point and averaging with respect to the cluster-specific random variable Z_i produces the multivariate survival function for the ith cluster in the form

$$S(t_{i1},\ldots,t_{in_i}|\mathbf{X}_i) = \mathbf{L}\Big(\sum_{j=1}^{n_i} M_0(t_{ij})e^{\boldsymbol{\beta}'\mathbf{X}_{ij}}\Big)$$

$$= \exp\Big[\Big(\sum_{j=1}^{n_i} M_0(t_{ij})e^{\boldsymbol{\beta}'\mathbf{X}_{ij}}\Big)^{\gamma}\Big]$$

$$= \exp\Big[\Big(\sum_{j=1}^{n_i} \big(-\ln S(t_{ij}|\mathbf{X}_{ij})\big)^{1/\gamma}\Big)^{\gamma}\Big]$$

where the last relation is a consequence of equation (3.42). Focusing on frailty models with fixed cluster size of two ($n_i = 2$, $i = 1,\ldots,n$), the joint survival function simplifies to

$$S(t_1,t_2) = \exp\Big[\Big(\big(-\ln S_1(t_1)\big)^{1/\gamma} + \big(-\ln S_2(t_2)\big)^{1/\gamma}\Big)^{\gamma}\Big], \qquad (4.7)$$

where the cluster index i is dropped but a single dichotomous covariate X is assumed representing two strata-specific baseline hazard functions. This results in two different marginal survival functions for the observations in each pair.

A bivariate parametric shared positive stable frailty model with Weibull baseline hazard function was used by Manatunga and Oakes (1999). The authors applied the model to the Diabetic Retinopathy Study, which examined the effectiveness of laser photocoagulation in delaying the onset of blindness in patients with diabetic retinopathy. One eye of each patient was randomly selected for photocoagulation treatment, and the other eye was left untreated. The positive stable frailty allows for proportional hazards in both the marginal and the conditional model.

4.6 Shared Compound Poisson/PVF Frailty Model

The compound Poisson distribution is a convenient frailty distribution because it includes the gamma and the inverse normal distribution, two important special cases. As already discussed in the univariate model, it allows a part of the study population to be not susceptible with respect to the event under investigation. And last but not least, its explicit form of the Laplace transform qualifies it also for use in a shared frailty model, allowing simple maximum likelihood estimation in the parametric model. The shared compound Poisson and PVF frailty model was considered, for example, by Hougaard (2000) and Duchateau and Janssen (2008). Because the PVF model is a special case of the compound Poisson model just with a restriction of the parameter space for the parameter γ, the shared PVF frailty model is not considered separately here. All formulas are similar in both cases.

The Laplace transform of a compound Poisson-distributed random variable with mean one, variance σ^2, and parameter γ is given by (3.53)

$$\mathbf{L}(u) = \exp\left[\frac{1-\gamma}{\gamma\sigma^2}\left(1 - \left(1 + \frac{\sigma^2 u}{1-\gamma}\right)^\gamma\right)\right].$$

Assuming a compound Poisson distribution for the frailty, averaging with respect to the cluster-specific random variable Z_i produces the multivariate survival function for the ith cluster

$$S(t_{i1}, \ldots, t_{in_i}|\mathbf{X}_i) \tag{4.8}$$

$$= \mathbf{L}\left(\sum_{j=1}^{n_i} M_0(t_{ij})e^{\boldsymbol{\beta}'\mathbf{X}_{ij}}\right)$$

$$= \exp\left[\frac{1-\gamma}{\gamma\sigma^2}\left(1 - \left(1 + \frac{\sigma^2}{1-\gamma}\sum_{j=1}^{n_i} M_0(t_{ij})e^{\boldsymbol{\beta}'\mathbf{X}_{ij}}\right)^\gamma\right)\right]$$

$$= \exp\left[\frac{1-\gamma}{\gamma\sigma^2}\left(1 - \left(1 + \sum_{j=1}^{n_i}\left(1 - \frac{\gamma\sigma^2}{1-\gamma}\ln S(t_{ij}|\mathbf{X}_{ij})\right)^{1/\gamma} - n_i\right)^\gamma\right)\right]$$

where the last relation is a consequence of equation (3.54). Similar to the gamma model, we focus on bivariate frailty models ($n_i = 2$, $i = 1, \ldots, n$), where the joint survival function simplifies to

$$S(t_1, t_2) =$$

$$\exp\left[\frac{1-\gamma}{\gamma\sigma^2}\left(1 - \left(\left(1 - \frac{\gamma\sigma^2}{1-\gamma}\ln S_1(t_1)\right)^{1/\gamma} + \left(1 - \frac{\gamma\sigma^2}{1-\gamma}\ln S_2(t_2)\right)^{1/\gamma} - 1\right)^\gamma\right)\right],$$

where cluster index i is dropped, but a single binary covariate X is assumed representing two strata-specific baseline hazard functions. This results in two different marginal survival functions for the partners in each pair.

4.7 Shared Frailty Models More General

One of the major drawbacks of the shared frailty approach is the fact that only positive association can be modeled. To overcome this strong limitation, Gordon (2000) suggests the reciprocal frailty model with negatively dependent competing risks. Negative dependence enters by means of individual-specific frailty that simultaneously increases the hazard for one risk while decreasing the hazard for the second. He introduced the model by assuming that the individual-specific hazard function for one risk is directly proportional to the heterogeneity term, while that of the second is inversely proportional, that is, $\mu_1(t_1|Z) = Z\mu_{01}(t_1)$ and $\mu_2(t_2|Z) = \frac{1}{Z}\mu_{02}(t_2)$. The conditional bivariate survival function is

$$S(t_1, t_2|Z) = \exp\left\{-ZM_{01}(t_1) - \frac{M_{02}(t_2)}{Z}\right\}.$$

Integrating with respect to the frailty distribution (here assumed to be a gamma distribution $\Gamma(\lambda, \lambda)$), we obtain the unconditional bivariate survival function

$$S(t_1, t_2) = \frac{2\lambda^\lambda}{\Gamma(\lambda)}\left[\left(\frac{M_{02}(t_2)}{M_{01}(t_1) + \lambda}\right)^{\lambda/2} K_\lambda(D(t_1, t_2))\right],$$

where $K_\lambda(\cdot)$ is the order λ modified Bessel function of the second kind, and

$$D(t_1, t_2) = 2\sqrt{M_{01}(t_1)M_{02}(t_2) + \lambda M_{02}(t_2)}.$$

Because of the complicated form of the unconditional survival function, this model was not further investigated in the literature.

An alternative for multivariate event times with dependence structures that are more general than in the symmetric shared frailty model is given by Hougaard (1986b). He considered the lifetimes of a monozygotic twin pair and a third sibling with equal marginal distributions. Let Z be common in the family, and let Y_1, Y_2 be terms shared by individuals with identical genes. Then, conditionally on Z, Y_1, Y_2, the hazard of each of the twins is $ZY_1\mu_0(t)$, and for the third individual it is $ZY_2\mu_0(t)$. Consequently,

$$S(t_1, t_2, t_3|Z, Y_1, Y_2) = \mathbf{P}(T_1 > t_1, T_2 > t_2, T_3 > t_3|Z, Y_1, Y_2)$$
$$= e^{-ZY_1(M_0(t_1)+M_0(t_2))-ZY_2M_0(t_3)}.$$

If Y_1 and Y_2 are independent stable distributed with parameter γ, and Z^γ is stable distributed with parameter κ, they can be integrated out by using the method of conditional means, giving

$$S(t_1, t_2, t_3) = e^{-((M_0(t_1)+M_0(t_2))^\gamma + M_0(t_3)^\gamma)^\kappa}.$$

This model allows for a stronger association between the lifetimes of the twins compared to the association between a twin and the third sibling in the family. Such kind of nonsymmetric correlation structure is considered in more detail in Chapter 5.

A shared frailty model with log-skew-t distribution of the frailty (including the log-normal distribution along with many other heavy-tailed distributions, such as log-Cauchy or log t-distribution) is considered by Sahu and Dey (2004). A shared gamma frailty model which is based on a Box–Cox transformation is investigated by Yin and Ibrahim (2005).

A completely different approach to bivariate frailty modeling was used by Bandyopadhyay and Basu (1990), and Gupta and Gupta (1990). The key idea of their (more specific) model is a bivariate hazard model in the form

$$\mu(t_1, t_2 | Z) = Z\mu_0(t_1, t_2).$$

Here the two lifetimes are not conditionally independent given the frailty. There are two types of dependencies. Dependence is caused by the bivariate hazard model $\mu_0(t_1, t_2)$ as well as by the shared frailty Z, which has to be integrated out. Similar models based on different bivariate extensions of the Weibull distribution are considered by Hanagal (2009). The advantage of such models is that dependence between lifetimes is still present even if frailty as a measure of heterogeneity is absent. Such models could be an alternative to the frailty models considered here in this monograph. As opposed to these models, multivariate frailty models simplify to univariate models (without frailty) if the frailty variance approaches zero. Consequently, correlation and unobserved heterogeneity are not completely separated in multivariate frailty models. Without unobserved heterogeneity, indicated by $\sigma^2 = 0$, there exists no correlation between lifetimes. This problem will be considered in more detail in Section 5.9.

4.8 Dependence measures

It is difficult to compare the degree of dependence between different frailty models. Often the variance of the frailty is used as a dependence measure, but this measure is useless in case of frailty distributions without existing second moments such as the positive stable distribution. Correlation coefficients (with respect to the observed event times) are tricky to obtain because of censored observations. Furthermore, they are often dependent on the time scale, which makes them difficult to compare. Kendall's τ can be used to quantify dependence because it is independent of transformations on the time scale and the frailty model used. It is a rank-based dependence measure. We consider bivariate data, for example, the times to blindness of n pairs of eyes.

Then, the uncensored data is given by $(T_{11}, T_{12}), (T_{21}, T_{22}), \ldots, (T_{n1}, T_{n2})$, where the first index denotes the cluster (patient), and the second index denotes the eye. Here τ is defined as

$$\tau = \mathbf{E}\big(\mathbf{sign}\{(T_{i1} - T_{j1})(T_{i2} - T_{j2})\}\big), \tag{4.9}$$

with $\mathbf{sign}\{t\}$ equal to -1 for negative values, 1 for positive values, and 0 if $t = 0$ $(i, j = 1, \ldots, n; i \neq j)$. Another formula is based on the Laplace transform:

$$\tau = 4 \int s \mathbf{L}''(s)\mathbf{L}(s)\, ds - 1. \tag{4.10}$$

To keep the notation simple, here and in the following all integrals are defined over the interval $[0, \infty)$ because lifetimes as well as frailties are nonnegative variables. In the next paragraph we will derive relation (4.10). Starting from definition (4.9), the conditional probability $T_{i1} < T_{j1}$ $(i, j = 1, \ldots, n; i \neq j)$ given the frailty vector (Z_i, Z_j) is calculated

$$
\begin{aligned}
\mathbf{P}(T_{i1} < T_{j1}|Z_i, Z_j) &= \frac{\int\int_{t_i < t_j} f(t_i, t_j, Z_i, Z_j)\, dt_i\, dt_j}{f(Z_i, Z_j)} \\
&= \frac{\int\int_{t_i < t_j} f(t_i, Z_j)f(t_i, Z_j)\, dt_i\, dt_j}{f(Z_i)f(Z_j)} \\
&= \frac{\int f(t, Z_1)S(t, Z_2)\, dt}{f(Z_1)f(Z_2)} \\
&= \int f(t|Z_i)S(t|Z_j)\, dt \\
&= \int \mu(t|Z_i)S(t|Z_i)S(t|Z_j)\, dt \\
&= Z_i \int \mu_0(t)e^{-(Z_i+Z_j)M_0(t)}\, dt \\
&= \frac{Z_i}{Z_i + Z_j}. \tag{4.11}
\end{aligned}
$$

For the last relation it is necessary that $M_0(t)$ be a nondegenerated cumulative hazard converging toward infinity as time approaches infinity. Hence, the difference of the event times $T_{i1} - T_{j1}$ is negative with probability $\frac{Z_i}{Z_i+Z_j}$, and positive with probability $\frac{Z_j}{Z_i+Z_j}$ (conditional on (Z_i, Z_j)). Because the function $\mathbf{sign}\{\cdot\}$ can take on only the two values minus and plus one (because of the condition $i \neq j$ zero can only occur with probability zero), it holds that

$$\mathbf{E}\big((\mathbf{sign}\{(T_{i1} - T_{j1})\})|Z_i, Z_j\big) = \frac{Z_j - Z_i}{Z_i + Z_j},$$

where the expectation is conditional on (Z_i, Z_j). An equivalent relationship holds for the second observations in the pairs:

$$\mathbf{E}\big((\mathbf{sign}\{(T_{i2} - T_{j2})\})|Z_i, Z_j\big) = \frac{Z_j - Z_i}{Z_i + Z_j}.$$

The lifetimes are independent given the frailties, which means

$$\begin{aligned}
\tau &= \mathbf{E}\big(\mathbf{sign}\{(T_{i1} - T_{j1})(T_{i2} - T_{j2})\}\big) \\
&= \mathbf{E}\Big(\mathbf{E}\big((\mathbf{sign}\{(T_{i1} - T_{j1})\})|Z_i, Z_j\big)\mathbf{E}\big((\mathbf{sign}\{(T_{i2} - T_{j2})\})|Z_i, Z_j\big)\Big) \\
&= \mathbf{E}\Big(\frac{Z_j - Z_i}{Z_i + Z_j}\Big)^2.
\end{aligned}$$

In the following we consider the integral $\int_0^\infty se^{-sx}\,ds$. Using integration by parts it holds that

$$\begin{aligned}
\int se^{-sx}\,ds &= -\frac{s}{x}e^{-sx}\Big|_0^\infty + \frac{1}{x}\int e^{-sx}\,ds \\
&= \frac{1}{x}\int e^{-sx}\,ds \\
&= \frac{-1}{x^2}e^{-sx}\Big|_0^\infty \\
&= \frac{1}{x^2}.
\end{aligned}$$

Applying this relation yields

$$\tau = \mathbf{E}\big(\frac{Z_j - Z_i}{Z_i + Z_j}\big)^2 = \int\int\int se^{-s(z_i + z_j)}(z_j - z_i)^2 f(z_i)f(z_j)\,dz_j\,dz_i\,ds.$$

Using

$$\begin{aligned}
\int e^{-sz_j}(z_j - z_i)^2 f(z_j)\,dz_j &= \int z_j^2 e^{-sz_j} f(z_j)\,dz_j \\
&\quad - 2z_i \int z_j e^{-sz_j} f(z_j)\,dz_j \\
&\quad + z_i^2 \int e^{-sz_j} f(z_j)\,dz_j \\
&= \mathbf{L}''(s) + 2z_i\mathbf{L}'(s) + z_i^2\mathbf{L}(s)
\end{aligned}$$

we obtain

$$
\tau = \int \int \int s e^{-s(z_i+z_j)}(z_j - z_i)^2 f(z_i) f(z_j) \, dz_j dz_i ds
$$
$$
= \int \int s\mathbf{L}''(s) e^{-sz_i} f(z_i) \, dz_i ds
$$
$$
+ 2 \int \int s\mathbf{L}'(s) z_i e^{-sz_i} f(z_i) \, dz_i ds
$$
$$
+ \int \int s\mathbf{L}(s) z_i^2 e^{-sz_i} f(z_i) \, dz_i ds
$$
$$
= \int s\mathbf{L}''(s)\mathbf{L}(s) \, ds - 2 \int s(\mathbf{L}'(s))^2 \, ds + \int \int s\mathbf{L}(s)\mathbf{L}''(s) \, ds
$$
$$
= 2 \int s\mathbf{L}''(s)\mathbf{L}(s) \, ds - 2 \int s(\mathbf{L}'(s))^2 \, ds. \tag{4.12}
$$

As a consequence of integration by parts it holds that

$$
\int s\mathbf{L}''(s)\mathbf{L}(s) \, ds = \mathbf{L}'(s) s\mathbf{L}(s) \Big|_0^\infty - \int \mathbf{L}'(s)(\mathbf{L}(s) + s\mathbf{L}'(s)) \, ds
$$
$$
= - \int s(\mathbf{L}'(s))^2 \, ds - \int \mathbf{L}'(s)\mathbf{L}(s) \, ds. \tag{4.13}
$$

Using integration by parts again we see that

$$
\int \mathbf{L}'(s)\mathbf{L}(s) \, ds = (\mathbf{L}(s))^2 \Big|_0^\infty - \int \mathbf{L}'(s)\mathbf{L}(s) \, ds,
$$

resulting in

$$
2 \int \mathbf{L}'(s)\mathbf{L}(s) \, ds = -1. \tag{4.14}
$$

Combining (4.13) and (4.14) implies

$$
\int s(\mathbf{L}'(s))^2 \, ds = - \int s\mathbf{L}''(s)\mathbf{L}(s) \, ds + \frac{1}{2}.
$$

Substituting this expression in (4.12) yields relation (4.10). This can be used to calculate Kendall's τ for shared frailty models with different frailty distributions. In the case of the shared gamma frailty model, by using (3.14) and (3.15) with $\lambda = k = 1/\sigma^2$, it holds that

$$\int s\mathbf{L}''(s)\mathbf{L}(s)\,ds = \int s(1+\sigma^2)(1+\sigma^2 s)^{-\frac{1}{\sigma^2}-2}(1+\sigma^2 s)^{-\frac{1}{\sigma^2}}\,ds$$

$$= (1+\sigma^2)\int s(1+\sigma^2 s)^{-\frac{2}{\sigma^2}-2}\,ds$$

$$= \frac{1+\sigma^2}{2+\sigma^2}\int (1+\sigma^2 s)^{-\frac{2}{\sigma^2}-1}\,ds$$

$$= \frac{1+\sigma^2}{-2(2+\sigma^2)}(1+\sigma^2 s)^{-\frac{2}{\sigma^2}}\Big|_0^\infty$$

$$= \frac{1+\sigma^2}{2(2+\sigma^2)}.$$

Consequently,

$$\tau = 4\int s\mathbf{L}''(s)\mathbf{L}(s)\,ds - 1 = \frac{\sigma^2}{\sigma^2+2}.$$

For the shared positive stable frailty model, Kendall's τ can be also easily calculated using (3.41)

$$\int s\mathbf{L}''(s)\mathbf{L}(s)\,ds = \int -\gamma(\gamma-1)s^{\gamma-1}e^{-2s^\gamma} + \gamma^2 s^{2\gamma-1}e^{-2s^\gamma}\,ds. \qquad (4.15)$$

The first expression of (4.15) gives

$$\int -\gamma(\gamma-1)s^{\gamma-1}e^{-2s^\gamma}\,ds = -\frac{\gamma-1}{2},$$

and using integration by parts it holds for the second expression of (4.15) that

$$\int \gamma^2 s^{2\gamma-1}e^{-2s^\gamma}\,ds = -\frac{1}{2}\gamma s^\gamma e^{-2s^\gamma}\Big|_0^\infty + \frac{1}{2}\gamma^2\int s^{\gamma-1}e^{-2s^\gamma} = \frac{\gamma}{4}.$$

Finally,

$$\tau = 4\int s\mathbf{L}''(s)\mathbf{L}(s)\,ds - 1$$

$$= 4\left(-\frac{\gamma-1}{2}+\frac{\gamma}{4}\right) - 1$$

$$= 1 - \gamma.$$

Unfortunately, for most other frailty distributions, Kendall's τ does not have such an explicit and simple form.

4.9   Limitations of the Shared Frailty Model

Shared frailty explains correlations within clusters. A cluster can consist of individuals from the same group, such as a family, litter, clinic, community; or of multiple or recurrent events from the same individual. However, it does have some limitations. In the following, we use some of the arguments already discussed by Xue and Brookmeyer (1996).

First, the concept of shared frailty forces the unobserved factors to be the same within the cluster, which is often not appropriate. For example, in general, it may be inappropriate to assume that both partners in a twin pair or all relatives in a family share all of their unobserved risk factors.

Second, in most cases, shared frailty will only induce positive associations within clusters (for exceptions see Joe 1993). However, in some situations the survival times for subjects within the same cluster are negatively associated. For example, growth rates of animals living in the same cage with limited food are probably negatively associated. Another example are transplantation studies, which found out that generally the longer an individual must wait for a transplantation, the shorter the chances of survival after the transplantation. Thus, the waiting and the survival time may be negatively associated. As another example, suppose a patient is repeatedly admitted to hospital for the same disease. The sicker the patient is, the higher the risk of readmission, and the lower the 'risk' (chance) of discharge. Therefore, the duration of the stays inside the hospital, on the one hand, and outside the hospital, on the other hand, are expected to be negatively associated. An additional example is provided by competing risk scenarios, where the reduction of the risk of dying from one disease increases the risk of dying from another disease.

Third, the dependence between survival times within the cluster is based on marginal distributions of survival times. To see this, when covariates are present in a proportional hazards model with a gamma-distributed frailty, the dependence parameter and the population heterogeneity are confounded (Clayton and Cuzick 1985b), meaning that the joint event time distribution can be identified from the marginal distributions (Hougaard 1986a). Elbers and Ridder (1982) show that this problem exists for any frailty distribution with a finite mean. However, "shared frailty" in multivariate models differs from "individual frailty" used in the case of univariate data. Originally, this difference in the notions of frailty was not clearly understood. But it is worth noting that the value of σ^2 estimated from univariate data may, in fact, has nothing to do with association. Indeed, consider two hypothetical bivariate data sets with different associations between lifespans of related individuals, for example, the lifetimes of men and their sons, and between the same men and their grandsons. In both situations the value of the variance parameter σ^2 will be the same estimated from the data on the group of men (grandfathers), despite the fact that associations between lifespans of grandfathers and their grandsons, and grandfathers and their sons are different. The use of other association measure such as Kendall's τ does not really help in this situation because it is a function of the frailty variance.

This last, and maybe most important, limitation of shared frailty models is a consequence of identifiability of the univariate frailty model with observed covariates. Hence, it is an inherent feature to all shared frailty models with a finite mean of frailty distribution. To overcome this problem, Hougaard (1986a, 1987) suggests the shared positive stable frailty model. In this case the univariate model with observed covariates is not identifiable because the mean of the positive stable distribution is infinite. So one can expect more flexibility from a shared frailty model with positive stable distribution than from models with gamma frailty. The bivariate survival function in the shared positive stable frailty model is given by (4.7)

$$S(t_1, t_2) = \exp\left[\left(\left(-\ln S_1(t_1)\right)^{1/\gamma} + \left(-\ln S_2(t_2)\right)^{1/\gamma}\right)^{\gamma}\right]. \qquad (4.16)$$

When single covariates X_i $(i = 1, 2)$ are observed, and the conditional hazard is (3.2), then the univariate survival functions are

$$S_i(t) = \exp\left(-M_{0i}^{\gamma}(t)e^{\gamma\beta_i X_i}\right) = \exp\left(-M_i^*(t)e^{\beta_i^* X_i}\right),$$

where $\beta_i^* = \gamma\beta_i$ and $M_i^*(t) = M_{0i}^{\gamma}(t)$. Using a shared positive stable frailty model it is possible to estimate both association parameter γ and regression coefficients β_i from data on related individuals. One problem remains yet unsolved: the interpretation of regression parameters β_i. To illustrate this problem, let $\beta = \beta_1 = \beta_2$ for two groups of relatives, for example, MZ and DZ twins. It is clear that the association parameter γ is different for MZ and DZ twins. Hence the values of parameter $\beta^* = \gamma\beta$ and $M^*(t)$ in equation (4.16) are also different for MZ and DZ twins, which contradicts the natural assumption that the survival of these individuals conditioned on observed covariates follow the same survival model. If the parameters $\beta^* = \gamma\beta$ are assumed to be the same for MZ and DZ twins, then the parameters β and the baseline hazards $\mu_0(t)$ should be different for these pairs of individuals, which creates a problem for the interpretation of the conditional hazard (3.2) for this model.

The problem can be described in a more general way. The main feature of the shared frailty approach is its symmetry. In multicenter clinical trials it is reasonable to assume a symmetric relationship between all possible pairs of patients in a study center because patients in a center are exchangeable. It makes no sense to assume a nonsymmetric correlation structure inside the centers. The situation changes dramatically when considering family studies with relatives of different relationship. Applying a shared frailty model would imply the same relationship (correlation) between any pairs of relatives in the family. This is, of course, not a reasonable assumption. Furthermore, it contradicts the assumption of different relationships in families, which is the basis for genetic studies.

To avoid such methodological problems, correlated frailty models have been developed for the analysis of multivariate failure time data. We will focus here mainly on bivariate models because generalizations of correlated frailty models to the multivariate case are not straightforward, and these will be discussed later on in more detail in some specific situations. Bivariate correlated frailty models have two associated random variables (Z_1, Z_2) that characterize the frailty effect for each cluster. One random variable, for example, is assigned to individual 1 and one to individual 2 so that they are no longer constrained by having a common frailty. The two random variables (Z_1, Z_2) are associated and jointly distributed; therefore, knowing one of them does not necessarily imply the other. Also, the two variables may be negatively associated, and this would induce a negative association between survival times. Similar to the univariate case as well as to shared frailty, the choice of frailty distribution is important for the modeling and will be considered in more detail later on.

Between shared and correlated frailty models (sometimes called univariate and bivariate frailty models with respect to the dimension of the frailty, but both models are considered here to deal with bivariate time-to-event data), there is an intermediate approach in which two variables are assigned to each cluster (of size two) to count for heterogeneity but are generated from one common random variable. An example are bivariate survival times (T_1, T_2) with Z_1 to account for the heterogeneity of T_1 and Z_2 to account for T_2, where Z_1 and Z_2 are defined by

$$Z_1 = e^{\alpha_1 W} \quad \text{and} \quad Z_2 = e^{\alpha_2 W}, \tag{4.17}$$

where W is a random variable, and α_1 and α_2 are parameters to be estimated. This model has been used frequently (Flinn and Heckman 1982, Clayton and Cuzick 1985b, Heckman and Walker 1990, Huang and Wolfe 2002) and is named one-factor loading specification in the econometric literature (van den Berg 2001). This approach is more flexible than that of assuming shared frailty for T_1 and T_2, and to some extent it allows for a negative association by allowing different signs of α_1 and α_2. However, it still imposes a linkage between the variance and the correlation, and also the expectation and the variance of the frailties. The overall hazard for the population (rather than the individual hazard), in consequence, is forced to move between restricted ranges. Therefore, Lindeboom and van den Berg (1994) conclude that it is hazardous to estimate bivariate survival models where the mixing distribution is parameterized univariately because a univariate random variable may not be able to account for both the dependence of the survival times and the change in the composition of the sample due to unobserved heterogeneity caused by covariates not being included in the analysis. Clearly, such kinds of problems do not arise in a genuine bivariate approach in which the dependence between T_1 and T_2 can be changed without changing the marginal distributions of T_1 and T_2. This will be the topic of the following chapter.

Chapter 5

Correlated Frailty Models

In the last chapter we focused on the shared frailty model as a way of modeling associations between event times. The concept of shared frailty goes back to Clayton (1978), and was extensively studied in books by Hougaard (2000), and Duchateau and Janssen (2008). The shared frailty approach has proven to be a useful and popular extension of the Cox model when observations from subjects are not statistically independent of each other. As discussed in Section 4.9, the shared frailty model is especially useful for clustered event time data when the correlation structure in the clusters is symmetric and not of special interest as, for example, in multicenter clinical trials.

Similar to the univariate and shared frailty model, the correlated frailty model is a mixture model because frailty for each individual is assumed to be random. This is also known as the concept of random hazards. The model is based on the assumption that event times in a cluster are independent, given the vector of frailties. In other words, it is a conditional independence model where the frailty variables are correlated but not necessarily common for all individuals in a cluster, and therefore, responsible for dependence between event times. The shared frailty model is a special case of the correlated frailty model with correlations between the frailties equal to one. A correlated frailty model can be considered as a mixed (random effects) model in survival analysis, with group and individual variation both included in the distribution of the frailty vector. Therefore, correlated frailty models contain association characteristics of frailty (correlation coefficients) among other parameters, which makes them especially convenient for genetic studies of relatives with event-time outcome. In particular, questions about the role of genes and environment in susceptibility to diseases and death can be addressed. Here, the correlation between frailties is of key interest. This is different from many other applications where correlation is treated as a nuisance to be adjusted for in the model, and not of special interest. Consequently, we will focus, the applications of the correlated frailty model, mainly on twin and family event-time data. In such kinds of applications, the researcher is usually faced with small cluster sizes. Special focus is on the bivariate case.

It is assumed that there is independence between observations from different clusters. If variances of the frailty variables are zero, this implies independence between event times in the clusters. The structure of the model makes them convenient for application of the EM algorithm, allowing for semiparametric estimation. The model can also be used to model dependent competing risks. Whereas the correlated gamma frailty model can only cover positive dependence between event times, the log-normal correlated frailty model offers a wider range of dependence between event times in the clusters. Hence, this approach has become a very attractive tool, with a flexibility in modeling correlation structures known from mixed models.

For the popular shared frailty model, many theoretical and practical results exist in the literature on frailty models. The model is implemented in many statistical packages, and, therefore accessible even to nonspecialists. For the correlated frailty model, there exist only a few papers, and software is practically not available. This has changed with the reformulation of the frailty model as a random effects/mixed model and with the application of recent results already achieved in this research area. Furthermore, during the last few years, powerful and user-friendly software solutions have become available for mixed models with normal distributed random effects. This opens new avenues for research in the field of correlated frailty models which is the topic of the present chapter. The similarity to mixed models is of special importance for correlated frailty models and will be exploited throughout this chapter.

Some history exists behind the development of correlated frailty models. Aalen (1987) discusses multivariate mixing distributions applied on a Markov chain. Marshall and Olkin (1988) discussed various multivariate correlated frailty distributions. Their work was continued by Yashin et al. (1993, 1995), Pickles et al. (1994), Yashin and Iachine (1997, 1999a,b), Petersen (1998), Iachine et al. (1998), and Iachine (2002), who mainly considered the bivariate correlated gamma frailty model and applied it to twin survival data. This approach forms the starting point for different extensions discussed in more detail in this monograph later on. Some of the results are already published in Wienke et al. (2000, 2001, 2002, 2003a,b, 2004, 2005a,b, 2006a,b, 2010). Another approach with an interesting real data example can be found in van den Berg et al. (2008), who combine twin data with economic information to analyze the influence of the economic situation at year of birth on later developments of cause-specific mortality. Xue and Brookmeyer (1996) deal with the bivariate correlated log-normal frailty model, developed in more general cases by Ripatti and Palmgren (2000), and Vaida and Xu (2000).

In the following section the main ideas of the correlated frailty concept are outlined, independent of frailty distribution. This more general part is followed by a detailed description and discussion of the correlated gamma frailty model in Section 5.2. The correlated log-normal frailty model as a very flexible model is considered in Section 5.3. A MCMC estimation procedure for the correlated log-normal frailty model is presented in Section 5.4. The newly suggested correlated compound Poisson frailty in Section 5.5 contains the correlated gamma and the correlated inverse Gaussian frailty model as special cases. It allows single individuals in the cluster to be at no risk (frailty equal to zero) for the event of interest.

5.1 The Concept of Correlated Frailty

The correlated frailty model is the second important concept in the area of multivariate frailty models. It is a natural extension of the shared frailty approach on the one hand, and of the univariate frailty model on the other. In the correlated frailty model, the frailties of individuals in a cluster are correlated but not necessarily shared. It enables the inclusion of additional correlation parameters, which then allows the addressing of questions about associations between event times. Furthermore, associations are no longer forced to be the same for all pairs of individuals in a cluster. This makes the model especially appropriate for situations where the association between event times is of special interest, for example, genetic studies of event times in families. We will come back to such applications later on. For introductory reasons we will discuss bivariate models first. The conditional survival function in the bivariate case (here without observed covariates) looks like

$$S(t_1, t_2|Z_1, Z_2) = S_1(t_1|Z_1)S_2(t_2|Z_2) = e^{-Z_1 M_{01}(t_1)} e^{-Z_2 M_{02}(t_2)},$$

where Z_1 and Z_2 are two correlated frailties. The distribution of the random vector (Z_1, Z_2) needs to be specified and determines the association structure of the event times in the model.

Consider some bivariate event times – for example, the lifetimes of twins, or age at onset of a disease in spouses, time to blindness in the left and right eye, or time to failure in the left and right kidney of patients. In the (bivariate) correlated frailty model, the frailty of each individual in a pair is defined by a measure of relative risk, that is, exactly as it was defined in the univariate case. For two individuals in a pair, frailties are not necessarily the same, as they are in the shared frailty model. We are assuming that the frailties are acting multiplicatively on the baseline hazard function (proportional hazards model) and that the observations in a pair are conditionally independent, given the frailties. Hence, the hazard of the individual j ($j = 1, 2$) in pair i ($i = 1, \ldots, n$) has the form

$$\mu(t|\mathbf{X}_{ij}, Z_{ij}) = Z_{ij}\mu_{0j}(t)e^{\boldsymbol{\beta}' \mathbf{X}_{ij}}, \tag{5.1}$$

where t denotes age or time, $\mathbf{X}_{ij}$ is a vector of observed covariates, $\boldsymbol{\beta}$ is a vector of regression parameters describing the effect of the covariates $\mathbf{X}_{ij}$, $\mu_{0j}(\cdot)$ are baseline hazard functions, and Z_{ij} are frailties. Bivariate correlated frailty models are characterized by the joint distribution of a two-dimensional vector of frailties (Z_{i1}, Z_{i2}). If the two frailties are independent, the resulting lifetimes are independent, and no clustering is present in the model. If the two frailties are equal, the shared frailty model is obtained as a special case of the correlated frailty model with correlation one between the frailties.

Any method in this context is based on likelihood functions. In order to derive a marginal likelihood function, the assumption of conditional independence of lifespans, given the frailty, is used. Let δ_{ij} be a censoring indicator for individual j ($j = 1, 2$) in pair i ($i = 1, \ldots, n$). Indicator δ_{ij} is 1 if the individual has experienced the event of interest, and 0 otherwise. According to (5.1), the conditional survival function of the jth individual in the ith pair is

$$S(t|\mathbf{X}_{ij}, Z_{ij}) = e^{Z_{ij} M_{0j}(t) e^{\boldsymbol{\beta}' \mathbf{X}_{ij}}},$$

with $M_{0j}(t)$ denoting the cumulative baseline hazard function. Here and in the following, S is used as a generic symbol for a survival function. The contribution of individual j ($j = 1, 2$) in pair i ($i = 1, \ldots, n$) to the conditional likelihood is given by

$$\left(Z_{ij} \mu_{0j}(t_{ij}) e^{\boldsymbol{\beta}' \mathbf{X}_{ij}} \right)^{\delta_{ij}} e^{Z_{ij} M_{0j}(t_{ij}) e^{\boldsymbol{\beta}' \mathbf{X}_{ij}}},$$

where t_{ij} stands for observation time of individual j from pair i. Assuming the conditional independence of lifespans, given the frailty, and integrating out the frailty, we obtain the marginal likelihood function

$$\prod_{i=1}^{n} \iint_{R^+ \times R^+} \left(z_{i1} \mu_{01}(t_{i1}) e^{\boldsymbol{\beta}' \mathbf{X}_{i1}} \right)^{\delta_{i1}} e^{z_{i1} M_{01}(t_{i1}) e^{\boldsymbol{\beta}' \mathbf{X}_{i1}}} \tag{5.2}$$

$$\times \left(z_{i2} \mu_{02}(t_{i2}) e^{\boldsymbol{\beta}' \mathbf{X}_{i2}} \right)^{\delta_{i2}} e^{z_{i2} M_{02}(t_{i2}) e^{\boldsymbol{\beta}' \mathbf{X}_{i2}}} f(z_{i1}, z_{i2}) \, dz_{i1} \, dz_{i2},$$

where $f(\cdot, \cdot)$ is the probability density function of the corresponding frailty distribution. All these formulas can be easily extended to the multivariate case, but need a specification of the correlation structure between individuals in a cluster in terms of the multivariate density function, which complicates analysis. An example is investigations dealing with family data. Here, the correlation structure is given by the degree of kinship. This remains relatively easy if only kernel families are considered (father–mother–child, for example), but becomes much more difficult if relatives of any degree are included such as half-sibs, grand–parents, nieces, and nephews, etc. Furthermore, the varying family size may also causes additional nontrivial technical problems in the estimation procedure.

Similar to univariate and shared frailty models, the choice of the frailty distribution is of great importance for modeling specific features of the joint survival distribution. Next, correlated frailty models with different frailty distribution are considered.

5.2   Correlated Gamma Frailty Model

This model was introduced by Yashin et al. (1993, 1995) and applied to related lifetimes in many different settings, for example, by Pickles et al. (1994), Yashin and Iachine (1995a,b, 1997, 1999a,b), Yashin et al. (1996), Zahl (1997), Iachine et al. (1998), Iachine (2002), Petersen (1998), Wienke et al. (2000, 2001, 2002, 2003a,b, 2004, 2005a), Zdravkovic et al. (2002, 2004), Kheiri et al. (2005), and van den Berg et al. (2008). The model has a very convenient representation of the survival function in closed form expressions, which allows nice interpretation of the model parameters. Here we restrict again to the bivariate model first.

Let k_0, k_1, k_2 be some nonnegative real-valued numbers. Set $\lambda_1 = k_0 + k_1$ and $\lambda_2 = k_0 + k_2$. Let Y_0, Y_1, Y_2 be independent, gamma-distributed random variables with parameters $Y_0 \sim \Gamma(k_0, \lambda_0)$, $Y_1 \sim \Gamma(k_1, \lambda_1)$, and $Y_2 \sim \Gamma(k_2, \lambda_2)$. Consequently,

$$Z_1 = \frac{\lambda_0}{\lambda_1} Y_0 + Y_1 \sim \Gamma(k_0 + k_1, \lambda_1) \tag{5.3}$$

$$Z_2 = \frac{\lambda_0}{\lambda_2} Y_0 + Y_2 \sim \Gamma(k_0 + k_2, \lambda_2) \tag{5.4}$$

and $\mathbf{E}Z_1 = \mathbf{E}Z_2 = 1, \mathbf{V}(Z_1) = \frac{1}{\lambda_1} := \sigma_1^2, \mathbf{V}(Z_2) = \frac{1}{\lambda_2} := \sigma_2^2$. Then the following relation holds

$$\begin{aligned}
\mathbf{cov}(Z_1, Z_2) &= \mathbf{cov}(\frac{\lambda_0}{\lambda_1} Y_0 + Y_1, \frac{\lambda_0}{\lambda_2} Y_0 + Y_2) \\
&= \frac{\lambda_0^2}{\lambda_1 \lambda_2} \mathbf{V}(Y_0) \\
&= \frac{\lambda_0^2}{\lambda_1 \lambda_2} \frac{k_0}{\lambda_0^2} \\
&= \frac{k_0}{(k_0 + k_1)(k_0 + k_2)}
\end{aligned}$$

This leads to the correlation

$$\rho = \frac{\mathbf{cov}(Z_1, Z_2)}{\sqrt{\mathbf{V}(Z_1)\mathbf{V}(Z_2)}} = \frac{k_0}{\sqrt{(k_0 + k_1)(k_0 + k_2)}}.$$

Consequently, because of the relation $k_0 + k_i = \lambda_i = \frac{1}{\sigma_i^2}$ ($i = 1, 2$), it holds that $k_0 = \frac{\rho}{\sigma_1 \sigma_2}$ and $k_i = \frac{1}{\sigma_i^2} - k_0 = \frac{1 - \frac{\sigma_i}{\sigma_j}\rho}{\sigma_i^2}$ ($i, j = 1, 2; i \neq j$). Now we can derive the unconditional survival function, applying the Laplace transform of gamma-distributed random variables. Hence,

$$
\begin{aligned}
S(t_1, t_2) &= \mathbf{E}S(t_1, t_2 | Z_1, Z_2) \\
&= \mathbf{E}S_1(t_1 | Z_1)S_2(t_2 | Z_2) \\
&= \mathbf{E}e^{-Z_1 M_{01}(t_1)}e^{-Z_2 M_{02}(t_2)} \\
&= \mathbf{E}e^{-(\frac{\lambda_0}{\lambda_1}Y_0+Y_1)M_{01}(t_1)}e^{-(\frac{\lambda_0}{\lambda_2}Y_0+Y_2)M_{02}(t_2)} \\
&= \mathbf{E}e^{-Y_0(\frac{\lambda_0}{\lambda_1}M_{01}(t_1)+\frac{\lambda_0}{\lambda_2}M_{02}(t_2))-Y_1 M_{01}(t_1)-Y_2 M_{02}(t_2)} \\
&= (1 + \frac{1}{\lambda_0}(\frac{\lambda_0}{\lambda_1}M_{01}(t_1) + \frac{\lambda_0}{\lambda_2}M_{02}(t_2)))^{-k_0} \\
&\quad \times (1 + \frac{1}{\lambda_1}M_{01}(t_1))^{-k_1}(1 + \frac{1}{\lambda_2}M_{02}(t_2))^{-k_2} \\
&= (1 + \sigma_1^2 M_{01}(t_1) + \sigma_2^2 M_{02}(t_2))^{\frac{-\rho}{\sigma_1\sigma_2}} \\
&\quad \times (1 + \sigma_1^2 M_{01}(t_1))^{\frac{-1+\frac{\sigma_1}{\sigma_2}\rho}{\sigma_1^2}}(1 + \sigma_2^2 M_{02}(t_2))^{\frac{-1+\frac{\sigma_2}{\sigma_1}\rho}{\sigma_2^2}}, \qquad (5.5)
\end{aligned}
$$

which results in the following representation of the correlated gamma frailty model

$$
S(t_1, t_2) = \frac{S_1(t_1)^{1-\frac{\sigma_1}{\sigma_2}\rho}S_2(t_2)^{1-\frac{\sigma_2}{\sigma_1}\rho}}{(S_1(t_1)^{-\sigma_1^2} + S_2(t_2)^{-\sigma_2^2} - 1)^{\frac{\rho}{\sigma_1\sigma_2}}}, \qquad (5.6)
$$

using independence of the gamma-distributed variables Y_0, Y_1, Y_2 and (3.17). This representation is called here the *copula representation*, because it reveals that the correlated gamma frailty model can be considered as a copula, but this copula is not an Archimedian copula as in the shared gamma frailty model. Copula representations allow separation of the marginal part of the model (univariate distributions) from the correlation structure of the model. Besides the fact that frailty models and copulas look very similar, it is important to note that there are also differences between both approaches that are often overlooked. For more details regarding this exciting aspect, we refer the interested reader to the paper by Goethals et al. (2008) and Chapter 6 in this monograph.

The possible range of the correlation between frailties depends on the values of σ_1 and σ_2:

$$
0 \leq \rho \leq \min\{\frac{\sigma_1}{\sigma_2}, \frac{\sigma_2}{\sigma_1}\}.
$$

Hence, if $\sigma_1 \neq \sigma_2$, the correlation between the frailties is always less than one. This property can be a serious limitation, especially when the values of σ_1 and σ_2 differ strongly.

Partial derivatives of the bivariate survival function (which are necessary for the likelihood) are given in Appendix A.2. The log-likelihood contribution of the ith pair in the parametric case without censoring, truncation, and observed covariates is given by

$$
\begin{aligned}
\log L_i(\boldsymbol{\theta}, \sigma^2, \rho) = {} & \frac{\rho}{\sigma_1 \sigma_2} \ln(S_1(t_{i1}; \boldsymbol{\theta})^{-\sigma_1^2}) + \frac{\rho}{\sigma_1 \sigma_2} \ln(S_2(t_{i2}; \boldsymbol{\theta})^{-\sigma_2^2}) \\
& - (\frac{\rho}{\sigma_1 \sigma_2} + 2) \ln(S_1(t_{i1}; \boldsymbol{\theta})^{-\sigma_1^2} + S_2(t_{i2}; \boldsymbol{\theta})^{-\sigma_2^2} - 1) \\
& + \ln \left(1 - \frac{\sigma_1}{\sigma_2}\rho - \frac{\sigma_2}{\sigma_1}\rho + \rho^2 + (1 - \frac{\sigma_2}{\sigma_1}\rho)S_1(t_{i1}; \boldsymbol{\theta})^{-2\sigma_1^2} \right. \\
& + (1 - \frac{\sigma_1}{\sigma_2}\rho)S_2(t_{i2}; \boldsymbol{\theta})^{-2\sigma_2^2} \\
& + (2 - \frac{\sigma_1}{\sigma_2}\rho - \frac{\sigma_2}{\sigma_1}\rho + \sigma_1 \sigma_2 \rho + \rho^2)S_1(t_{i1}; \boldsymbol{\theta})^{-\sigma_1^2} S_2(t_{i2}; \boldsymbol{\theta})^{-\sigma_2^2} \\
& + (-2 + \frac{\sigma_1}{\sigma_2}\rho + 2\frac{\sigma_2}{\sigma_1}\rho - \rho^2)S_1(t_{i1}; \boldsymbol{\theta})^{-\sigma_1^2} \\
& \left. + (-2 + \frac{\sigma_2}{\sigma_1}\rho + 2\frac{\sigma_1}{\sigma_2}\rho - \rho^2)S_2(t_{i2}; \boldsymbol{\theta})^{-\sigma_2^2} \right).
\end{aligned}
$$

In the following we apply the correlated gamma frailty model to cause-specific mortality data of Danish twins, described in Example 1.4. The assumption of conditional independence plays an important role in genetic analysis of event times. Under this assumption, the frailty variable becomes the only carrier of genetic influence on durations. It means that the underlying hazard represents only nongenetic influence on the event time. Univariate frailty models do not have such a property.

Example 5.1

Age at death by cancer (all types of cancer combined) and age at death by stroke in twin pairs are the event times of interest. Because of the symmetric structure of the twin data, we use the simplifications $S(t) = S_1(t) = S_2(t)$ and $\sigma^2 = \sigma_1^2 = \sigma_2^2$. A parametric approach with a Gompertz baseline hazard $\mu_0(t) = \lambda e^{\varphi t}$ is fitted, resulting in the univariate marginal survival function

$$
S(t) = (1 + \sigma^2 \frac{\lambda}{\varphi}(e^{\varphi t} - 1))^{-\frac{1}{\sigma^2}}.
$$

The data is right censored, and left truncated, which has to be included into the likelihood. The results of the maximum likelihood parameter estimation procedure are given in Table 5.1.

For each cause of death, a separate analysis of the same data was performed, treating all other causes of death as independent censored observations. To allow a combined analysis of monozygotic (MZ) and dizygotic (DZ) twins, we include two correlation coefficients into the model, ρ_{MZ} and ρ_{DZ}, respectively. These correlations between MZ and DZ twins provide important information about genetic and environmental influences on frailty (susceptibility) within

Table 5.1:   Parameter estimates in the correlated gamma frailty model applied to Danish twin pairs

	males		females	
	cancer	stroke	cancer	stroke
σ^2	3.388 (0.572)	5.146 (1.373)	7.194 (1.197)	1.794 (0.793)
ρ_{MZ}	0.350 (0.088)	0.706 (0.160)	0.245 (0.065)	0.688 (0.316)
ρ_{DZ}	0.194 (0.068)	0.208 (0.119)	0.076 (0.041)	0.407 (0.254)
λ	4.4e-6 (1.5e-6)	5.8e-8 (3.9e-8)	7.3e-6 (2.8e-6)	1.0e-7 (5.6e-8)
φ	0.118 (0.006)	0.160 (0.010)	0.111 (0.007)	0.144 (0.008)

individuals (see Appendix A.6). For both causes of death and both sexes, the estimates of correlation of frailty for MZ twins (ρ_{MZ}) are higher than that for DZ twins (ρ_{DZ}). These higher correlations in MZ twins compared to DZ twins indicate the importance of genetic factors involved in susceptibility (frailty) to cause-specific mortality. Estimates of correlations range between 0.08 (cancer, DZ female twins) and 0.71 (stroke, MZ male twins). The differences in the estimates of the frailty variance σ^2 indicate different levels of heterogeneity. The shared gamma frailty model $\rho = 1$ is sometimes applied to twin data, but results in different estimates of σ^2 for MZ and DZ twins (Hougaard 2000). This contradicts the observation that univariate (marginal) lifetimes of MZ and DZ twins are similar.

Parameter estimates were obtained using a selfwritten GAUSS routine. The routine is based on constrained maximum likelihood estimation, maximizing the parametric likelihood function under user-specified constraints on the parameters. The likelihood function for left-truncated and right-censored bivariate data is given in Appendix A.1 and A.2. We will reanalyze the data again in the following example with the emphasis on obtaining quantitative results about the heritability of cause-specific mortality.   □

Example 5.2

This example deals with an extension of the above correlated gamma frailty model which allows the integration of genetic models (see Appendix A.6). In this approach, the correlations between the frailties of family members are substituted by their respective variance components. In the present case of MZ and DZ twins, relation (A.8) can be used. In ACE models containing additive genetic factors (A), common environment (C), and unique environment (E), the corresponding variance components are denoted by a^2, c^2, and e^2. Using this reparameterization of the model, the data from Example 5.1 are analyzed again in Table 5.2. The main interest is in the estimation of the heritability (a^2), which quantifies the importance of genetic factors on a trait. Here, the trait of interest is susceptibility to death caused by cancer and stroke, respectively. Again, a Gompertz baseline hazard is used.

Table 5.2: Heritability of cause of death. Parameter estimates in the correlated gamma frailty model applied to Danish twin pairs

	males		females	
	cancer	stroke	cancer	stroke
σ^2	3.388 (0.572)	4.956 (1.360)	7.233 (1.198)	1.791 (0.796)
a^2	0.311 (0.215)	0.635 (0.150)	0.211 (0.052)	0.564 (0.678)
c^2	0.038 (0.158)	0.000 (-)	0.000 (-)	0.126 (0.509)
e^2	0.650 (0.088)	0.365 (0.150)	0.789 (0.052)	0.311 (0.316)
λ	4.4e-6 (1.5e-6)	6.3e-8 (4.1e-8)	7.2e-6 (2.8e-6)	1.0e-7 (6.0e-8)
φ	0.118 (0.006)	0.159 (0.010)	0.111 (0.007)	0.144 (0.008)

Heritability estimates differ by gender and cause of death, ranging from 0.21 (cancer in females) to 0.63 (stroke in males). At least moderate heritability is usually the basis for further linkage and association studies to identify risk genes.

This approach from event history analysis permits accounting for censoring and truncation present in the data. The method is combined with variance component models from genetic epidemiology. For such a combined analysis, we apply the correlated gamma frailty model, which takes into account the dependence of lifespans of relatives. This enables the estimation of the effect of genetic factors in susceptibility to cancer and stroke. The approach allows the combination of data on age of death and cause of death and for overcoming the drawbacks of the traditional concordance analysis usually applied in twin studies with time-to-event data. For each twin partner two competing risks of latent times (with respect to death due to cancer or stroke, and with respect to death due to all other diseases including censoring) are modeled. In addition, we assume that these competing risks are independent. ⬚

In the following, an adaption of the bivariate correlated gamma frailty model to a three-dimensional approach in genetics is considered. This model was introduced by Korsgaard and Andersen (1998). It is based on the idea of correlated gamma frailty but with pre-specified correlations between family members. In one of their examples, the authors consider families of size three with a father (F), a mother (M), and one child (C). Let V_1 represent the part of the father's genome affecting frailty that is transmitted to the child, and V_2 the corresponding part of the father's genome not transmitted to the child. Similarly, V_3 represents the part of the mother's genome affecting frailty transmitted to the child, and V_4 the corresponding part of the mother's genome not transmitted to the child. Assuming that the father and mother are unrelated, additive genetic gamma frailties for the father, Z_F, the mother, Z_M, and the child, Z_C, are given by

$$Z_F = V_1 + V_2 \quad Z_M = V_3 + V_4 \quad Z_C = V_1 + V_3.$$

Here, it is necessary to mention that the interpretation of frailty in the present model is different from the interpretation of frailty in the foregoing correlated frailty model applied to twin data to estimate heritability of specific traits. In the Korsgaard and Andersen model, frailty only represents genetic factors, whereas in the correlated frailty model used in Example 5.2, frailty represents genetic as well as environmental factors.

Assuming that the V_i's are i.i.d., with $V_i \sim \Gamma(\frac{\lambda}{2}, \lambda)$, so that $\mathbf{E}(V_i) = \frac{1}{2}$ and $\mathbf{V}(V_i) = \frac{1}{2\lambda}$, then $\mathbf{E}(Z_F) = \mathbf{E}(Z_M) = \mathbf{E}(Z_C) = 1$ and

$$\mathbf{V}(Z_F, Z_M, Z_C) = \frac{1}{\lambda} \begin{pmatrix} 1 & 0 & \frac{1}{2} \\ 0 & 1 & \frac{1}{2} \\ \frac{1}{2} & \frac{1}{2} & 1 \end{pmatrix}.$$

The correlation between the frailty of the father Z_F or the mother Z_F and frailty of the child Z_C is one half due to the fact that the two individuals share half of their genes. The frailties of the father and mother in each family are assumed to be independent. It is assumed that the baseline hazard functions were unknown (semiparametric model). In the bivariate cases (father – child or mother – child), the genetic frailty model is a correlated frailty model with correlation equals to one half. This can be seen from the trivariate survival function of the model (with reparameterization $\sigma^2 = 1/\lambda$)

$$\begin{aligned} S(t_1, t_2, t_3) &= \mathbf{E}e^{-Z_F M_1(t_1)} e^{-Z_M M_2(t_2)} e^{-Z_C M_3(t_3)} \\ &= \mathbf{E}e^{-(V_1+V_2)M_{01}(t_1) - (V_3+V_4)M_{02}(t_2) - (V_1+V_3)M_3(t_3)} \\ &= \mathbf{E}e^{-V_1(M_{01}(t_1)+M_3(t_3))} e^{-V_3(M_{02}(t_2)+M_3(t_3))} e^{-V_2 M_{01}(t_1)} e^{-V_4 M_{02}(t_2)} \\ &= (1 + \frac{1}{\lambda}(M_{01}(t_1) + M_3(t_3)))^{-\frac{\lambda}{2}} (1 + \frac{1}{\lambda}(M_{02}(t_2) + M_3(t_3)))^{-\frac{\lambda}{2}} \\ &\quad \times (1 + \frac{1}{\lambda}M_{01}(t_1))^{-\frac{\lambda}{2}} (1 + \frac{1}{\lambda}M_{02}(t_2))^{-\frac{\lambda}{2}} \\ &= \left(S_1(t_1)^{-\sigma^2} + S_3(t_3)^{-\sigma^2} - 1\right)^{-\frac{1}{2\sigma^2}} \\ &\quad \times \left(S_2(t_2)^{-\sigma^2} + S_3(t_3)^{-\sigma^2} - 1\right)^{-\frac{1}{2\sigma^2}} S_1(t_1)^{\frac{1}{2}} S_2(t_2)^{\frac{1}{2}} \end{aligned}$$

using the Laplace transform of a gamma distributed random variable (3.17). Obviously, the following relations hold:

$$S(t_1, t_2, 0) = S_1(t_1)S_2(t_2)$$
$$S(t_1, 0, t_3) = \left(S_1(t_1)^{-\sigma^2} + S_3(t_3)^{-\sigma^2} - 1\right)^{-\frac{1}{2\sigma^2}} S_1(t_1)^{\frac{1}{2}} S_3(t_3)^{\frac{1}{2}}$$
$$S(0, t_2, t_3) = \left(S_2(t_2)^{-\sigma^2} + S_3(t_3)^{-\sigma^2} - 1\right)^{-\frac{1}{2\sigma^2}} S_2(t_2)^{\frac{1}{2}} S_3(t_3)^{\frac{1}{2}}.$$

The first equation reflects the fact that the frailties of the parents are assumed to be uncorrelated. This results in independent event times. The second and third function, respectively, are survival functions of the correlated gamma frailty model with correlation $\rho = 0.5$ (see equation (5.6)). Korsgaard and Andersen (1998) apply their model to data from the Danish adoptee register. Each of the 792 families, as well as the father and mother of each family, are assumed to be unrelated. It seems reasonable to assume that no environmental correlations between lifetimes are present. No environmental correlations exist between the child and its biological father and mother because the child is adopted very soon after birth. It is therefore very likely that the parents did not live together, and thus, it is reasonable to assume that the environmental correlation is absent between the lifetimes of the parents. The (bivariate) correlated gamma frailty model was used to perform a goodness-of-fit test of the (trivariate) additive genetic gamma frailty model. Further extensions by including genetic marker information can be found in a series of papers by Li (1999, 2002), Li and Zhong (2002), Zhong and Li (2004), and Jonker et al. (2009). A more general multivariate correlated gamma frailty is considered at the end of this section.

It is necessary to keep in mind that parameter ρ describes the correlation between the frailties in a pair and *not* the correlation of the related lifetimes. Lindeboom and van den Berg (1994) analyzed the relationship of correlations between frailties and between lifetimes. They derive explicit expressions for the correlation between the survival times, and examined the properties of this correlation in the special case of a constant baseline hazard function. Unfortunately, in general situations, such explicit results are not available. One possibility would be to simulate noncensored event-time data following the estimated model and using it to estimate the correlation between the event times directly.

Up to now only the case without observed covariates was considered. This situation is common in demographic applications with large register data. In many demographic studies, only information about gender and year of birth is available. However, especially in medical applications, covariates are usually available and need to be included into the model. This can be done in a natural way similar to the univariate and shared frailty model. The correlated gamma frailty model with observed covariates is a simple extension of (5.6):

$$S(t_1, t_2 | \mathbf{X}_1, \mathbf{X}_2) = \frac{S_1(t_1 | \mathbf{X}_1)^{1 - \frac{\sigma_1}{\sigma_2}\rho} S_2(t_2 | \mathbf{X}_2)^{1 - \frac{\sigma_2}{\sigma_1}\rho}}{(S_1(t_1 | \mathbf{X}_1)^{-\sigma_1^2} + S_2(t_2 | \mathbf{X}_2)^{-\sigma_2^2} - 1)^{\frac{\rho}{\sigma_1 \sigma_2}}},$$

where $\mathbf{X}_1$ and $\mathbf{X}_2$ are the covariate vectors of the partners in the pair. Again, the marginal survival functions are assumed to be identical in the following applications to twin data by $S(t|\mathbf{X}) = S_1(t|\mathbf{X}) = S_2(t|\mathbf{X})$ and $\sigma^2 = \sigma_1^2 = \sigma_2^2$ yielding:

$$S(t|\mathbf{X}) = \left(1 + \sigma^2 M_0(t) e^{\boldsymbol{\beta}' \mathbf{X}}\right)^{-\frac{1}{\sigma^2}}. \tag{5.7}$$

Example 5.3

In the following we present an application of the bivariate correlated gamma frailty model with observed covariates to the lifetimes of MZ and DZ Danish twins with respect to coronary heart disease (CHD). We analyze the influence of smoking, body mass index (BMI), gender, and birth year (using the variable transformation birth year minus 1890 because the oldest twins are born in 1890) on the susceptibility to death by CHD.

Table 5.3: Correlated gamma frailty model with covariates

parameter	Weibull	exponential	Gompertz
σ^2	0.467 (0.196)	0.107 (0.032)	0.622 (0.214)
ρ_{MZ}	1.000 (-)	1.000 (-)	1.000 (-)
ρ_{DZ}	0.884 (0.428)	0.889 (0.425)	0.689 (0.306)
λ	1.7e-20 (4.4e-20)	0.397 (0.213)	3.5e-6 (2.4e-6)
ν	10.362 (0.590)		
φ			0.131 (0.008)
cigarette smokers	0.451 (0.144)	0.337 (0.150)	0.465 (0.149)
other smokers	0.167 (0.139)	0.142 (0.147)	0.184 (0.144)
former smokers	0.168 (0.147)	0.162 (0.154)	0.186 (0.152)
BMI < 22	0.213 (0.139)	0.155 (0.147)	0.228 (0.144)
BMI > 28	0.073 (0.122)	0.014 (0.133)	0.081 (0.127)
gender (female)	-0.734 (0.120)	-0.728 (0.149)	-0.783 (0.126)
birthyear	-0.022 (0.008)	-0.136 (0.016)	-0.022 (0.009)
likelihood	-2733.98424	-2929.10475	-2729.89782

Parametric models with different cumulative baseline hazards $M_0(t)$ in (5.7) were fitted. The results are given in Table 5.3. The Gompertz model shows the best fit to the data (based on the likelihood) compared to the other two models and should be preferred. The correlation for MZ twins ($\rho_{MZ} = 1$) is on the boundary of the parameter space, whereas DZ twins show a smaller correlation ($\rho_{DZ} = 0.689$). Cigarette smokers have a significant higher risk to die from CHD, with $\beta = 0.465$ (0.149), compared to nonsmokers. Other smokers and former smokers show a small but nonsignificant risk increase compared to nonsmokers. Twins with small or high BMI have a slightly worse prognosis compared to twins in the reference category with BMI between 22 and 28 kg/m^2. Women show a significant better survival with $\beta = -0.783$ (0.126) compared to males, and later birth is related to a decreasing risk. □

An interesting extension of the bivariate correlated gamma frailty model is given in a recent paper by van den Berg et al. (2008). Here, information about the economic situation at birth time and the seasonality of birth is included into the analysis of lifetimes of Danish twins with special interest in mortality caused by cardiovascular diseases.

The bivariate correlated gamma frailty model can be extended to the multivariate case with p related lifespans, which results in the gamma-distributed frailty case in the multivariate survival times

$$S(t_1, \ldots, t_p) = \prod_{i=1}^{p} S_i(t_i)^{1-\rho} \Big(\sum_{i=1}^{p} S_i(t_i)^{-\sigma^2} - p + 1 \Big)^{-\rho/\sigma^2}.$$

In this model, identical distributions are used for the frailties of the subjects in a cluster, and the correlations between frailties in a cluster are unique and given by ρ. Further extensions of this model with different frailty variances can be found in Yashin and Iachine (1999a), but need additional requirements, which are rather restrictive for real applications. A major disadvantage of the model is that it becomes very complex with increasing cluster size. In the foregoing twin example the likelihood consists of four terms caused by the different possibilities for censoring plus one term for truncation (see Appendix (A.2)). With cluster size three, the number of terms increases to nine; with cluster size four, 17 terms have to be calculated. These terms include derivatives of the survival function of the order of the cluster size. This limits multivariate extensions of the correlated gamma frailty model to cluster sizes of three or at most four. This inflexibility was the main reason why this model was not considered further in the literature, for example, to model family data. For such kind of applications (cluster size larger than two), the correlated log-normal frailty model considered in the following chapter is much more appropriate because of the flexibility of multivariate normal distribution.

In the applications of the correlated gamma frailty model presented here, a parametric approach is used. Similar to shared frailty models, semiparametric approaches are sometimes preferable to prevent assumptions about the form of the baseline hazard function. For the bivariate correlated gamma frailty model, an EM algorithm for a semiparametric approach was suggested by Iachine (1995), but software is not publicly available for this model. Further developments in this direction are restricted by the problems with extensions of the bivariate correlated gamma frailty model to the larger cluster sizes discussed earlier. The main problem in comparison with the shared frailty model is that the number of frailties per cluster to be estimated in the EM algorithm is determined by the number of observations in the cluster. This causes severe problems with larger cluster size.

Parner (1998) extends results from Murphy (1994,1995) from the shared gama frailty model and shows consistency and asymptotic normality of the nonparametric maximum likelihood estimator in the multivariate correlated gamma frailty model with observed covariates.

The correlated gamma frailty model can also be applied to current status data. In the case of bivariate event times the likelihood function is given by (4.7). Information about identifiability, consistency, and asymptotic normality in the correlated gamma frailty model with current status data is given in the paper by Chang et al. (2007). In the following results of a small simulation study are presented to check the performance of the estimation procedure. One thousand samples of 1000 pairs each are generated using the bivariate correlated gamma frailty model with frailty variance $\mathbf{V}(Z) = \sigma^2$, expectation $\mathbf{E}Z = 1$, and Gompertz baseline. We consider the two scenarios similar to that of the shared gamma frailty model in Section 4.3.3.

Scenario 1: Both censoring/monitoring times c_1, c_2 are independent.

Table 5.4: Simulation (Scenario 1) of correlated gamma frailty ($\rho = 0.5$) with current status data

parameter	true	current status	right censored
σ^2	1.000	1.442 (1.332)	1.030 (0.379)
ρ	0.500	0.636 (0.290)	0.596 (0.241)
λ_1	0.100	0.105 (0.136)	0.099 (0.008)
φ_1	0.120	0.436 (0.990)	0.143 (0.103)
λ_2	0.100	0.112 (0.134)	0.100 (0.008)
φ_2	0.120	0.435 (0.981)	0.143 (0.102)

Each data set is analyzed under two different censoring mechanisms – once as right-censored lifetimes, and once as current status data. The correlated gamma frailty model is much more complex than the shared gamma frailty model because of the additional correlation parameter ρ in the model. In this model the parameter estimates based on right-censored data are much closer to the true parameter values and with much smaller standard errors compared to the estimates based on the current status data. Especially, the parameter estimates for φ_1, φ_2 are strongly biased upward with the current status data, as are the estimates of σ^2 and ρ. Consequently, switching from right-censored lifetime data to current status data causes an important information loss. However, further simulations with increasing sample size (results are not shown) imply that parameters can be estimated consistently based on event-time data as well as current status data.

Scenario 2: Both censoring/monitoring times are equal.
We consider this situation in detail here because it holds for the real data example considered later. Correlation coefficients of $\rho = 0.25, 0.5, 0.75$, and 1 are simulated. The results are similar to that of the situation of independent censoring. For the current status data, the upwards bias in the parameter estimates of $\varphi_1, \varphi_2, \sigma^2$ is more pronounced; also, the standard errors are larger. Obviously, the upwards bias becomes less pronounced for larger values of the correlation ρ (see Tables 5.5-5.8). The correlated gamma frailty model with parametric baseline hazard is identifiable with current status data and gives better results with larger sample size (results are not shown).

Table 5.5:   Simulation Scenario 2 with $\rho = 0.25$

parameter	true	current status	right censored
σ^2	1.000	1.904 (2.140)	1.249 (0.978)
ρ	0.250	0.378 (0.326)	0.382 (0.309)
λ_1	0.100	0.168 (0.882)	0.099 (0.012)
φ_1	0.120	0.912 (2.175)	0.286 (0.724)
λ_2	0.100	0.120 (0.465)	0.100 (0.023)
φ_2	0.120	0.918 (2.208)	0.285 (0.741)

Table 5.6:   Simulation Scenario 2 with $\rho = 0.5$

parameter	true	current status	right censored
σ^2	1.000	1.489 (1.592)	1.020 (0.346)
ρ	0.500	0.606 (0.292)	0.585 (0.230)
λ_1	0.100	0.108 (0.141)	0.100 (0.008)
φ_1	0.120	0.531 (1.799)	0.138 (0.091)
λ_2	0.100	0.100 (0.052)	0.100 (0.008)
φ_2	0.120	0.539 (1.865)	0.138 (0.092)

Table 5.7:   Simulation Scenario 2 with $\rho = 0.75$

parameter	true	current status	right censored
σ^2	1.000	1.228 (0.805)	1.023 (0.201)
ρ	0.750	0.764 (0.212)	0.769 (0.156)
λ_1	0.100	0.102 (0.078)	0.100 (0.008)
ψ_1	0.120	0.252 (0.623)	0.131 (0.050)
λ_2	0.100	0.101 (0.038)	0.100 (0.008)
φ_2	0.120	0.250 (0.600)	0.131 (0.050)

Table 5.8:   Simulation Scenario 2 with $\rho = 1$

parameter	true	current status	right censored
σ^2	1.000	1.164 (0.320)	1.061 (0.099)
ρ	1.000	0.916 (0.110)	0.950 (0.071)
λ_1	0.100	0.099 (0.016)	0.100 (0.008)
φ_1	0.120	0.173 (0.185)	0.136 (0.027)
λ_2	0.100	0.102 (0.127)	0.099 (0.008)
φ_2	0.120	0.174 (0.173)	0.136 (0.027)

Example 5.4

Here, the hepatitis A and B current status data from Example 1.7 are analyzed in detail. In the second column of Table 5.9, a correlated gamma frailty model with different frailty variances σ_1^2 and σ_2^2 for hepatitis A and B, respectively, is presented (correlated I). In the third column, a model with equal variances $\sigma_1^2 = \sigma_2^2$ is used (correlated II). The fourth column contains a shared gamma frailty model ($\rho = 1$), and column five contains the univariate frailty model ($\rho = 0$). There is no reason to assume per se that the frailty variance with

Table 5.9: Analysis of hepatitis A and B current status data with the correlated gamma frailty model

parameter	correlated I	correlated II	shared	univariate
σ_1^2	2.668 (0.572)	2.600 (0.553)	0.522 (0.028)	2.018 (0.510)
σ_2^2	1.472 (2.528)	2.600 (0.553)	0.522 (0.028)	10.037 (8.821)
ρ	0.653 (1.938)	0.485 (0.038)	1.000 (–)	0.000 (–)
λ_1	0.007 (0.001)	0.007 (0.001)	0.012 (0.001)	0.008 (0.001)
φ_1	0.105 (0.017)	0.103 (0.016)	0.037 (0.002)	0.085 (0.016)
λ_2	0.002 (0.001)	0.002 (0.001)	0.002 (0.001)	0.002 (0.001)
φ_2	0.002 (0.032)	0.002 (0.007)	-0.001 (0.007)	0.015 (0.142)
log-likelihood	-2826.7159	-2826.7918	-2843.5100	-2841.4151

respect to hepatitis A is similar to the frailty with respect to hepatitis B. That is why a correlated frailty model with different variances is applied, but the model with equal variances is supported by the log-likelihood. A further simplification of the model to the shared gamma frailty model implies a significant worsening in the fit ($p < 0.0001$). The univariate frailty models treats time-to-infection by hepatitis A and B, respectively, as independent. It allows for different variances and shows a log-likelihood similar to the one in the shared frailty model. A Gompertz baseline hazard was used in all models.

Besides the good fit of the correlated gamma frailty model compared to the shared frailty model, it provides a nice interpretation of the parameters. Here, σ_1^2 and σ_2^2 are measures of population heterogeneity in the susceptibility to hepatitis A and B, respectively. These parameters yield implications for further programs to prevent infections, as the critical vaccination coverage is higher for more heterogeneous populations. Furthermore, the parameter ρ provides a correlation measure. The analysis of bivariate infection data allows study of the association between the acquisition of both infections. The correlation indicates similar transmission routes (correlation near one) or reflects to what extent a latent process, such as the social or hygienic behavior of people, drives the more general infection process (Hens et al. 2009). □

5.3 Correlated Log-normal Frailty Model

The correlated log-normal frailty model is much more flexible than the gamma model because it is not based on the additive composition of the frailties as used in (5.3) and (5.4). However, the log-normal distribution does not allow us to integrate out the frailties with an explicit representation of the likelihood. This requires more sophisticated estimation strategies. The distribution can be obtained by assuming a bivariate normal distribution on the logarithm of the frailty vector,

$$\begin{pmatrix} \ln Z_1 \\ \ln Z_2 \end{pmatrix} = \begin{pmatrix} W_1 \\ W_2 \end{pmatrix} \sim \mathrm{N}\left(\begin{pmatrix} m \\ m \end{pmatrix}, \begin{pmatrix} s^2 & rs^2 \\ rs^2 & s^2 \end{pmatrix} \right),$$

with N denoting the bivariate normal distribution whose parameters are some functions of the frailty parameters σ^2 and ρ, similar to the univariate log-normal frailty model in (3.36) and (3.37):

$$\mu = \mathbf{E}Z_j = e^{m+\frac{s^2}{2}}$$

$$\sigma^2 = \mathbf{V}(Z_j) = e^{2m+s^2}(e^{s^2} - 1)$$

$$\rho = \mathbf{corr}(Z_1, Z_2) = \frac{e^{rs^2} - 1}{e^{s^2} - 1}.$$

Again, the restriction $m = 0$ is used to guarantee identifiability of the model parameters. This means that the random effects W_j $(j = 1, 2)$ (log frailties) have an expectation of zero.

Xue and Brookmeyer (1996) were the first authors to consider the correlated log-normal frailty model and applied it to mental health data to evaluate the health policy effects for inpatient psychiatric care. Yau and McGilchrist (1997) used a generalized linear mixed model approach to analyze data from litter-matched tumorigenesis experiments in rats with help of the correlated log-normal model. Cook et al. (1999) used a correlated log-normal frailty in two-state mixed renewal processes for chronic diseases. Other examples can be found in Ripatti and Palmgren (2000) and Ripatti et al. (2002). Based on correlated log-normal frailty models, Pankratz et al. (2005) perform genetic analysis of age at onset in breast cancer in a large familial cohort. Their method is based on a Laplace approximation similar to the approach by Ripatti and Palmgren (2000).

Example 5.5
The correlated log-normal frailty model is applied to the mortality of Danish twins. The duration of interest is lifetime with respect to CHD; that means lifetimes with respect to other causes of death are considered as censoring

Table 5.10: Correlated log-normal frailty model with covariates

parameter	without covariates	with covariates
s^2	6.520 (3.263)	2.394 (1.210)
ρ_{MZ}	0.509 (0.108)	0.575 (0.190)
ρ_{DZ}	0.359 (0.097)	0.426 (0.141)
λ	2.8e-11 (1.1e-10)	9.6e-9 (1.9e-8)
φ	0.249 (0.045)	0.195 (0.024)
cigarette smokers		0.556 (0.192)
other smokers		0.265 (0.182)
former smokers		0.247 (0.192)
BMI < 22		0.312 (0.184)
BMI > 28		0.149 (0.161)
gender (female)		-0.966 (0.194)
birthyear		0.006 (0.010)
log-likelihood	-2797.45474	-2761.61131

times. The results in Table 5.10 are difficult to compare with Example 5.3, where a correlated gamma frailty model was applied. The variances σ^2 of the gamma and s^2 of the log-normal model are not directly comparable. The same problem holds for the correlations in both models. The analysis indicates a nonsignificant mortality increase for twins with BMI less than 22 kg/m^2 with $\beta = 0.312\,(0.184)$ and BMI more than 28 kg/m^2 with $\beta = 0.149\,(0.161)$, respectively. The reference group are twins with BMI between 22 kg/m^2 and 28 kg/m^2. Cigarette smoking shows a significant influence on CHD mortality with $\beta = 0.556\,(0.192)$, whereas pipe/cigar smokers $\beta = 0.32\,(0.23)$ and former smokers $\beta = 0.48\,(0.26)$ experience only a nonsignificant increase in risk. The reference group are the nonsmokers. Females have a significant better survival $\beta = -0.966\,(0.194)$ compared to males. The birth year shows no significant association with CHD death in this sample. Analysis was performed with SAS NLMIXED.

In twin studies, the main focus is on the correlations between MZ and DZ twins and not on the covariates. The effect of covariates may be better evaluated in studies of singletons. Correlations are of special interest for the quantification of the influence of genetic and environmental factors. A comparison between models without and with covariates allows conclusions about the nature of the covariates (genetic vs. environment). The inclusion of the covariates reduces the frailty variance. This is expected because these covariates are included in the frailty in the model without covariates. By explicit modeling as observed covariates in the analysis, these covariates are no longer included in the frailty (as a proxy for unobserved covariates). It implies the reduction in the frailty variance from 6.520 (3.263) to 2.394 (1.210). In contrast, the correlations change only slightly between the two models. This point is further discussed in the next example. □

Example 5.6

In this example, an extension of the correlated log-normal frailty model is presented, which allows the integration of genetic models (see Appendix A.6). In this approach the correlations between family members are substituted by the respective variance components. In the case of MZ and DZ twins relation (A.8) can be used. In an ACE model including additive genetic factors (A), common environment (C), and unique environment (E), the corresponding variance components are denoted by a^2, c^2, and e^2. This reparameterization is used to analyze the data from Example 5.3 again. The main interest is in the estimation of the heritability (a^2), which quantifies the importance of genetic factors on a trait. Here, the trait of interest is lifetime with respect to CHD. Again, a Gompertz baseline hazard is used (semiparametric approach).

Table 5.11: Correlated log-normal frailty model with covariates

parameter	without covariates	with covariates
s^2	7.875 (3.505)	2.500 (1.182)
a^2	0.295 (0.261)	0.464 (0.365)
c^2	0.223 (0.198)	0.151 (0.276)
e^2	0.482 (0.097)	0.384 (0.171)
λ	5.9e-12 (2.3e-11)	8.5e-9 (1.6e-8)
φ	0.267 (0.045)	0.197 (0.023)
cigarette smokers		0.595 (0.196)
other smokers		0.249 (0.183)
former smokers		0.247 (0.193)
BMI < 22		0.257 (0.184)
BMI > 28		0.146 (0.162)
gender (female)		-0.996 (0.194)
birthyear		0.006 (0.010)
log-likelihood	-2797.41765	-2761.36539

Former studies from the Danish (Harvald and Hauge 1970) and Swedish (de Faire 1975, Marenberg et al. 1994) twin registries found a genetic component in the susceptibility to death from coronary heart disease. The advantage of the approach presented here is the combination of methods from survival analysis with methods from genetic epidemiology. This allows the estimation of the effect of genetic factors in susceptibility to CHD and the evaluation as to what extent smoking, BMI, and susceptibility to CHD are all influenced by common genetic factors. For each individual, two independent, underlying, competing risks of latent times – lifetime with respect to death due to CHD and lifetime with respect to death due to all other causes including censoring events – are assumed.

Both, smoking and BMI, are influenced by genes with heritability estimates in the range $0.35 - 0.75$ (smoking) and $0.5 - 0.8$ (BMI) (Bouchard 1994, Heath and Madden 1995, Herskind et al. 1996b). However, whether common genes influence these phenotypic traits as well as susceptibility to CHD is an open question. In a different situation Fisher (1958) suggested that the association between smoking and lung cancer is spurious and reflects only the circumstance that the same genes influence both smoking habits and lung cancer. This was the starting point for a long debate on genetic confounding.

The main result of the present analysis is that the inclusion of smoking and BMI do not cause any substantial decrease in the heritability estimate. Consequently, no evidence was found for common genetic factors acting on smoking and susceptibility to CHD or BMI, and susceptibility to CHD. This study confirms the earlier finding that the genetic influence on susceptibility to CHD is not mediated through genetic influence on smoking and BMI. Similar results were found by Zdravkovic et al. (2004) in Swedish twins. The approach here is different from the common study design in many medical applications. Usually the investigator is interested in the effect of covariates on the outcome, adjusted for the correlation in clustered observations, treating the correlation as a nuisance parameter. In genetic epidemiology, the main interest is in the correlations, adjusted for the effect of covariates.

As expected, the inclusion of covariates decreases the heterogeneity in the study population, which can be seen in the decline of the frailty variance from $s^2 = 7.875$ (3.505) to $s^2 = 2.500$ (1.182). This underlines that frailty depends on the model, and it describes factors not included in the model.

When covariates are included in the model, the relative importance of environmental factors is reduced, leading to an increase in the heritability estimate observed in the present analysis. This is a result of the heritability coefficient as a variance proportion. The variance of the random effects can be decomposed as follows: $s^2 = s^2_{genes} + s^2_{environment}$. Focusing on heritability only one does not know whether the heritability increases due to an increase in the genetic variance or due to a decrease in the environmental variance. In the present case, the increase was largely due to the latter. By including smoking and BMI, the genetic variance was reduced from $s^2_{genes} = 2.32$ to $s^2_{genes} = 1.16$. The reduction of the environmental heterogeneity is more pronounced, for example, from $s^2_{environment} = 5.55$ to $s^2_{environment} = 1.34$. This result underlines that both factors primarily represent environmental sources of variation for age at CHD death, despite the role that genetics may play for the specific factors. A comprehensive discussion of variance components can be found in Hopper (1993). Genetic confounding would lead to a decrease in heritability estimates after the inclusion of observed covariates because, in that case, genetic factors contribute predominantly to the observed covariates rather than to the unobserved covariates included in the frailty. Our results are similar to the results obtained in a study of Swedish twins (Zdravkovic et al. 2004). More details in a slightly different analysis of the same data are given in Wienke et al. (2005a).   ☐

5.4 MCMC Methods for the Correlated Log-normal Frailty Model

Any distribution of nonnegative random variables can be adapted to model frailty. The gamma distribution has been widely applied in different fields (Sections 3.3 and 5.2). The gamma distribution is a very convenient choice from a mathematical point of view because of the simplicity of the Laplace transform, which allows for the use of maximum likelihood procedures in the parameter estimation. Another possibility is to assume that frailty is log-normally distributed (Sections 3.4 and 5.3). The log-normal approach is much more flexible than the gamma model in creating correlated but distinct frailties as required in the correlated frailty model. Unfortunately, with a log-normal assumption, it is impossible to derive the marginal likelihood function in an explicit form, and parameter estimation has to be performed with the help of more sophisticated estimation strategies.

There are four main methods for parameter estimation in frailty models: maximum likelihood methods (only applicable in parametric models), the EM algorithm, penalized partial likelihood, and Markov Chain Monte Carlo (MCMC) methods. Yashin et al. (1995) and Wienke et al. (2003a,b) applied procedures based on maximum likelihood methods in the gamma context, where an explicit representation of the likelihood function is available. The maximum likelihood procedure has also been adopted in log-normal frailty models by different numerical approximation algorithms (McGilchrist and Aisbett 1991, McGilchrist 1993, Lillard 1993, Lillard et al. 1995, Ripatti and Palmgren 2000, Ripatti et al. 2002). For example, such routines are implemented in the aML software package (Lillard and Panis 2000) and in newer versions of SAS.

In the present section, based on Locatelli (2003) and Locatelli et al. (2004), we consider an example of how to apply MCMC methods to the parametric bivariate correlated log-normal frailty model with Gompertz baseline hazard, as described in Section 5.3, with parameterization $\mathbf{E}Z = 1$ and $\sigma_1^2 = \sigma_2^2 = \sigma^2$ because of the symmetry of the twin data, which is used as an illustrative example here. A similar analysis can be found in Kheiri et al. (2005), who use a piecewise constant baseline hazard function.

Bayesian MCMC methods have been developed by Clayton (1991), and based on this work, implemented in WinBUGS by Spiegelhalter et al. (1996). Further applications of Bayesian methods, especially in shared frailty models are given by Sahu et al. (1997) and Sinha and Dey (1997) but also in the case of correlated frailty models by Xue and Ding (1999). The Bayesian approach is in fact natural when dealing with conditionally independent observations and when working with hierarchical models, with the frailty variables at an intermediate stage between the observations and the hyperparameters. In the Bayesian context, the frailty distribution represents a "prior" of the model, and its parameters (hyperparameters) are considered as random variables following some noninformative distribution, meaning a distribution with huge variance. The MCMC method consists of generating a set of Markov chains whose joint stationary distribution corresponds to the joint posterior of the model, this one being, in the Bayesian framework, the distribution of the random parameters given the observed data. In most hierarchical models, the posterior distribution is often very difficult to work with and hardly ever possible to integrate out in order to find the marginal posterior of each of the random parameters. By MCMC methods we can circumvent this problem. The posterior of each parameter is approximated by the empirical distribution of the values of the corresponding Markov chain, and empirical summary statistics calculated along each chain can be used to make inferences about the true value of the corresponding parameter (see Gilks et al. 1996). The Gibbs sampling (Geman and Geman 1984) is one of the algorithms that have been created in order to obtain Markov chains with the desired stationary distribution. The basic idea behind the Gibbs sampling is to successively sample from the conditional distribution of each random node, given all the other nodes in the model. These distributions are known as "full conditional distributions". It can be shown that, under broad conditions, this process eventually provides samples from the joint posterior distribution of the unknown quantities.

In this section, MCMC methods have been adopted to estimate correlated log-normal frailty models. Calculations are performed within the software WinBUGS (Spiegelhalter et al. 1999). This is a package that enables the researcher to solve Bayesian hierarchical models, essentially using the Gibbs sampling algorithm. The correlated log-normal frailty model applied here can be represented as a Bayesian hierarchical three–level model in the following way:

1. Likelihood function:

$$L(\lambda, \varphi | \mathbf{W}) = \prod_{i=1}^{n} \prod_{j=1}^{2} (e^{W_{ij}} \lambda e^{\varphi t_{ij}})^{\delta_{ij}} e^{-e^{W_{ij}} \frac{\lambda}{\varphi} (e^{\varphi t_{ij}} - 1)}$$

2. Priors:

   (i) $\begin{pmatrix} W_{i1} \\ W_{i2} \end{pmatrix} \sim N\left(\begin{pmatrix} -\frac{1}{2} \ln(\sigma^2 + 1) \\ -\frac{1}{2} \ln(\sigma^2 + 1) \end{pmatrix}, \begin{pmatrix} \ln(\sigma^2 + 1) & \ln(\rho\sigma^2 + 1) \\ \ln(\rho\sigma^2 + 1) & \ln(\sigma^2 + 1) \end{pmatrix} \right)$

   (ii) $\lambda \sim \Gamma(0.01, 0.01)$

   (iii) $\varphi \sim \Gamma(0.01, 0.01)$

3. Hyperpriors:

   (i) $\sigma^2 \sim \Gamma(0.01, 0.01)$ (ii) $\rho \sim U(-1, 1)$

with $\mathbf{W} = (W_{11}, W_{12}, W_{21}, W_{22}, ..., W_{n1}, W_{n2})$. Γ and U denote the gamma and uniform distribution, respectively, and λ and φ are parameters of the Gompertz baseline hazard. The prior (i), assigned to the vector (W_{i1}, W_{i2}), is chosen in order to have a vector of log-normal frailties $(Z_{i1}, Z_{i2}) = (e^{W_{i1}}, e^{W_{i2}})$ with mean equal to one:

$$\begin{pmatrix} Z_{i1} \\ Z_{i2} \end{pmatrix} \sim \ln \mathrm{N} \left(\begin{pmatrix} 1 \\ 1 \end{pmatrix}, \begin{pmatrix} \sigma^2 & \rho\sigma^2 \\ \rho\sigma^2 & \sigma^2 \end{pmatrix} \right).$$

Finally, noninformative priors are assigned to the parameters of the Gompertz curve and to the frailty parameters. The full conditional distributions can be obtained because they are proportional to the joint distribution of all the random quantities of the model. In our case, this joint distribution takes the form

$$\pi(t, \delta, \mathbf{W}, \lambda, \varphi, \sigma^2, \rho) = L(\lambda, \varphi|\mathbf{W}) \prod_{i=1}^{n} \left[\prod_{j=1}^{2} \pi(W_{ij}|\sigma^2, \rho) \right] \pi(\lambda)\pi(\varphi)\pi(\sigma^2)\pi(\rho),$$

where $\pi(\cdot)$ indicates the density function of the corresponding argument.

Gibbs sampling is an algorithm to generate a sequence of samples from the joint probability distribution of two or more random variables. The purpose of such a sequence is to approximate the unknown joint distribution. The Gibbs sampling algorithm generates an instance from the distribution of each variable in turn, conditional on the current values of the other variables. It can be shown that the sequence of samples constitutes a Markov chain, and the stationary distribution of that Markov chain is just the sought-after joint distribution.

A slice-sampler algorithm is used in WinBUGS for nonlog-concave densities defined on a restricted range (Neal 1997). It has an adaptive phase of 500 iterations, which are discarded from all summary statistics. A Metropolis within Gibbs algorithm based on a symmetric normal proposal distribution is applied in the case of nonlog-concave densities defined on an unrestricted range (Metropolis et al. 1953, Hastings 1970, Besag and Green 1993).

Example 5.7
The results of applying the correlated log-normal frailty model to the Swedish breast cancer data using MCMC methods as described before are presented in Table 5.12. The study population consists of 12,568 female twin pairs of the old and middle cohort. Estimated parameters include the Gompertz parameters λ and φ and the variance of the frailty distribution σ^2, which can be seen as the extent of population heterogeneity with respect to age at onset of breast cancer, and estimates of the correlation coefficient for both MZ twins (ρ_{MZ}) and DZ twins (ρ_{DZ}). Two estimates for each parameter are given in terms of the mean and the median of the correspondent Markov chain. In all cases, both values are very close to each other. This means

Table 5.12:   Correlated log-normal frailty model

parameter	mean	median	sdv	MC error	CSRF
σ^2	45.19	41.50	17.05	0.824	1.055
ρ_{MZ}	0.311	0.299	0.046	0.005	1.008
ρ_{DZ}	0.104	0.097	0.108	0.002	1.005
λ	2.54e-5	2.52e-5	3.24e-6	7.92e-8	1.002
φ	0.072	0.072	0.003	8.94e-5	1.006

that empirical estimates of the marginal posterior densities (kernel density estimates) are approximately symmetric. For each parameter, the sample standard deviation and an estimate of the standard error of the mean are also given. This one is obtained following Roberts' (1996) batch means method. In the last column, the value of the corrected scale reduction factor (CSRF) for each parameter is reported. This value corresponds to the Gelman–Rubin convergence statistic (Gelman and Rubin 1992), as modified by Brooks and Gelman (1998), and is based on a comparison of the inter- and intra-chain variance for each variable. When values of this diagnostic are approximately equal to one, the sample must have arisen from the stationary distribution. In this case, descriptive statistics are valid estimates of the unknown parameters.

According to the foregoing model, the population is largely heterogenous (σ^2) in terms of susceptibility toward breast cancer. The estimated correlation between frailties is larger for MZ than for DZ twins. This means that MZ individuals who genetically are more similar than DZ twins also present a larger correlation in terms of frailty toward breast cancer. This finding suggests that there is a genetic influence on breast cancer propensity.   ☐

The WinBUGS package proved to be useful and flexible enough to estimate correlated frailty models. With this software it is easy to modify the hypothesis on frailty distribution. Different assumptions about frailty distribution and the shape of the baseline hazard can be compared using an information criterion (DIC) which was introduced by Spiegelhalter et al. (2002) in order to compare Bayesian models in terms of adequacy and complexity.

A disadvantage of Bayesian methods is the time required for parameter estimation. In fact, we are working with models that include a very large number of parameters, especially when dealing with large data sets. This means that every MCMC algorithm that updates parameters one by one (like the Gibbs Sampling used in WinBUGS) is very time consuming. To solve this problem, an algorithm that enables the updating of parameters all together (or groups of parameters) at the same time should be adopted. The MCMC procedure in SAS 9.2. opens new avenues in this direction and provides a very user-friendly environment in the SAS package. This makes MCMC methods easier available for a large community of researchers, who are not familiar with the very specific WinBUGS package.

5.5   Correlated Compound Poisson Frailty Model

The model is an extension of the correlated PVF frailty model (sometimes called three-parameter frailty model) suggested by Yashin et al. (1999a) and Iachine (2002). It is based on a bivariate extension of the compound Poisson frailty model introduced to univariate survival analysis by Aalen (1988, 1992). It is also related to the correlated gamma frailty cure model in Section 5.8, which allows for a nonsusceptible fraction in the study population, as well as the compound Poisson frailty models with a random scale considered by Moger et al. (2004b) and Moger and Aalen (2005).

Let be k_0, k_1 nonnegative variables, and Y_0, Y_1, Y_2 independently compound Poisson-distributed random variables with distributions $Y_0 \sim cP(\gamma, k_0, \lambda)$, $Y_1 \sim cP(\gamma, k_1, \lambda)$, and $Y_2 \sim cP(\gamma, k_1, \lambda)$. Consequently, using an additive structure for the frailties similar to (5.3), it holds that

$$Z_1 = Y_0 + Y_1 \sim cP(\gamma, k_0 + k_1, \lambda)$$

$$Z_2 = Y_0 + Y_2 \sim cP(\gamma, k_0 + k_1, \lambda).$$

For simplicity, we shall present only the symmetric case here, where the two lifetimes are interchangeable. Consequently, the following assumptions are made in the model:

$$\mathbf{E}Z_1 = \mathbf{E}Z_2 = 1, \mathbf{V}(Z_1) = \mathbf{V}(Z_2) = \sigma^2.$$

This implies (compare relations (3.51) and (3.52)) that $(k_0 + k_1)\lambda^{\gamma-1} = 1$ and $(k_0 + k_1)(1 - \gamma)\lambda^{\gamma-2} = \sigma^2$. Consequently, $(k_0 + k_1)\lambda^{\gamma-2} = 1/\lambda$, and $(k_0 + k_1)\lambda^{\gamma-2} = \frac{\sigma^2}{1-\gamma} = \frac{1}{\lambda}$. Hence, $\lambda = \frac{1-\gamma}{\sigma^2}$, which results in

$$(k_0 + k_1)\lambda^\gamma = \lambda = \frac{1 - \gamma}{\sigma^2}. \tag{5.8}$$

It holds

$$\mathbf{cov}(Z_1, Z_2) = \mathbf{cov}(Y_0 + Y_1, Y_0 + Y_2) = \mathbf{V}(Y_0) = k_0(1 - \gamma)\lambda^{\gamma-2}.$$

This leads to the correlation

$$\begin{aligned}
\rho &= \frac{\mathbf{cov}(Z_1, Z_2)}{\sqrt{\mathbf{V}(Z_1)\mathbf{V}(Z_2)}} \\
&= \frac{k_0(1 - \gamma)\lambda^{\gamma-2}}{(k_0 + k_1)(1 - \gamma)\lambda^{\gamma-2}} \\
&= \frac{k_0}{k_0 + k_1}.
\end{aligned} \tag{5.9}$$

Consequently, because of (5.8) and (5.9),

$$k_0 \lambda^\gamma = \frac{k_0}{k_0 + k_1}(k_0 + k_1)\lambda^\gamma = \rho \frac{1 - \gamma}{\sigma^2}. \tag{5.10}$$

Now we can derive the unconditional model, applying the Laplace transform of compound Poisson-distributed random variables (3.53). Hence,

$$
\begin{aligned}
S(t_1, t_2) &= \mathbf{E} S(t_1, t_2 | Z_1, Z_2) \\
&= \mathbf{E} S(t_1 | Z_1) S(t_2 | Z_2) \\
&= \mathbf{E} e^{-Z_1 M_0(t_1)} e^{-Z_2 M_0(t_2)} \\
&= \mathbf{E} e^{-(Y_0 + Y_1) M_0(t_1)} e^{-(Y_0 + Y_2) M_0(t_2)} \\
&= \mathbf{E} e^{-Y_0(M_0(t_1) + M_0(t_2)) - Y_1 M_0(t_1) - Y_2 M_0(t_2)} \\
&= e^{-\frac{k_0}{\gamma}((\lambda + M_0(t_1) + M_0(t_2))^\gamma - \lambda^\gamma)} \\
&\quad \times e^{-\frac{k_1}{\gamma}((\lambda + M_0(t_1))^\gamma - \lambda^\gamma)} e^{-\frac{k_1}{\gamma}((\lambda + M_0(t_2))^\gamma - \lambda^\gamma)}. \tag{5.11}
\end{aligned}
$$

The three terms are considered in detail. For the marginal survival function, it holds that

$$S(t) = e^{-\frac{k_0 + k_1}{\gamma}((\lambda + M_0(t))^\gamma - \lambda^\gamma)}, \tag{5.12}$$

which implies

$$\lambda + M_0(t) = (\lambda^\gamma - \frac{\gamma}{k_0 + k_1} \ln S(t))^{1/\gamma}. \tag{5.13}$$

Hence, using (5.9) and (5.12),

$$
\begin{aligned}
e^{-\frac{k_1}{\gamma}((\lambda + M_0(t))^\gamma - \lambda^\gamma)} &= e^{-\frac{k_1}{k_0 + k_1} \frac{k_0 + k_1}{\gamma}((\lambda + M_0(t))^\gamma - \lambda^\gamma)} \\
&= e^{-(1-\rho)\frac{k_0 + k_1}{\gamma}((\lambda + M_0(t))^\gamma - \lambda^\gamma)} \\
&= \left(e^{-\frac{k_0 + k_1}{\gamma}((\lambda + M_0(t))^\gamma - \lambda^\gamma)}\right)^{1-\rho} \\
&= S(t)^{1-\rho}.
\end{aligned}
$$

The first of the three terms in (5.11) can be rewritten because of (5.13):

$$
\begin{aligned}
e^{-\frac{k_0}{\gamma}((\lambda + M_0(t_1) + M_0(t_2))^\gamma - \lambda^\gamma)} & \\
&= e^{-\frac{k_0}{\gamma}((\lambda + M_0(t_1) + \lambda + M_0(t_2) - \lambda)^\gamma - \lambda^\gamma)} \\
&= e^{-\frac{k_0}{\gamma}(((\lambda^\gamma - \frac{\gamma}{k_0 + k_1} \ln S(t_1))^{1/\gamma} + (\lambda^\gamma - \frac{\gamma}{k_0 + k_1} \ln S(t_2))^{1/\gamma} - \lambda)^\gamma - \lambda^\gamma)} \\
&= e^{\frac{k_0 \lambda^\gamma}{\gamma}(1 - ((1 - \frac{\gamma}{(k_0 + k_1)\lambda^\gamma} \ln S(t_1))^{1/\gamma} + (1 - \frac{\gamma}{(k_0 + k_1)\lambda^\gamma} \ln S(t_2))^{1/\gamma} - 1)^\gamma)},
\end{aligned}
$$

which results because of (5.8) and (5.10) in the following representation of the correlated model

$$S(t_1, t_2) = S(t_1)^{1-\rho} S(t_2)^{1-\rho} \tag{5.14}$$

$$\times \exp\left(\frac{\rho(1-\gamma)}{\gamma\sigma^2}\left[1 - \left(\left(1 - \frac{\gamma\sigma^2}{1-\gamma}\ln S(t_1)\right)^{\frac{1}{\gamma}} + \left(1 - \frac{\gamma\sigma^2}{1-\gamma}\ln S(t_2)\right)^{\frac{1}{\gamma}} - 1\right)^{\gamma}\right]\right).$$

This model includes both the gamma and the inverse Gaussian correlated frailty model as a special case; and the gamma model corresponds to $\gamma = 0$, and the inverse Gaussian model has $\gamma = 0.5$. The correlated inverse Gaussian model was considered by Zahl (1994) analyzing excess hazards of cancer patients, and by Kheiri et al. (2007) using a piecewise constant baseline hazard and a Bayesian approach. For $\gamma \geq 0$, the correlated PVF frailty model is obtained, which was introduced by Yashin et al. (1999a). For $\gamma < 0$, the correlated compound Poisson frailty model is obtained, including a fraction of individuals in the population with zero frailty.

Example 5.8

The model is applied to breast cancer incidence of MZ and DZ female Swedish twins born 1886 – 1925 (Wienke et al. 2006a, 2010), described in detail in Example 1.6. A parametric model with Gompertz baseline hazard function is used with parameters λ and φ. The data is left truncated, because only breast cancer cases are included that occurred after the foundation of the cancer register. This truncation is adjusted for in the analysis. The results are given in Table 5.13.

Table 5.13: Analysis of time to breast cancer in Swedish twins

parameter	gamma	inverse Gaussian	compound Poisson
σ^2	32.78 (7.776)	17.62 (14.22)	15.94 (8.273)
ρ_{MZ}	0.154 (0.052)	0.343 (0.131)	0.154 (0.053)
ρ_{DZ}	0.126 (0.040)	0.299 (0.106)	0.130 (0.041)
γ	0 (-)	0.5 (-)	-0.617 (0.905)
λ	1.3e-5 (1.0e-5)	1.8e-4 (5.7e-5)	2.5e-5 (1.9e-5)
φ	0.099 (0.016)	0.047 (0.008)	0.080 (0.016)
susceptible	100%	100%	15.2%
log-likelihood	-5122.31549	-5130.58558	-5121.23195

The model in the first column is the correlated gamma frailty model (5.2). Parameter σ^2 is a measure of heterogeneity, which is estimated to be large in this data, and all individuals of the population are assumed to be susceptible to breast cancer. The correlated gamma frailty model is a special case of the correlated compound Poisson/PVF frailty model with $\gamma = 0$.

In the second model, inverse Gaussian distributed frailty is used to account for heterogeneity in the population and to model dependence between times to onset of breast cancer in twin pairs. Parameter estimates are different from those in the gamma case with smaller heterogeneity and larger correlations. As in the gamma model, all women are assumed to be susceptible to breast cancer. The correlated inverse Gaussian frailty model is a special case of the correlated compound Poisson/PVF frailty model with $\gamma = 0.5$.

The most interesting parameter in the compound Poisson model is γ, which is negative $\gamma = -0.617$ (0.905) and indicates the existence of a fraction of individuals nonsusceptible to breast cancer. The size of the susceptible fraction is calculated by $1 - e^{\frac{1-\gamma}{\gamma \sigma^2}}$ and is around 15.2%. This estimate is slightly smaller than the value of 22% found by Chatterjee and Shih (2001) in a study population that is completely different, and in Section 5.8 applying a correlated gamma frailty cure model to the same data set. The compound Poisson model fits the data better than the two submodels but at the cost of an additional parameter. Compared to the gamma model, the improvement is not significant based on the likelihood ratio test.

Additionally, the size of the susceptible fraction in the correlated compound Poisson frailty model is not that far from the range of the figures obtained by Farewell et al. (1977) for different combinations of four risk factors. The authors found that, if none of the risk factors is present, the fraction of females susceptible to breast cancer is around 1.5%. If all risk factors are present, the estimate increases to 27.2%.

In all models, correlations in MZ pairs are higher than in DZ pairs, but the differences are small. This is in line with the well-known fact that the influence of genetic factors on susceptibility to breast cancer is small (5–10%). A disadvantage of the compound Poisson/PVF model is that it is not able to handle negative dependencies.

The correlated compound Poisson/PVF frailty model offers a very elegant approach to integrating the concept of cure models into frailty modeling. The likelihood function is explicitly available in a very simple form, which is the most important advantage of the model compared to the model suggested by Moger and Aalen (2005). Popular frailty models such as the correlated and shared gamma model ($\gamma = 0$) and inverse Gaussian model ($\gamma = 0.5$) are included in this model family, which provides a great flexibility to the model. Because of the extension to negative values of γ, the gamma distribution ($\gamma = 0$) as one of the most popular frailty distributions is no longer on the border of the parameter space. Consequently, standard tests can be applied to test hypotheses about the frailty distribution (for example, $H_0 : \gamma = 0$ versus $H_A : \gamma \neq 0$). Simulation studies show a good performance of the parameter estimates in this model with nearly no bias. $\square$

Another bivariate compound Poisson frailty model with Weibull baseline hazard functions is suggested by Hanagal (2010).

5.6 Correlated Quadratic Hazard Frailty Model

As already shown in the foregoing sections, the correlated frailty model is a powerful tool in the analysis of bivariate survival data. The unconditional survival function has an explicit form in frailty models based on the gamma or the more general compound Poisson distribution. Otherwise, multivariate event time models with gamma or compound Poisson distributed frailty are less flexible in specifying multivariate correlations needed in the analysis of family data compared to frailty models based on the (log)normal distribution. To join the flexibility of the multivariate normal distribution in the analysis of event time data on related individuals with the benefits of frailty distributions allowing for an explicit representation of the unconditional survival and finally the likelihood function, the correlated quadratic hazard model considered by Aalen (1987), Iachine and Yashin (1999), and Iachine (2002) can be used. The conditional bivariate survival function in this model is given by

$$S(t_1, t_2|Z_1, Z_2) = S(t_1|Z_1)S(t_2|Z_2)$$
$$= e^{-Z_1 M_0(t_1)} e^{-Z_2 M_0(t_2)}$$
$$= e^{-W_1^2 M_0(t_1)} e^{-W_2^2 M_0(t_2)},$$

with $Z_j = W_j^2$ $(j = 1, 2)$. A bivariate normal distribution of the random effects (W_1, W_2) with parameters m_1, m_2, s_1^2, s_2^2, and r is assumed. The unconditional bivariate survival function is

$$S(t_1, t_2) = \mathbf{E}S(t_1, t_2|Z_1, Z_2)$$
$$= \frac{1}{2\pi s_1 s_2 \sqrt{1 - r^2}} \iint e^{-w_1^2 M_0(t_1)} e^{-w_2^2 M_0(t_2)}$$
$$\times e^{-\frac{1}{(1-r^2)}\left(\frac{(w_1 - m_1)^2}{2s_1^2} - r\frac{(w_1 - m_1)(w_2 - m_2)}{s_1 s_2} + \frac{(w_2 - m_2)^2}{2s_2^2}\right)} dw_1 dw_2.$$

It turns out that this integral has an explicit solution but requires some lengthy calculations. Therefore, the calculation of the unconditional survival function has been moved to the Appendix A.4. The survival function is

$$S(t_1, t_2) \tag{5.15}$$
$$= \frac{1}{\sqrt{1 + 2s_1^2 M_0(t_1) + 2s_2^2 M_0(t_2) + 4(1 - r^2)s_1^2 s_2^2 M_0(t_1)M_0(t_2)}}$$
$$\times \exp\left\{-\frac{m_1^2 M_0(t_1)(1 + 2s_2^2 M_0(t_2)) + m_2^2 M_0(t_2)(1 + 2s_1^2 M_0(t_1))}{1 + 2s_1^2 M_0(t_1) + 2s_2^2 M_0(t_2) + 4(1 - r^2)s_1^2 s_2^2 M_0(t_1)M_0(t_2)}\right\}$$
$$\times \exp\left\{\frac{4rm_1 m_2 s_1 s_2 M_0(t_1)M_0(t_2)}{1 + 2s_1^2 M_0(t_1) + 2s_2^2 M_0(t_2) + 4(1 - r^2)s_1^2 s_2^2 M_0(t_1)M_0(t_2)}\right\}.$$

In the case of independence ($r = 0$), this simplifies to the expressions in the univariate case (compare with (3.55)):

$$S(t_1, t_2) = \frac{1}{\sqrt{1 + 2s_1^2 M_0(t_1)}} e^{\frac{-M_0(t_1)m_1^2}{1+2s_1^2 M_0(t_1)}} \frac{1}{\sqrt{1 + 2s_2^2 M_0(t_2)}} e^{\frac{-M_0(t_2)m_2^2}{1+2s_2^2 M_0(t_2)}}.$$

For identifiability reasons, it is necessary to place restrictions on the parameters of the frailty distribution, for example, $s_1^2 = s_2^2 = 1$ as considered by Aalen (1987) and Iachine and Yashin (1999). The latter authors also provide a semiparametric EM algorithm for parameter estimation in the model. The flexibility of the multivariate normal distribution in modeling correlations can be used, but even in this case the range of the correlation between W_1^2 and W_2^2 depends on m_1 and m_2 and does not cover the full range between -1 and 1. Especially, the modeling of negative correlations is still problematic. For more details in a more general case, see the paper by Aalen (1987). For mathematical convenience, here we assume $m_1 = m_2 = 0$. This restricts the correlation between the frailties to be nonnegative, and is different from the usual convention $\mathbf{E}Z_1 = \mathbf{E}Z_2 = 1$, which would lead to very complicated expressions. Furthermore, the restriction $m_1 = m_2 = 0$ implies a gamma distribution with $\Gamma(\frac{1}{2}, \frac{1}{2s_j^2})$ ($j = 1, 2$) for the margins of the frailties. In this case, the unconditional survival function simplifies to

$$S(t_1, t_2) = \frac{1}{\sqrt{1 + 2s_1^2 M_0(t_1) + 2s_2^2 M_0(t_2) + 4(1 - r^2)s_1^2 s_2^2 M_0(t_1)M_0(t_2)}}.$$

We are now interested in the correlation between the frailties $Z_1 = W_1^2$ and $Z_2 = W_2^2$. First, we need the mixed second moment $\mathbf{E}W_1^2 W_2^2$. To calculate this moment, we rewrite the density of the two-dimensional normal distribution of the random effects:

$\mathbf{E}W_1^2 W_2^2$

$$= \frac{1}{2\pi s_1 s_2 \sqrt{1 - r^2}} \iint w_1^2 w_2^2 e^{-\frac{1}{(1-r^2)}\left(\frac{w_1^2}{2s_1^2} - r\frac{w_1 w_2}{s_1 s_2} + \frac{w_2^2}{2s_2^2}\right)} dw_1 dw_2$$

$$= \frac{1}{2\pi s_1 s_2 \sqrt{1 - r^2}} \iint w_1^2 w_2^2 e^{-\frac{1}{2(1-r^2)}\left(\frac{w_1^2}{s_1^2} - 2\frac{rw_2}{s_1 s_2}w_1\right)} e^{-\frac{w_2^2}{2(1-r^2)s_2^2}} dw_1 dw_2$$

$$= \int w_2^2 \frac{1}{2\pi s_1 s_2 \sqrt{1 - r^2}} \int w_1^2 e^{-\frac{1}{2(1-r^2)}\left(\frac{w_1^2}{s_1^2} - 2\frac{rw_2}{s_1 s_2}w_1\right)} dw_1 e^{-\frac{w_2^2}{2(1-r^2)s_2^2}} dw_2$$

$$= \int w_2^2 I(w_2) e^{-\frac{w_2^2}{2(1-r^2)s_2^2}} dw_2 \tag{5.16}$$

with

$$I(w_2) = \frac{1}{2\pi s_1 s_2 \sqrt{1 - r^2}} \int w_1^2 e^{-\frac{1}{2(1-r^2)}\left(\frac{w_1^2}{s_1^2} - 2\frac{rw_2}{s_1 s_2}w_1\right)} dw_1.$$

In the following, we first calculate the inner integral $I(w_2)$ and then the outer integral in a second step:

$$I(w_2) = \frac{1}{\sqrt{2\pi}s_1\sqrt{1-r^2}} \int_{-\infty}^{\infty} w_1^2 e^{-\frac{1}{2(1-r^2)}\left(\frac{w_1^2}{s_1^2} - 2\frac{rw_2}{s_1 s_2}w_1\right)} dw_1$$

$$= \frac{1}{\sqrt{2\pi}s_1\sqrt{1-r^2}} \int_{-\infty}^{\infty} w_1^2 e^{-\frac{w_1^2 - 2r\frac{s_1}{s_2}w_2 w_1}{2(1-r^2)s_1^2}} dw_1$$

$$= \frac{1}{\sqrt{2\pi}s_1\sqrt{1-r^2}} \int_{-\infty}^{\infty} w_1^2 e^{-\frac{(w_1 - r\frac{s_1}{s_2}w_2)^2}{2(1-r^2)s_1^2}} dw_1 e^{-\frac{-r^2\frac{s_1^2}{s_2^2}w_2^2}{2(1-r^2)s_1^2}}$$

$$= \left((1-r^2)s_1^2 + r^2\frac{s_1^2}{s_2^2}w_2^2\right) e^{-\frac{-r^2 s_1^2 w_2^2}{2(1-r^2)s_1^2 s_2^2}}.$$

Here, the last equation holds because the integral is the expectation of a random variable W^2, with W following a normal distribution with expectation $r\frac{s_1}{s_2}w_2$ and variance $(1-r^2)s_1^2$. Now we are solving the second integral with respect to w_2

$$EW_1^2 W_2^2 = \frac{(1-r^2)s_1^2}{\sqrt{2\pi}s_2} \int_{-\infty}^{\infty} w_2^2 e^{-\frac{w_2^2}{2(1-r^2)s_2^2}} e^{-\frac{-r^2 s_1^2 w_2^2}{2(1-r^2)s_1^2 s_2^2}} dw_2$$

$$+ \frac{r^2\frac{s_1^2}{s_2^2}}{\sqrt{2\pi}s_2} \int_{-\infty}^{\infty} w_2^4 e^{-\frac{w_2^2}{2(1-r^2)s_2^2}} dw_2$$

$$= \frac{(1-r^2)s_1^2}{\sqrt{2\pi}s_2} \int_{-\infty}^{\infty} w_2^2 e^{-\frac{w_2^2}{2s_2^2}} dw_2 + \frac{r^2\frac{s_1^2}{s_2^2}}{\sqrt{2\pi}s_2} \int_{-\infty}^{\infty} w_2^4 e^{-\frac{w_2^2}{2s_2^2}} dw_2$$

$$= (1-r^2)s_1^2 EW_2^2 + r^2\frac{s_1^2}{s_2^2}EW_2^4$$

$$= (1-r^2)s_1^2 s_2^2 + r^2\frac{s_1^2}{s_2^2}3s_2^4$$

$$= (1+2r^2)s_1^2 s_2^2.$$

Using the relations $\mathbf{V}(W_j^2) = EW_j^4 - (EW_j^2)^2 = 3s_j^4 - s_j^4 = 2s_j^4$ $(j = 1, 2)$, we can now calculate the correlation between $Z_1 = W_1^2$ and $Z_2 = W_2^2$

$$\mathbf{corr}(W_1^2, W_2^2) = \frac{EW_1^2 W_2^2 - EW_1^2 EW_2^2}{\sqrt{\mathbf{V}(W_1^2)\mathbf{V}(W_2^2)}} = \frac{(1+2r^2)s_1^2 s_2^2 - s_1^2 s_2^2}{\sqrt{4s_1^4 s_2^4}} = r^2.$$

Consequently, the correlation between the frailties $Z_1 = W_1^2$ and $Z_2 = W_2^2$ in the pairs is just the square of the correlation between the random effects W_1, W_2. Consequently, the correlation in this model is always nonnegative, even if the correlation between W_1 and W_2 is negative. Negative correlations between the frailties are possible if restrictions other than $m_1 = m_2 = 0$ are used in the model. This was considered in Aalen (1987).

We are now interested in a copula representation of the unconditional survival function similar to the correlated gamma and compound Poisson frailty model. The univariate survival functions are given by the relation $S_j(t) = \frac{1}{\sqrt{1+2s_j^2 M_0(t)}}$ $(j = 1, 2)$. Substituting $2s_1^2 M_0(t_1)$ and $2s_2^2 M_0(t_2)$ into the expression

$$S(t_1, t_2) = \frac{1}{\sqrt{1 + 2s_1^2 M_0(t_1) + 2s_2^2 M_0(t_2) + 4(1 - r^2)s_1^2 s_2^2 M_0(t_1)M_0(t_2)}}$$

results in

$$S(t_1, t_2) = \frac{1}{\sqrt{S_1^{-2}(t_1)S_2^{-2}(t_2) - r^2(S_1^{-2}(t_1) - 1)(S_2^{-2}(t_2) - 1)}}. \qquad (5.17)$$

This is a very interesting relation because the bivariate copula depends only on the correlation parameter, and not on the variances of the frailties. This is different compared to the correlated gamma and compound Poisson frailty model. From the interpretational point of view, this is an advantage of the model because only the correlation parameter influences the bivariate copula, whereas the frailty variances as heterogeneity parameters influence only the marginal distributions.

The model contains an interesting special case. Consider the case of a shared quadratic hazard frailty model ($r = 1, s^2 = s_1^2 = s_2^2$). In that case, the bivariate copula representation is of the form

$$S(t_1, t_2) = (S_1^{-2}(t_1) + S_2^{-2}(t_2) - 1)^{-1/2}. \qquad (5.18)$$

This is the copula representation in the shared gamma frailty model with $\sigma^2 = 2$ (see (4.3)). Both frailty models are equal if $s^2 = 2$ holds. In general, the marginal survival functions in (5.18) depend on s^2, a parameter that can vary freely and influences the marginal distributions. Interestingly, in this shared quadratic hazard frailty model, the copula representation of the lifetimes is independent of the variance of the random effects s^2. This underlines the fact that it is misleading to use the frailty variance as an association measure, as is often done in shared frailty models.

5.7 Other Correlated Frailty Models

A more general correlated frailty model can be introduced with the help of frailties generated by nonnegative Lévy processes. Aalen and Hjort (2002) considered such frailty distributions in the univariate setting, see Section 3.10. Let $Z_1 = D(u_0) + D_1(u)$ and $Z_2 = D(u_0) + D_2(u)$ be frailties with respect to two correlated lifetimes. Here it is assumed that there were three damage processes running prior to the follow-up. The first process describes damage shared by both partners in a pair and is running until time point u_0. $D_1(u)$ and $D_2(u)$ are two independent and identically distributed versions of the process D covering the unique damage experience of each partner. Both processes are assumed to run until time u in parallel to the shared process $D(u_0)$. The univariate unconditional survival function is given by

$$S(t) = \mathbf{E}S(t|Z_j) = \mathbf{E}e^{-(D(u_0)+D_j(u))M_0(t)} = e^{-(u_0+u)\psi(M_0(t))},$$

where ψ denotes the characteristic exponent of the Lévy process ($j = 1, 2$). Consequently, after some simple algebra, the cumulative baseline hazard can be represented in the form

$$M_0(t) = \psi^{-1}\left(\frac{-\ln S(t)}{u_0 + u}\right).$$

Hence,

$$S(t_1, t_2) = \mathbf{E}e^{-D(u_0)(M_0(t_1)+M_0(t_2))-D_1(u)M_0(t_1)-D_2(u)M_0(t_2)}$$
$$= e^{-u_0\psi(M_0(t_1)+M_0(t_2))}e^{-u\psi(M_0(t_1))}e^{-u\psi(M_0(t_2))}$$
$$- e^{-u_0\psi\left(\psi^{-1}(\frac{-\ln S(t_1)}{u_0+u})+\psi^{-1}(\frac{-\ln S(t_2)}{u_0+u})\right)}S(t_1)^{\frac{u}{u_0+u}}S(t_2)^{\frac{u}{u_0+u}}.$$

Using the variance formula for Lévy processes $\mathbf{V}(D(u)) = u\mathbf{V}(D(1) - D(0))$ assuming finite second moments of $D(0)$ and $D(1)$ and because of the independence of $D(u_0)$, $D_1(u)$ and $D_2(u)$ it holds for the correlation between the two frailty variables

$$\rho = \mathbf{corr}(Z_1, Z_2)$$
$$= \frac{\mathbf{cov}\left(D(u_0) + D_1(u), D(u_0) + D_2(u)\right)}{\sqrt{\mathbf{V}\left(D(u_0) + D_1(u)\right)\mathbf{V}\left(D(u_0) + D_2(u)\right)}}$$
$$= \frac{\mathbf{V}\left(D(u_0)\right)}{\mathbf{V}\left(D(u_0) + D_1(u)\right)}$$
$$= \frac{u_0}{u_0 + u}. \tag{5.19}$$

Applying relation (5.19) we get the final form in the general correlated frailty model

$$S(t_1, t_2) = S(t_1)^{1-\rho} S(t_2)^{1-\rho} e^{-u_0 \psi \left(\psi^{-1} \left(\frac{-\ln S(t_1)}{u_0 + u} \right) + \psi^{-1} \left(\frac{-\ln S(t_2)}{u_0 + u} \right) \right)} \qquad (5.20)$$

The correlated gamma frailty model can be obtained from (5.20) as a special case by substituting the characteristic exponent from (3.59) $\psi(u) = k \ln(1 + \frac{u}{\lambda})$ and its inverse $\psi^{-1}(u) = \lambda(e^{\frac{u}{k}} - 1)$

$$
\begin{aligned}
S(t_1, t_2) &= S(t_1)^{1-\rho} S(t_2)^{1-\rho} e^{-u_0 \psi \left(\psi^{-1} \left(\frac{-\ln S(t_1)}{u_0 + u} \right) + \psi^{-1} \left(\frac{-\ln S(t_2)}{u_0 + u} \right) \right)} \\
&= S(t_1)^{1-\rho} S(t_2)^{1-\rho} e^{-u_0 k \ln \left(1 + 1/\lambda \left[\psi^{-1} \left(\frac{-\ln S(t_1)}{u_0 + u} \right) + \psi^{-1} \left(\frac{-\ln S(t_2)}{u_0 + u} \right) \right] \right)} \\
&= S(t_1)^{1-\rho} S(t_2)^{1-\rho} \left(S(t_1)^{-\frac{1}{k(u_0 + u)}} + S(t_2)^{-\frac{1}{k(u_0 + u)}} - 1 \right)^{-u_0 k}.
\end{aligned}
$$

Applying the standard constraints $\mathbf{E}Z_1 = \mathbf{E}Z_2 = 1$, reparameterization $\lambda = k(u_0 + u) = 1/\sigma^2$, and (5.19) results in the bivariate survival function of the symmetric correlated gamma frailty model

$$S(t_1, t_2) = S(t_1)^{1-\rho} S(t_2)^{1-\rho} \left(S(t_1)^{-\sigma^2} + S(t_2)^{-\sigma^2} - 1 \right)^{-\rho/\sigma^2}.$$

The correlated compound Poisson frailty model from Section 5.5 can be obtained in a similar way. Another special case is the shared positive stable frailty model, considered by Hougaard (1986a,b, 1995), Lam and Kuk (1997), and Qiou et al. (1999). Mallick et al. (2008) suggest a bivariate positive stable frailty model, but the correlation structure between the frailties in this model is complicated.

A different approach is suggested by Henderson and Shimakura (2003). They used their correlated frailty model with gamma-distributed frailty to model longitudinal count data instead of event time data. Their main idea is the derivation of a multivariate frailty with gamma distributed marginals and a suitable correlation matrix allowing the association between event counts in different time interval to depend on the distance between the intervals. Applying their concept of gamma-distributed frailty to bivariate lifetimes, the survival function is

$$S(t_1, t_2) = \left[S(t_1)^{-\sigma^2} S(t_2)^{-\sigma^2} - \rho \left(S(t_1)^{-\sigma^2} - 1 \right) \left(S(t_2)^{-\sigma^2} - 1 \right) \right]^{-1/\sigma^2},$$

which is another correlated gamma frailty model, but not based on the additive decomposition of the gamma-distributed frailties as the model in Section 5.2. In the case of $\sigma^2 = 2$ the survival function of the correlated quadratic hazard model in (5.17) is obtained. Furthermore, the shared gamma frailty model from Section 4.3 is also a special case of the model introduced by Henderson and Shimakura (2003) with $\rho = 1$.

5.8 Bivariate Frailty Cure Models

A bivariate frailty cure model for familiar association in onset of diseases was established by Chatterjee and Shih (2001), which is an extension of the univariate frailty cure model in (3.62). For a pair of individuals we define

$$
Y_j = \begin{cases} 1 & : \text{ if the } j^{\text{th}} \text{ individual is susceptible} \\ 0 & : \text{ otherwise,} \end{cases} \tag{5.21}
$$

and let T_j denote the age at onset of the disease for the jth individual when $Y_j = 1$ ($j = 1, 2$). Then the bivariate survival function is of the form

$$
S^*(t_1, t_2) = \phi_{00} + \phi_{10} S(t_1) + \phi_{01} S(t_2) + \phi_{11} S(t_1, t_2), \tag{5.22}
$$

with the relations $\phi_{11} = \mathbf{P}(Y_1 = 1, Y_2 = 1)$, $\phi_{10} = \mathbf{P}(Y_1 = 1, Y_2 = 0)$, $\phi_{01} = \mathbf{P}(Y_1 = 0, Y_2 = 1)$, and $\phi_{00} = \mathbf{P}(Y_1 = 0, Y_2 = 0)$. $S(t_1, t_2)$ denotes the bivariate survival function of pairs with both individuals susceptible to the event under study. $S(t_1) = S(t_1, 0)$ and $S(t_2) = S(0, t_2)$ are the (here for ease of presentation as equal assumed) marginal survival functions. Plugging this survival function into the general bivariate likelihood (A.1), the likelihood function of the ith pair in the parametric model $S(t_1, t_2) = S(t_1, t_2; \boldsymbol{\theta})$ yields

$$
\begin{aligned}
L_i(\boldsymbol{\theta}) = {} & \delta_{i1}\delta_{i2}\phi_{11} S_{t_{i1}, t_{i2}}(t_{i1}, t_{i2}; \boldsymbol{\theta}) \\
& + \delta_{i1}(1 - \delta_{i2})\big(\phi_{11} S_{t_{i1}}(t_{i1}, t_{i2}; \boldsymbol{\theta}) + \phi_{10} S_{t_{i1}}(t_{i1}; \boldsymbol{\theta})\big) \\
& + (1 - \delta_{i1})\delta_{i2}\big(\phi_{11} S_{t_{i2}}(t_{i1}, t_{i2}; \boldsymbol{\theta}) + \phi_{01} S_{t_{i2}}(t_{i2}; \boldsymbol{\theta})\big) \\
& + (1 - \delta_1)(1 - \delta_2)\big(\phi_{11} S(t_1, t_2; \boldsymbol{\theta}) + \phi_{10} S(t_1; \boldsymbol{\theta}) + \phi_{01} S(t_2; \boldsymbol{\theta}) + \phi_{00}\big),
\end{aligned}
$$

This bivariate survival is often given as a copula. Chatterjee and Shih (2001) considered three different copulas: the shared gamma frailty model (Claytons model), Frank's copula, and Hougaard's shared positive stable frailty model. For more details about copulas see Chapter 6. Chatterjee and Shih (2001) applied a two-step estimation procedure to breast cancer using the kinship data from the Washington Ashkenazi Study, but by ignoring the dependency among different pairs within the same family. Their model can be extended by substituting the shared gamma frailty model by the symmetric correlated gamma frailty model (Wienke et al. 2003a)

$$
S(t_1, t_2) = S(t_1)^{1-\rho} S(t_2)^{1-\rho} (S(t_1)^{-\sigma^2} + S(t_2)^{-\sigma^2} - 1)^{\frac{\rho}{\sigma^2}}.
$$

In the following analysis a parametric model with Gompertz baseline hazard was used, for example,

$$
S(t) = S(0, t) = S(t, 0) = \left(1 + \sigma^2 \frac{\lambda}{\varphi}(e^{\varphi t} - 1)\right)^{-\frac{1}{\sigma^2}}.
$$

Example 5.9

The model was applied to the breast cancer incidence data of MZ and DZ Swedish female twin pairs from the old cohort of the Swedish Twin Registry. The results are given in Table 5.14.

Table 5.14: Correlated gamma frailty models with and without cure fraction applied to breast cancer in Swedish twins

parameter	gamma frailty without cure	gamma frailty with cure[1]	gamma frailty with cure[2]
σ^2	32.78 (7.759)	4.438 (1.709)	2.508 (3.032)
ρ_{MZ}	0.154 (0.052)	1.000 (-)	1.000 (-)
ρ_{DZ}	0.126 (0.040)	0.932 (0.361)	0.960 (0.454)
λ	1.3e-5 (5.2e-6)	7.7e-5 (4.8e-5)	1.2e-4 (1.2e-4)
φ	0.099 (0.016)	0.091 (0.012)	0.086 (0.015)
ϕ_{11}	1.000 (-)	0.050 (-)	0.038 (0.021)
ϕ_{10}	0.000 (-)	0.173 (-)	0.134 (0.059)
ϕ_{00}	0.000 (-)	0.604 (-)	0.695 (0.138)
ϕ	1.000 (-)	0.223 (0.046)	0.172[3] (-)
log-likelihood	-5122.31549	-5120.17769	-5120.06055

[1] constrained by $\phi_{11} = \phi^2$, $\phi_{10} = \phi_{01} = \phi(1 - \phi)$, $\phi_{00} = (1 - \phi)^2$
[2] constrained by $\phi_{10} = \phi_{01}$, $\phi_{11} + \phi_{10} + \phi_{01} + \phi_{00} = 1$
[3] calculated as $\phi = \phi_{11} + \phi_{10}$

We consider two different cases of cure models. In the first case, it is assumed that the susceptible status of the individuals in a pair is independent, for example, $\mathbf{P}(Y_1 = p_1, Y_2 = p_2) = \mathbf{P}(Y_1 = p_1)\mathbf{P}(Y_2 = p_2)$ with $p_1, p_2 \in \{0, 1\}$. The size of the cure fraction is uniquely described by the univariate probability $\phi = \mathbf{P}(Y_1 = 1) = \mathbf{P}(Y_2 = 1)$, which results in $\phi_{10} = \phi_{01} = \phi(1 - \phi)$, $\phi_{11} = \phi^2$, and $\phi_{00} = (1 - \phi)^2$. In the second case, which is an extension of the first one, the restriction of independence between the susceptibility status of the partners in a pair is relaxed and substituted by the weaker constraints $\phi_{10} = \phi_{01}$, $\phi_{11} + \phi_{10} + \phi_{01} + \phi_{00} = 1$. When comparing the likelihoods, it turns out that the cure model with an independent susceptible status of the partners shows a significantly better fit compared to the model without a cure fraction. The more complicated cure model without assuming independence between the susceptible status of the twin partners shows no significant improvement compared to the cure model assuming independence. Interestingly, the estimate of the size of a susceptible fraction (due to breast cancer) with $\phi = 0.223$ (0.046) is close to the estimate $\phi = 0.22$ (0.0093) in the shared gamma frailty model found by Chatterjee and Shih (2001) in a study population that is completely different from the one used here. Nevertheless, the estimates of the susceptible fraction in both models in Table 5.14 are in the range of the results obtained by Farewell et al. (1977) for different combinations of four risk factors. If none of the risk factors is present, the susceptible fraction is around 0.015; if all risk factors are present, the estimate increases to 0.272.

A simulation study was performed to check the properties of the estimates in the proposed gamma frailty model. All simulations involve generating gamma-distributed frailties, bivariate lifetimes, censoring times, as well as the inclusion of a cured fraction in the study population. A total of 5000 twin pairs are simulated in each data set. Samples are generated to mimic the structure of the data analyzed in Table 5.14:

- Generate frailty variables using gamma-distributed random variables.

- Generate lifetimes given the frailties using $S(t|Z) = e^{-Z\frac{\lambda}{\varphi}(e^{\varphi t}-1)}$.

- Define cured individuals by using a random variable.

- Birth years are generated by using a uniform distribution on $[1886,1925]$.

- Censored lifetimes are generated by using year 2000 as end of study.

The data sets are simulated assuming dependence between the susceptibility status of the partners (second column in Table 5.14), but in the estimation procedure, the more general model with independent susceptibility status was applied (third column in Table 5.14). There were 1000 data sets simulated. The mean of the parameter estimates and their standard errors are presented in Table 5.15, in comparison with the true values. There appears to be only moderate bias in the parameter estimates, and the overall performance is very good. More information about this study is given in Wienke et al. (2003a).

Table 5.15: Parameter estimation in the simulation study

parameter	true	mean	s.e.
σ^2	4.000	4.461	2.117
ρ_{MZ}	0.800	0.751	0.250
ρ_{DZ}	0.600	0.570	0.278
λ	1.00e-5	1.23e-5	1.14e-5
φ	0.120	0.121	0.022
ϕ_{11}	0.040	0.042	0.014
ϕ_{10}	0.160	0.161	0.029
ϕ_{00}	0.640	0.619	0.094

Another approach to include a cure fraction into a bivariate frailty model is the correlated compound Poisson model in Section 5.5. □

5.9　Comparison of Different Estimation Strategies

In this section, we examine bivariate correlated frailty models, especially the behavior of parameter estimates when using different estimation strategies. We consider three different correlated frailty models: the gamma model and two versions of the log-normal model. The traditional maximum likelihood estimation procedure in the gamma case with explicitly available likelihood function is compared with maximum likelihood methods based on numerical integration and a Bayesian approach using MCMC methods by means of a comprehensive simulation study. We investigate the correlation between the two parameter estimates of the variance and the correlation of the frailties in the bivariate correlated frailty model with equal variances, and analyze it in detail.

Throughout this section we will refer to the correlated gamma frailty model as Model 1. The second frailty model considered in detail in this section is the log-normal model. Two variants of the log-normal model are analyzed. We assume a normally distributed random variable W to generate frailty $Z = e^W$. The variants of the model are given by the constraints $\mathbf{E}W = 0$ (Model 2) and $\mathbf{E}Z = 1$ (Model 3). Unfortunately, no explicit form of the unconditional likelihood exists in log-normal frailty models. Consequently, estimation strategies based on numerical integration of the random effects in the maximum likelihood approach are required.

To check whether the dependence between the variance and correlation parameters is related to the estimation strategy or the choice of the frailty distribution, we use the bivariate models mentioned above and apply three different estimation strategies. First, we perform a traditional maximum likelihood estimation procedure (only possible in the gamma model); second, we use a maximum likelihood approach based on numerical integration; and finally, we apply MCMC methods as a Bayesian approach.

Parameter estimation in the gamma model is straightforward. The frailty term can be integrated out, and an explicit representation of the unconditional bivariate survival function (5.5) exists to calculate the likelihood function.

Unfortunately, the integrals in expression (5.2) have no explicit solution in the log-normal model. Several estimation methods for bivariate log-normal frailty models in consequence have been suggested within a non-Bayesian framework. Various modifications of the maximum likelihood procedure are applicable. Ripatti and Palmgren (2000) derived an estimating algorithm based on the penalized partial likelihood (PPL). Xue and Brookmeyer (1996) suggested a modified EM algorithm for log-normal frailty models. Sastry (1997) developed the modified EM algorithm for the multiplicative two-level gamma frailty model. The same method can be applied to bivariate log-normal frailty models. Ripatti et al. (2002) present yet another method for EM-like algorithms in log-normal frailty models.

In the present section we use numerical integration procedures. Integrals over univariate and multivariate normal distributions can be approximated in different ways. One possibility is to use Gauss–Hermite quadratures (Naylor and Smith 1982, Smith et al. 1987). Similar ideas are employed in various applications of mixed models in survival analysis (Lillard 1993, Lillard et al. 1995, Panis and Lillard 1995). The methods are implemented in the aML software package (Lillard and Panis 2000).

Several examples on the application of Bayesian methods to multivariate frailty models exist. Bolstad and Manda (2001) considered the gamma frailty model. Gibbs' sampler for the bivariate log-normal frailty model with an exponential baseline hazard is given in Xue and Ding (1999). Korsgaard et al. (1998) present a Bayesian inference in the log-normal frailty model with a semiparametric baseline hazard.

In the Bayesian framework the correlated frailty model takes the form of a *hierarchical* model, with the frailty variables at an intermediate stage between observations and hyperparameters. The conditional likelihood represents the first level of the model and is given by

$$L(\boldsymbol{\beta}, \lambda, \varphi | \mathbf{Z}) = \prod_{i=1}^{n} \prod_{j=1}^{2} \left(Z_{ij} \mu_0(t_{ij}) e^{\boldsymbol{\beta}' \mathbf{X}_{ij}} \right)^{\delta_{ij}} e^{-Z_{ij} M_0(t_{ij}) e^{\boldsymbol{\beta}' \mathbf{X}_{ij}}},$$

with $\mathbf{Z} = (Z_{11}, Z_{12}, Z_{21}, Z_{22}, \ldots, Z_{n1}, Z_{n2})$ and λ, φ being the parameters of the Gompertz baseline hazard function.

By definition of the model, the vector of frailties (Z_{i1}, Z_{i2}) $(i = 1, \ldots, n)$ in each pair is assumed to follow a bivariate log-normal distribution, with variances $\sigma_1^2 = \sigma_2^2 = \sigma^2$ and correlation coefficient ρ. The parameters of the baseline hazard, regression coefficients $\boldsymbol{\beta}$, σ^2, and ρ (the latter two being the hyperparameters) are assumed to follow a noninformative distribution. We adopt uniform priors over the intervals [1e-7, 0.005], [0.05, 0.15] and [-1,1] for λ, φ and ρ, respectively. Furthermore, log-normal priors with mean 0.5 and variance 0.25 for σ^2 and multivariate normal priors for $\boldsymbol{\beta}$ are used. More details about the MCMC approach can be found in Section 5.4.

We estimated Model 1 following a maximization procedure, and Models 2 and 3 using a numerical integration procedure (Gauss–Hermite quadrature). MCMC methods are employed in all three models. We generated data sets with different frailty distributions. First, we used $\sigma^2 = 1$ and $\rho = 0.7$. Second, we used parameters $\sigma^2 = 0.3$ and $\rho = 0.2$. In both cases, $\lambda = 0.003$, $\varphi = 0.07$, $\boldsymbol{\beta}' = (\beta_1, \beta_2)$, $\beta_1 = 0.1$, and $\beta_2 = -0.2$. Two types of covariates were used. One covariate was generated as binary variable

$$X_{ij1} = \begin{cases} 1 & \text{if } i \leq \frac{n}{2} \\ 0 & \text{if } i > \frac{n}{2}, \end{cases}$$

and the other as normal distributed variable $X_{ij2} \sim N(0, 1)$. Consequently, the first covariate is pair-specific, whereas the second covariate is individual specific. We used sample sizes of 500 and 5000 pairs and simulated 500 data sets in each case (50 data sets only for Bayesian methods because of time constraints). Only the case of complete event times (meaning no censoring) was considered here. Results are shown in Tables 5.16 – 5.18.

Table 5.16: Model 1 with two covariates, 500 simulated data sets (Bayes 50 data sets)

method	sample size	λ	φ	σ^2	ρ	β_1	β_2
true		3.00e-3	0.070	0.300	0.200	0.100	-0.200
ML	500	3.01e-3	0.070	0.294	0.222	0.105	-0.198
		(3.70e-4)	(0.004)	(0.087)	(0.194)	(0.082)	(0.042)
ML	5000	3.01e-3	0.070	0.299	0.197	0.099	-0.200
		(1.25e-4)	(0.001)	(0.027)	(0.069)	(0.026)	(0.013)
Bayes	5000	3.04e-3	0.070	0.292	0.208	0.093	-0.196
		(1.16e-4)	(0.001)	(0.024)	(0.059)	(0.027)	(0.013)
true		3.00e-3	0.070	1.000	0.700	0.100	-0.200
ML	500	2.99e-3	0.070	1.001	0.699	0.107	-0.202
		(4.03e-4)	(0.005)	(0.141)	(0.080)	(0.105)	(0.054)
ML	5000	3.01e-3	0.070	1.000	0.700	0.098	-0.199
		(1.34e-4)	(0.002)	(0.044)	(0.023)	(0.034)	(0.017)

ML - maximum likelihood estimation
Bayes - MCMC estimation

The three models show the same pattern. As expected, the estimations for the larger sample size are far more accurate. The most striking effect is the strong negative correlation between estimates of ρ and σ^2, independently of the model and the estimation procedure (see Table 5.19). Similar simulations were performed in the more general model with two different frailty variances (one for each of the two individuals). The results are similar to those with one frailty variance and are therefore omitted here.

As Bayesian methods are very time consuming, only 50 data sets with 5000 pairs each were generated for this analysis method. We run two parallel chains from different starting points and considered the first 4000 iterations for each chain as "burn-in".

The simulated values of parameters of random effects have auto-correlations close to unity in our case. The convergence of the Markov chain is very slow. Altogether, from 10000 up to 60000 iterations per chain were generated after the "burn-in" phase for each data set. The values of the Gelman–Rubin statistics are quite close to one (see Section 5.4), indicating convergence of the chains.

Table 5.17: Model 2 with two covariates, 500 simulated data sets (Bayes 50 data sets)

method	sample size	λ	φ	σ^2	ρ	β_1	β_2
true		3.00e-3	0.070	0.300	0.200	0.100	-0.200
ML*	500	3.02e-3	0.071	0.372	0.237	0.097	-0.203
		(8.23e-4)	(0.008)	(0.378)	(0.352)	(0.080)	(0.045)
ML*	5000	2.99e-3	0.070	0.308	0.204	0.099	-0.200
		(2.04e-4)	(0.002)	(0.077)	(0.083)	(0.025)	(0.013)
Bayes	5000	3.04e-3	0.070	0.300	0.218	0.095	-0.199
		(2.01e-4)	(0.002)	(0.067)	(0.089)	(0.022)	(0.012)
true		3.00e-3	0.070	1.000	0.700	0.100	-0.200
ML*	500	2.81e-3	0.075	1.283	0.689	0.113	-0.211
		(1.06e-3)	(0.014)	(0.731)	(0.186)	(0.118)	(0.059)
ML*	5000	3.07e-3	0.069	0.977	0.720	0.098	-0.199
		(3.44e-4)	(0.004)	(0.173)	(0.072)	(0.034)	(0.017)
Bayes	5000	3.12e-3	0.069	0.981	0.726	0.091	-0.198
		(3.93e-4)	(0.004)	(0.193)	(0.074)	(0.031)	(0.015)

ML* - maximum likelihood estimation with numerical integration
Bayes - MCMC estimation

Because of their simplicity and strengths, multivariate frailty models have become very popular over the last two decades. A wide range of papers has been published, dealing with different structures of multivariate models (shared vs. correlated frailty models), different distributions of frailty (gamma, log-normal, stable, PVF, etc.), different assumptions about the baseline hazard (parametric vs. semi-parametric models), and different estimation strategies (traditional maximum likelihood procedures, maximum likelihood procedures based on numerical integration, EM algorithm, MCMC methods). Having long time experience with correlated frailty models in real data applications, we recognized a striking negative correlation between the variance and the correlation estimates.

First, we tested whether the correlation of the estimates depends on the distribution of frailty. We used three very often used frailty distributions to answer this question: the gamma distribution and two different variants of the log-normal distribution (Models 1 – 3).

Second, we tested whether the observed effect was caused by the estimation strategy. This is why we used three different estimation strategies: traditional maximum likelihood estimation (using a self-written GAUSS code), maximum likelihood estimation based on numerical integration (using routines in aML and a self-written code), and MCMC methods in WinBUGS.

Table 5.18: Model 3 with two covariates, 500 simulated data sets (Bayes 50 data sets)

method	sample size	λ	φ	σ^2	ρ	β_1	β_2
true		3.00e-3	0.070	0.300	0.200	0.100	-0.200
ML*	500	3.01e-3	0.071	0.361	0.243	0.095	-0.204
		(4.22e-4)	(0.007)	(0.297)	(0.358)	(0.078)	(0.043)
ML*	5000	2.99e-3	0.070	0.308	0.204	0.099	-0.200
		(1.38e-4)	(0.002)	(0.075)	(0.082)	(0.025)	(0.013)
Bayes	5000	3.03e-3	0.070	0.302	0.218	0.095	-0.199
		(1.36e-4)	(0.002)	(0.070)	(0.092)	(0.022)	(0.012)
true		3.00e-3	0.070	1.000	0.700	0.100	-0.200
ML*	500	3.00e-3	0.075	1.323	0.683	0.107	-0.212
		(4.35e-4)	(0.015)	(0.998)	(0.160)	(0.117)	(0.064)
ML*	5000	3.00e-3	0.070	1.022	0.701	0.099	-0.201
		(1.46e-4)	(0.004)	(0.179)	(0.067)	(0.034)	(0.018)
Bayes	5000	3.02e-3	0.070	1.000	0.713	0.102	-0.199
		(1.30e-4)	(0.003)	(0.134)	(0.058)	(0.034)	(0.015)

ML* - maximum likelihood estimation with numerical integration

The results of the simulation study are very clear. The observed effect is stable over different frailty distributions and different estimation strategies. Moreover, different choices of parameters and sample sizes did not change the correlation.

The present study is limited to parametric correlated frailty models. An open question remains whether the observed negative correlation between the parameter estimates is also present in semiparametric correlated frailty models. This is a topic for future research.

A high correlation of parameter estimates could be a sign of identifiability problems in the model. Correlated frailty models were investigated in order to overcome the problems of the shared frailty models, which provide only one parameter to model variance and correlation. One idea was to include observed covariates into the models to improve identifiability characteristics. This is why all models were run both with and without observed covariates. The results in both cases are very similar. Consequently, we dropped results for models without observed covariates. Two types of covariates were used, one dichotomous and one continuous. However, no effect of the covariates on the correlation between the parameter estimates was detected.

Regarding identifiability, note that heterogeneity (variance of frailty) and correlation between frailties (implying dependence of lifetimes) are correlated in a frailty model based on conditional independence. To see this, assume that the variance of the frailty tends to zero. Obviously, this implies zero

Table 5.19: Models 1–3 with two covariates, 500 simulated data sets (Bayes 50 data sets)

model	method	sample size	corr(ρ, σ^2)	parameters
1	ML	500	-0.229**	$\sigma^2 = 0.3$, $\rho = 0.2$
1	ML	5000	-0.227**	
1	Bayes	5000	-0.331*	
1	ML	500	-0.431**	$\sigma^2 = 1$, $\rho = 0.7$
1	ML	5000	-0.396**	
2	ML*	500	-0.241**	$\sigma^2 = 0.3$, $\rho = 0.2$
2	ML*	5000	-0.414**	
2	Bayes	5000	-0.382**	
2	ML*	500	-0.789**	$\sigma^2 = 1$, $\rho = 0.7$
2	ML*	5000	-0.875**	
2	Bayes	5000	-0.921**	
3	ML*	500	-0.242**	$\sigma^2 = 0.3$, $\rho = 0.2$
3	ML*	5000	-0.409**	
3	Bayes	5000	-0.438**	
3	ML*	500	-0.717**	$\sigma^2 = 1$, $\rho = 0.7$
3	ML*	5000	-0.862**	
3	Bayes	5000	-0.854**	

* $p < 0.05$, ** $p < 0.01$
ML - maximum likelihood estimation
ML* - maximum likelihood estimation with numerical integration
Bayes - MCMC estimation

correlation. The assumption about the conditional independence of lifetimes given the frailty could be the reason for the correlation linking the estimates of variance (heterogeneity) and correlation between frailties. This would explain why the observed effect is stable over the considered models and different estimation procedures.

The conclusion to draw is that researchers should be cautious, and be aware of the problem presented in applying correlated frailty models. Nevertheless, this study shows that the models perform well and that there is nearly no bias in the parameter estimates. This supports the use of correlated frailty models for obtaining accurate parameter estimates and useful interpretations of these estimates. More detailed information about this study can be found in Wienke et al. (2005b).

5.10　Dependent Competing Risks in Frailty Models

In Section 5.2, cause-specific mortality data was analyzed using the correlated gamma frailty model, assuming independence between causes of death in a competing risk scenario. The assumption about independence between the competing risks allows treating other causes of death as censored observations, which makes analysis very easy. In this section we sketch an approach to removing this limitation. The model allows testing of the hypothesis on dependence between competing risks. To simplify description, we consider models limited to two competing risks (death by cause of interest and by other causes), but the model can easily be extended to the case of multiple competing risks.

Estimating correlations of durations is difficult because of censored data, which complicates the statistical analysis far more than does complete data. Using a bivariate survival model to estimate correlations among lifetimes can solve this problem. The correlated gamma frailty model can be used to fit the lifetime data and provide a specific parameter for the correlation among frailties. It was already used to analyze cause-specific mortality in twins under the assumption of independence between competing risks in Examples 5.1–5.3. However, the assumption of independence between competing risks is often questionable. Typically, in clinical and epidemiological studies, two different types of competing events (censoring) occur. The observations of certain individuals are censored because they are still alive at the end of the study. Other individuals drop from the follow-up for reasons not associated with the disease under study but through life events beyond the control of the researcher, such as migration.

If censoring can be assumed noninformative in regard to all different causes, then the traditional model applies, with the censoring times taken as the minimum of the hypothetical censoring times arising from the different causes of censoring. However, the situation becomes much more difficult if censoring arising from at least one of the competing risks needs to be assumed to be informative. Informative censoring means that the lifetimes and censoring times are dependent or, in case of their independence, the distribution of censoring times contains parameters of lifetime distribution.

Various approaches have been proposed to account for informative censoring. Link (1989) proposes a model for informative censoring in which censoring only occurs in a subpopulation defined by the frailty distribution. Emoto and Matthews (1990) assume a bivariate Weibull model for failure and censoring times. Zheng and Klein (1995) use a copula to study dependent competing risks. Carling and Jacobson (1995) modeled unemployment duration in a dependent competing risk framework by means of three different models. Their paper also contains considerations of the identifiability aspects of the models. Lin et al. (1996) use data collected after nonfatal failure events to model dependent censoring by death or selective patient withdrawal. Lee and Wolfe (1998) proposed a test for independent censoring. Their method involves further follow-up of a subpopulation of lost-to-follow-up censored subjects. Asymptotic results in a specific situation are obtained by Wienke (1998). All these methods deal with uncorrelated subjects only. The method described in this section deals with correlated subjects and was published first in an analysis about genetic factors influencing CHD by Wienke et al. (2002). Essentially, it understands correlated subjects as partial replicates for each other, and hence gains identifiability for informative censoring.

Two types of censoring are considered, one noninformative and the other informative. Let $(T_{i1}^*, Y_{i1}, C_{i1}, T_{i2}^*, Y_{i2}, C_{i2})$ $(i = 1, \ldots, n)$ be independent and identically distributed vectors of nonnegative random variables. The variables (T_{i1}^*, T_{i2}^*) denote the nonobservable cause-specific lifetimes with respect to the cause of death under investigation. The (Y_{i1}, Y_{i2}) are informative censoring times (for example, lifetimes with respect to causes of death not of special interest) and (C_{i1}, C_{i2}) are noninformative censoring times. The event times $T_{ij} = \min\{T_{ij}^*, Y_{ij}, C_{ij}\}$ $(i = 1, \ldots, n; j = 1, 2)$ are observed and

$$
\Delta_{ij} = \left\{
\begin{array}{rcl}
1 & : & \text{if } T_{ij}^* \leq \min\{C_{ij}, Y_{ij}\} \\
0 & : & \text{if } C_{ij} < \min\{T_{ij}^*, Y_{ij}\} \\
-1 & : & \text{if } Y_{ij} < \min\{T_{ij}^*, C_{ij}\},
\end{array}
\right. \tag{5.23}
$$

where $\Delta_{ij} = 1$ indicates no censoring, $\Delta_{ij} = 0$ noninformative censoring, and $\Delta_{ij} = -1$ informative censoring. Now we derive the four-dimensional survival function. The vector (T_1^*, Y_1, T_2^*, Y_2) is used as a shorthand for $(T_{i1}^*, Y_{i1}, T_{i2}^*, Y_{i2})$ $(i = 1, \ldots, n)$. Let (T_1^*, Y_1, T_2^*, Y_2) and (Z_1, Z_2, Z_3, Z_4) be the lifetimes and informative censoring times, and the frailties of two partners with respect to two causes of death. Their individual hazards are given by the proportional hazards model

$$
\begin{array}{ll}
T_1^* \sim \mu_1(t_1|Z_1) = Z_1\mu_{01}(t_1) & T_2^* \sim \mu_1(t_2|Z_3) = Z_3\mu_{01}(t_2) \\
Y_1 \sim \mu_2(y_1|Z_2) = Z_2\mu_{02}(y_1) & Y_2 \sim \mu_2(y_2|Z_4) = Z_4\mu_{02}(y_2),
\end{array} \tag{5.24}
$$

where $T \sim \mu$ means that μ is the hazard function of T. Hence, the baseline hazard of the lifetime of the first (T_1^*) and second partner (T_2^*) with respect to the first cause of death are assumed to be equal (denoted by μ_1). The same statement holds for the lifetime of the first (Y_1) and second partner (Y_2) regarding to the second cause of death (μ_2). The variables T_1^*, Y_1, T_2^*, and Y_2 are assumed to be independent, given the vector of frailties (Z_1, Z_2, Z_3, Z_4). Let $V_1, V_8 \sim \Gamma(k_1, \lambda_0)$, $V_2 \sim \Gamma(k_2, \lambda_1)$, $V_3 \sim \Gamma(k_3, \lambda_2)$, $V_4, V_7 \sim \Gamma(k_4, \lambda_2)$, $V_5, V_6 \sim \Gamma(k_5, \lambda_1)$ be independent gamma-distributed random variables with $k_1 + k_2 + k_5 := \lambda_1 = \frac{1}{\sigma_1^2}$ and $k_1 + k_3 + k_4 := \lambda_2 = \frac{1}{\sigma_2^2}$. The frailties and their correlations are depicted in Figure 5.1.

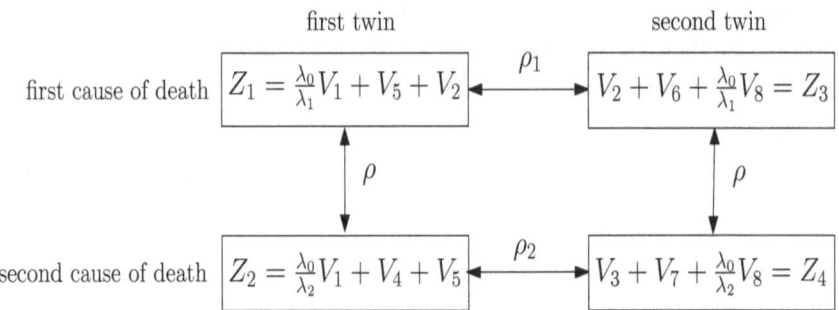

Figure 5.1: Cause-specific frailties and their correlations in a twin pair.

Z_1, Z_3 denote frailties with respect to the main cause of death (the cause under study) and Z_2, Z_4 are the frailties with respect to the second cause of death. The parameters ρ_1, ρ_2, and ρ describe correlations between the frailties: $\rho_1 = \mathbf{corr}(Z_1, Z_3)$, $\rho_2 = \mathbf{corr}(Z_2, Z_4)$, and $\rho = \mathbf{corr}(Z_1, Z_2) = \mathbf{corr}(Z_3, Z_4)$. The four-dimensional survival function is obtained by integrating out the conditional lifetimes with respect to the frailty distribution by using (5.24) and applying the Laplace transform of gamma-distributed random variables (see Appendix A.5):

$$S(t_1, y_1, t_2, y_2) \tag{5.25}$$
$$= \mathbf{E} S_1(t_1)^{Z_1} S_2(y_1)^{Z_2} S_1(t_2)^{Z_3} S_2(y_2)^{Z_4}$$
$$= \left(S_1(t_1)^{-\sigma_1^2} + S_1(t_2)^{-\sigma_1^2} - 1 \right)^{-\frac{\rho_1}{\sigma_1^2}} \left(S_2(y_1)^{-\sigma_2^2} + S_2(y_2)^{-\sigma_2^2} - 1 \right)^{-\frac{\rho_2}{\sigma_2^2}}$$
$$\times \left(S_1(t_1)^{-\sigma_1^2} + S_2(y_1)^{-\sigma_2^2} - 1 \right)^{-\frac{\rho}{\sigma_1 \sigma_2}} \left(S_1(t_2)^{-\sigma_1^2} + S_2(y_2)^{-\sigma_2^2} - 1 \right)^{-\frac{\rho}{\sigma_1 \sigma_2}}$$
$$\times S_1(t_1)^{1-\rho_1-\frac{\sigma_1}{\sigma_2}\rho} S_1(t_2)^{1-\rho_1-\frac{\sigma_1}{\sigma_2}\rho} S_2(y_1)^{1-\rho_2-\frac{\sigma_2}{\sigma_1}\rho} S_2(y_2)^{1-\rho_2-\frac{\sigma_2}{\sigma_1}\rho}$$

with the constraint $0 \le \rho \le \min\{\frac{\sigma_2}{\sigma_1}(1-\rho_1), \frac{\sigma_1}{\sigma_2}(1-\rho_2)\}$. Parameter ρ_1 denotes the correlation between Z_1 and Z_3. This parameter measures the correlation between frailties of partners in a pair with respect to the cause of death under investigation and is important for genetic analysis of susceptibility to cause-specific mortality. Parameter ρ_2 models the correlation between frailties regarding all other causes of death (combined to the second cause of death or, more general, informative censoring). Parameter ρ describes the association between the unobservable cause-specific lifetimes in each individual. This parameter allows to test the hypothesis of dependence between competing risks. S_1 and S_2 denote the marginal survival functions regarding the first and second cause of death. The likelihood function of the model can be found in Appendix A.5.

It is of interest to consider two special cases included in the above model to get deeper insight into the structure. Fixing $\rho = 0$ results in two separate correlated gamma frailty models for the two causes of death:

$$S(t_1, y_1, t_2, y_2) = S_1(t_1)^{1-\rho_1} S_1(t_2)^{1-\rho_1} (S_1(t_1)^{-\sigma_1^2} + S_1(t_2)^{-\sigma_1^2} - 1)^{-\frac{\rho_1}{\sigma_1^2}}$$
$$\times S_2(y_1)^{1-\rho_2} S_2(y_2)^{1-\rho_2} (S_2(y_1)^{-\sigma_2^2} + S_2(y_2)^{-\sigma_2^2} - 1)^{-\frac{\rho_2}{\sigma_2^2}}.$$

If $\rho_1 = 0$ and $\rho_2 = 0$ holds (unrelated individuals), the model simplifies to

$$S(t_1, y_1, t_2, y_2) = S_1(t_1)^{1-\frac{\sigma_1}{\sigma_2}\rho} S_2(y_1)^{1-\frac{\sigma_2}{\sigma_1}\rho} (S_1(t_1)^{-\sigma_1^2} + S_2(y_1)^{-\sigma_2^2} - 1)^{-\frac{\rho}{\sigma_1 \sigma_2}}$$
$$\times S_1(t_2)^{1-\frac{\sigma_1}{\sigma_2}\rho} S_2(y_2)^{1-\frac{\sigma_2}{\sigma_1}\rho} (S_1(t_2)^{-\sigma_1^2} + S_2(y_2)^{-\sigma_2^2} - 1)^{-\frac{\rho}{\sigma_1 \sigma_2}}.$$

Using cause-specific mortality data of relatives (for example, twins), it is possible to solve nonidentifiability problems in univariate censored lifetimes as investigated by Tsiatis (1975). The model enables dependencies between competing risks and allows to test for such dependencies.

The consistency and asymptotic normality of the estimators in this model are not proofed yet, but simulation results (not shown here) indicate the asymptotic validity of the proposed model.

The correlation coefficients between the frailties are always nonnegative, which is clearly a limitation of the proposed model. This restriction poses no problem when analyzing the lifetimes of relatives, where a positive association between lifetimes seems reasonable. However, it is not clear that the same holds for the competing risks in an individual. On the one hand, many major diseases have risk factors in common, and consequently, the presence of any one of these risk factors will increase the risk of death with respect to all diseases. On the other hand, everyone dies eventually, so it is only logical that if the risk of death from one cause is decreased, then the risk from another cause is increased. Furthermore, the parameter ρ is only identifiable in a "real" multivariate case (cluster size larger than two). Having pairs of unrelated individuals (e.g., $\rho_1 = \rho_2 = 0$), implying the univariate case, makes the parameter ρ nonidentifiable. The nature of dependencies among competing risks deserves further study.

A similar model for current state data was established in Giard (2001) and Giard et al. (2002). A more general approach compared to model (5.25) was investigated by Bandeen-Roche and Liang (1996). The difference in the models is in the observed data. In the model just shown only the minimum of two competing lifetimes in each individual is observed, whereas Bandeen-Roche and Liang (1996) assume that all lifetimes are observable. Another four-dimensional correlated gamma frailty model is proposed by Jonker and Boomsma (2010).

Huang and Wolfe (2002) based their model on log-normal frailty and (4.17), which means a model somewhere between shared and correlated frailty models. In a recent paper, Huang et al. (2004) suggested a test procedure to test the hypothesis of dependence between survival and censoring times in their model.

Chapter 6

Copula Models

Copula models are an attractive possibility to model clustered survival data. However, the application of such models requires unique cluster size for all clusters in the study population. This situation is illustrated in the twin data examples. Here the cluster size is always two. Other bivariate examples are event times in paired organs such as eyes and kidneys. Duchateau and Janssen (2008) give an interesting four-dimensional example with udder data. There are exactly four udder quarters for each cow, which is considered to be the cluster. Researcher are interested in the time until the occurrence of an infection. Typical examples of unique cluster size are family studies with fixed family size, for example, studies with kernel families of size three (father, mother, child).

The copula C is a function defined on $[0,1]^n$ and taking values in $[0,1]$. The copula establishes the link between the marginal survival functions to generate the joint survival function. Let $S_j(t_j)$ $(j = 1,\ldots,n)$ denote the marginal survival functions in clusters of size n. Then the joint survival function is given by $S(t_1,\ldots,t_n) = C(S_1(t_1),\ldots,S_n(t_n))$. The existence of the copula C follows from the theorem by Sklar (1959). For continuous marginal survival functions, a unique copula exists. For a comprehensive overview of copula models see Nelsen (2006). For survival data, the family of copulas is often restricted to the class of Archimedian copulas, described in detail by Genest and MacKay (1986):

$$S(t_1,\ldots,t_n) = p\big(q(S_1(t_1)) + \ldots + q(S_n(t_n))\big),$$

where p is a decreasing function defined on nonnegative numbers taking values in $[0,1]$ and $p(0) = 0$. Furthermore, it is assumed that $p(t)$ has a positive second derivative for all $t > 0$ and q denotes the inverse of p. A detailed discussion about the relation between Archimedian copulas and the shared frailty model can be found in Goethals et al. (2008) and Duchateau and Janssen (2008). In the following we will restrict our discussion to the bivariate case for ease of presentation. Higher-dimensional extensions are possible but they extend the length of the formulas. The copula of the shared gamma frailty model (the Clayton copula) will serve as a specific example to explain the basic ideas in Section 6.1. It will be helpful to derive the correlated gamma frailty copula in Section 6.2. Section 6.3 deals with a general correlated frailty copula and Section 6.4 considers the cross-ratio function.

6.1 Shared Gamma Frailty Copula

Clayton (1978), Cox and Oakes (1984), and Yashin and Iachine (1999a) pointed out that the bivariate survival function in the shared gamma frailty model (4.3) can also be derived using a radically different approach. In the next paragraph we will outline this approach and discuss its interpretational consequences in more detail.

Denote two possibly dependent event times by T_1, T_2, and let the expression $S(t_1, t_2) = \mathbf{P}(T_1 > t_1, T_2 > t_2)$ be their bivariate joint survival function that is absolutely continuous with margins $S_1(t_1) = S(t_1, 0)$ and $S_2(t_2) = S(0, t_2)$. Consequently, the conditional survival function of T_1 given $T_2 > t_2$ is

$$S(t_1 | T_2 > t_2) = \frac{S(t_1, t_2)}{S_2(t_2)}$$

and that of T_1 given $T_2 = t_2$ is

$$S(t_1 | T_2 = t_2) = \frac{\frac{\partial S(t_1, t_2)}{\partial t_2}}{\frac{\partial S_2(t_2)}{\partial t_2}}.$$

The respective conditional hazard functions are important for the following considerations. Using the relation $\mu(t) = -\frac{S'(t)}{S(t)}$ implies

$$\mu(t_1 | T_2 > t_2) = -\frac{\partial}{\partial t_1} \ln(S(t_1, t_2)) \tag{6.1}$$

and

$$\mu(t_1 | T_2 = t_2) = -\frac{\partial}{\partial t_1} \ln\left(-\frac{\partial}{\partial t_2} S(t_1, t_2)\right). \tag{6.2}$$

These hazards describe the risk of failure at age t_1 for the first individual, given the information about the event status of the second individual in the pair. The first hazard (6.1) uses the condition $\{T_2 > t_2\}$, and the second one (6.2) is conditional on $\{T_2 = t_2\}$. The deviation of the ratio of these hazards from one was used by Oakes (1989) as a measure of mutual dependence of the respective marginal lifetimes. The survival function of the shared gamma frailty model can now be obtained from the following relation between the above hazards

$$\mu(t_1 | T_2 = t_2) = (1 + \sigma^2)\mu(t_1 | T_2 > t_2), \tag{6.3}$$

where σ^2 denotes a nonnegative constant (without interpretation as a frailty variance). The advantage of model (6.3) is the fancy interpretation of the factor $(1 + \sigma^2)$ as the relative risk associated with a nonsurviving partner. This risk is always greater or equal to one because of the nonnegative dependence in the shared frailty model. The main advantage of this model is that the increase in risk with a nonsurviving partner is constant over time. Obviously, formula (6.3) is equivalent to a similar condition with the roles of T_1 and T_2 being interchanged. This relation defines the bivariate survival function (4.3) uniquely (but not the marginal distributions). For derivation we use definitions (6.1) and (6.2) and integrate both sides of the equation (Cox and Oakes 1984):

$$\mu(t_1|T_2 = t_2) = (1 + \sigma^2)\mu(t_1|T_2 > t_2)$$

$$\frac{\partial}{\partial t_1} \ln \left(\frac{-\partial}{\partial t_2} S(t_1, t_2) \right) = (1 + \sigma^2) \frac{\partial}{\partial t_1} \ln(S(t_1, t_2))$$

$$\int_0^{t_1} \frac{\partial}{\partial t} \ln \left(\frac{-\partial}{\partial t_2} S(t, t_2) \right) dt = (1 + \sigma^2) \int_0^{t_1} \frac{\partial}{\partial t} \ln(S(t, t_2)) \, dt.$$

Solving the integral and rearranging the terms, it holds that

$$\ln \left(\frac{-\partial}{\partial t_2} S(t_1, t_2) \right) - \ln \left(\frac{-\partial}{\partial t_2} S_2(t_2) \right) = (1 + \sigma^2) \left(\ln(S(t_1, t_2)) - \ln(S_2(t_2)) \right)$$

$$\ln \left(\frac{-\partial}{\partial t_2} S(t_1, t_2) \right) - \ln(S(t_1, t_2)^{1+\sigma^2}) = \ln \left(\frac{-\partial}{\partial t_2} S_2(t_2) \right) - \ln(S_2(t_2)^{1+\sigma^2})$$

$$\frac{\frac{\partial}{\partial t_2} S(t_1, t_2)}{S(t_1, t_2)^{1+\sigma^2}} = \frac{\frac{\partial}{\partial t_2} S_2(t_2)}{S_2(t_2)^{1+\sigma^2}}.$$

Integrating again implies the bivariate survival function

$$\int_0^{t_2} \frac{\frac{\partial}{\partial t} S(t_1, t)}{S(t_1, t)^{1+\sigma^2}} \, dt = \int_0^{t_2} \frac{\frac{\partial}{\partial t} S_2(t)}{S_2(t)^{1+\sigma^2}} \, dt$$

$$S(t_1, t_2)^{-\sigma^2} - S_1(t_1)^{-\sigma^2} = S_2(t_2)^{-\sigma^2} - 1$$

$$S(t_1, t_2) = \left(S_1(t_1)^{-\sigma^2} + S_2(t_2)^{-\sigma^2} - 1 \right)^{-\frac{1}{\sigma^2}}.$$

Thus, there are two ways of deriving formula (4.3) based on two radically different concepts: one uses the assumption (6.3), concerning proportionality of conditional hazards; the other uses the concept of gamma-distributed shared frailty. In the literature it has often been claimed that particular copulas can be deduced from frailty models by choosing the appropriate frailty distribution. This happens because the survival functions are similar in both approaches, at least at first sight. It is necessary to note that there exists one important difference between the survival functions resulting from both approaches. In the shared gamma frailty model, transformation (3.17) is used to generate the bivariate survival function. Consequently, the marginal survival functions

S_1 and S_2 include the frailty parameter σ^2, which is not the case in the approach using proportional conditional hazards (6.3). The latter model is a copula model. Consequently, it is necessary to make assumptions about the data generation mechanism. This is important for the interpretation of the data analysis; for more details see Goethals et al. (2008). The bivariate representation (6.3) was extended to the multivariate setting by Guo and Rodriguez (1992) and Guo (1993).

Fitting copula models is often performed by using a two-stage procedure (Shih and Louis 1995a, Glidden 2000, Andersen 2005). In the first stage the marginal survival functions are estimated without taking into account the clustering of the data. This can be done in a parametric or nonparametric way. A semiparametric approach is also possible by assuming a Cox model and therefore the inclusion of covariates (Glidden 2000, Andersen 2005). It turns out that these estimates are consistent (Spiekerman and Lin 1998) and can be used in the second step to estimate the copula parameters. Alternatively, the likelihood can also be maximized in a one-step procedure. In the next section we consider the copula of the correlated gamma frailty model to illustrate the difference between the copula and the frailty approach.

6.2 Correlated Gamma Frailty Copula

Starting from the conditional frailty model, the hazard of individual j in the ith pair is given by

$$\mu(t|Z_{ij}) = Z_{ij}\mu_{0j}(t),$$

omitting covariates for ease of presentation. The joint conditional survival function is then given by

$$S(t_1, t_2|Z_{i1}, Z_{i2}) = e^{-Z_{i1}M_{01}(t_1) - Z_{i2}M_{02}(t_2)}.$$

The joint survival function is now obtained by integrating out the random frailties

$$S(t_1, t_2) = \int e^{-z_1 M_{01}(t_1) - z_2 M_{02}(t_2)} f(z_1, z_2)\, dz_1\, dz_2$$

with respect to their density $f(z_1, z_2)$. This integral can be solved analytically, and the joint survival function of the correlated gamma frailty model is now (see 5.6)

$$S(t_1, t_2) = \frac{S_1(t_1)^{1-\frac{\sigma_1}{\sigma_2}\rho} S_2(t_2)^{1-\frac{\sigma_2}{\sigma_1}\rho}}{(S_1(t_1)^{-\sigma_1^2} + S_2(t_2)^{-\sigma_2^2} - 1)^{\frac{\rho}{\sigma_1\sigma_2}}}. \tag{6.4}$$

The joint survival function in the copula model looks completely the same. To understand the difference between the correlated gamma frailty model and the related copula, it is necessary to keep in mind how formula (6.4) was derived.

The formula is obtained by substituting the expressions $(1 + \sigma_j^2 M_{0j}(t_j))^{-\frac{1}{\sigma_j^2}}$ $(j = 1, 2)$ by the marginal survival functions $S_j(t_j)$ in (5.5) using (3.17). Consequently, in the frailty model, the survival functions $S_j(t_j)$ depend on the variance of the frailties σ_j^2. This is often overlooked when dealing with representation (6.4). In the copula approach the derivation in (5.5) is no longer of interest, formula (5.6) is just a bivariate survival function without any frailty interpretation. It should be noted that the copula in (6.4) is not an Archimedian copula in contrast to the Clayton copula, which is obtained as a special case with $\rho = 1$. Here, the marginal survival functions are completely unrestricted and can follow any distribution. That is the reason why a two-step procedure can be applied by estimating the marginal survival functions in the first step. The assumption that the marginal survival functions depend on the frailty variances is no longer used. As a consequence, in frailty models, such a two-step estimation procedure is impossible. In the frailty model the choice of the frailty distribution determines the functional form of the copula as well as the functional form of the marginal distributions, which is different compared to the copula model. It is important to understand the difference between the two approaches because the results and their interpretation will not be the same. We illustrate this problem in the following example by reanalyzing the data of male Danish twins in Example 5.1 with respect to cancer.

Example 6.1

Because of the symmetry in the twin data, the restrictions $S(t) = S_1(t) = S_2(t)$ and $\sigma^2 = \sigma_1^2 = \sigma_2^2$ are imposed. A parametric approach with a Gompertz baseline hazard function is considered. In the case of the gamma frailty models this results in

$$S(t) = (1 + \sigma^2 \frac{\lambda}{\varphi}(e^{\varphi t} - 1))^{-\frac{1}{\sigma^2}}.$$

In the copula approach, no restrictions about the form of the marginal survival functions exist. This can, for example, be incorporated into the model by the specification

$$S(t) = (1 + s^2 \frac{\lambda}{\varphi}(e^{\varphi t} - 1))^{-\frac{1}{s^2}},$$

where s^2 denotes a new parameter of the marginal distribution. In some sense, s^2 is interpretable as the variance of a univariate gamma-distributed frailty. The correlated gamma frailty model is characterized by the condition $\sigma^2 = s^2$. Consequently, using this parameterization, the frailty model is a special case of the copula model. Additionally, the semiparametric copula model is also applied to the data. The results of the maximum likelihood parameter estimation in all three models are given in Table 6.1.

Table 6.1: Correlated gamma frailty and copula models applied to lifetimes of Danish male twins with respect to cancer

parameter	frailty model	copula model	semip. copula
σ^2	3.388 (0.572)	5.911 (3.154)	5.707 (3.019)
ρ_{MZ}	0.350 (0.088)	0.275 (0.090)	0.269 (0.091)
ρ_{DZ}	0.194 (0.068)	0.148 (0.061)	0.148 (0.062)
λ	4.4e-6 (1.5e-6)	4.7e-6 (1.6e-6)	
φ	0.118 (0.006)	0.117 (0.006)	
s^2		3.264 (0.579)	
log-likelihood	-14283.1939	-14282.3678	

The difference between the models in the first two columns is obvious. In the copula model, σ^2 has no longer an interpretation as a frailty variance, and ρ is no longer interpretable as a correlation between frailties. Both ρ and σ^2 are parameters of the copula without any relation to random effects. In contrast, the parameter s^2 has an interpretation as variance of the univariate frailty in the marginal distributions. Consequently, the foregoing approach can be used to test whether the frailty model fits the data. If both parameters σ^2 and s^2 are similar, the frailty model provides a good fit. If there is a significant difference between the two parameters, this contradicts the frailty model and speaks in favor of the less restrictive copula model. In the situation considered here, the likelihood ratio test indicates no significant difference between the models, preferring the more simple frailty model. This fact is also supported by the large standard error of σ^2 in the copula model. Interestingly, semiparametric analysis (last column) reveals similar results compared to the parametric copula model. This speaks in favor of the hypothesis that the parametric analysis is not sensitive to the choice of the hazard function. In the semiparametric copula model, a one-step estimation procedure is used, where the Kaplan–Meier–estimator is plugged into the likelihood function to substitute the unknown marginal survival functions. Unfortunately, this approach is not possible in the frailty model, where the more demanding EM algorithm is needed to analyze the semiparametric model. The reason for this difference is the already mentioned dependence of the marginal survival functions on the frailty variance in the frailty model, which is not present in the copula approach. □

6.3 General Correlated Frailty Copulas

The question arises whether the correlated gamma frailty copula can also be derived without a frailty approach. Yashin and Iachine (1999a,b) gave such a derivation of this copula using a transformation of a well-known bivariate survival function. It turns out that this concept can also be used to generate copulas related to other correlated frailty models. Additionally, the authors extended the copula of the correlated gamma frailty model (6.4) to the case $\rho < 0$, and conditions are derived that guarantee negative associations of lifespans. Let T_1, T_2 be two dependent failure times, and $S(t_1, t_2)$ be their respective bivariate survival function. Any such function can be written in the form

$$S(t_1, t_2) = S_1(t_1) S_2(t_2) e^{A(t_1, t_2)}, \tag{6.5}$$

where $A(t_1, t_2) = \ln\left(\frac{S(t_1, t_2)}{S_1(t_1) S_2(t_2)}\right)$, and $S_j(t_j)$ $(j = 1, 2)$ are the marginal univariate survival functions. If the bivariate distribution of the survival times (T_1, T_2) is absolutely continuous, the above-introduced function $A(t_1, t_2)$ can be given using the representation $A(t_1, t_2) = \int_0^{t_1} \int_0^{t_2} \phi(u, v) \, du \, dv$ (Anderson et al. 1992). Expression (6.5) is called an exponential representation of a bivariate survival function with association function ϕ. It turns out (and will be proved in the following theorem) that the expression

$$\begin{aligned}
\tilde{S}(t_1, t_2) &= S_1(t_1) S_2(t_2) e^{\rho A(t_1, t_2)} \\
&= S_1(t_1) S_2(t_2) e^{\rho \ln\left(\frac{S(t_1, t_2)}{S_1(t_1) S_2(t_2)}\right)} \\
&= \left(S_1(t_1) S_2(t_2)\right)^{1-\rho} S(t_1, t_2)^{\rho} \tag{6.6}
\end{aligned}$$

determines for $0 \leq \rho \leq 1$ a bivariate survival function with exactly the same marginal distributions as in the original model $S(t_1, t_2)$. The new bivariate survival function $\tilde{S}(t_1, t_2)$ is a geometric mean of two survival functions. The first survival function corresponds to the independent case $S_1(t_1) S_2(t_2)$, whereas the second deals with dependent survival times given by $S(t_1, t_2)$. The parameter ρ may therefore be considered as an association describing the location of $\tilde{S}(t_1, t_2)$ between the survival functions $S_1(t_1) S_2(t_2)$ and $S(t_1, t_2)$.

Relation (6.6) is of great practical relevance. In general, each copula can be extended in this simple way while keeping the same marginal distributions. Here we are especially interested in the fact that each shared frailty copula can be generalized in a very simple way to a related correlated copula. This opens new avenues in the modeling of dependent event times by the copula approach.

THEOREM 6.1

(Yashin and Iachine 1999a) Let $S(t_1, t_2)$ be the joint survival function of T_1 and T_2 given by formula (6.5) with marginals $S_1(t_1)$ and $S_2(t_2)$. Furthermore, let $A(t_1, t_2) = \int_0^{t_1} \int_0^{t_2} \phi(u, v) du dv$, with $\phi(u, v) \geq 0$ for all $u \geq 0, v \geq 0$. Then, for any $0 \leq \rho \leq 1$,

$$\tilde{S}(t_1, t_2) = S_1(t_1) S_2(t_2) e^{\rho A(t_1, t_2)}$$

determines a survival function for survival times $\tilde{T}_1$ and $\tilde{T}_2$. The marginal distributions of T_j and $\tilde{T}_j$ $(j = 1, 2)$ are identical.

Proof: It follows from (6.6) that $\tilde{S}(t_1, 0) = S_1(t_1)$, and $\tilde{S}(0, t_2) = S_2(t_2)$, and that $\tilde{S}(t_1, \infty) = \tilde{S}(\infty, t_2) = \tilde{S}(\infty, \infty) = 0$. Hence, $\tilde{A}(t_1, t_2) = \rho A(t_1, t_2)$. To complete the proof, it is enough to show that $\tilde{S}_{t_1 t_2}(t_1, t_2) = \frac{\partial^2 \tilde{S}(t_1, t_2)}{\partial t_1 \partial t_2} \geq 0$. Using relation (6.6) we obtain

$$\tilde{S}_{t_1 t_2}(t_1, t_2) \qquad (6.7)$$

$$= S_1'(t_1) S_2'(t_2) e^{\rho A(t_1, t_2)}$$
$$+ S_1'(t_1) S_2(t_2) \rho A_{t_2}(t_1, t_2) e^{\rho A(t_1, t_2)}$$
$$+ S_1(t_1) S_2'(t_2) \rho A_{t_1}(t_1, t_2) e^{\rho A(t_1, t_2)}$$
$$+ S_1(t_1) S_2(t_2) \rho A_{t_1 t_2}(t_1, t_2) e^{\rho A(t_1, t_2)}$$
$$+ S_1(t_1) S_2(t_2) \rho^2 A_{t_1}(t_1, t_2) A_{t_2}(t_1, t_2) e^{\rho A(t_1, t_2)}$$
$$= \tilde{S}(t_1, t_2) \big[\mu_1(t_1) \mu_2(t_2) - \mu_1(t_1) \rho A_{t_2}(t_1, t_2)$$
$$- \mu_2(t_2) \rho A_{t_1}(t_1, t_2) + \rho A_{t_1 t_2}(t_1, t_2) + \rho^2 A_{t_1}(t_1, t_2) A_{t_2}(t_1, t_2) \big]$$
$$= \tilde{S}(t_1, t_2) \big[(\rho A_{t_1}(t_1, t_2) - \mu_1(t_1))(\rho A_{t_2}(t_1, t_2) - \mu_2(t_2)) + \rho A_{t_1 t_2}(t_1, t_2) \big],$$

where $\mu_i(t_i) = -\frac{S_i'(t_i)}{S_i(t_i)}$. Starting from relation $A(t_1, t_2) = \ln \frac{S(t_1, t_2)}{S_1(t_1) S_2(t_2)}$, the following holds:

$$A_{t_1}(t_1, t_2) = \frac{S_{t_1}(t_1, t_2)}{S(t_1, t_2)} - \frac{S_1'(t_1)}{S_1(t_1)} = \mu_1(t_1) - \mu_1(t_1, t_2)$$

and $A_{t_2}(t_1, t_2) = \mu_2(t_2) - \mu_2(t_1, t_2)$. Here, $\mu_i(t_1, t_2)$ denotes the hazard of individual i given the information that $\{T_j > t_j\}$ $(i, j = 1, 2; \ i \neq j)$. Taking into account that $A_{t_1 t_2}(t_1, t_2) = \phi(t_1, t_2)$, we can rewrite (6.7) in the form

$$\tilde{S}_{t_1 t_2}(t_1, t_2) = \tilde{S}(t_1, t_2) \big[((\rho - 1)\mu_1(t_1) - \rho \mu_1(t_1, t_2))$$
$$\times ((\rho - 1)\mu_2(t_2) - \rho \mu_2(t_1, t_2)) + \rho \phi(t_1, t_2) \big] \qquad (6.8)$$

which is always nonnegative, and this completes the proof. ∎

If $S(t_1, t_2)$ is be given by (4.2) (Clayton copula, copula of the shared gamma frailty model), then $\tilde{S}(t_1, t_2)$ is obtained as the survival function of the copula of the correlated gamma frailty model (6.4) with $\sigma_1^2 = \sigma_2^2$:

$$\tilde{S}(t_1, t_2) = \frac{S_1(t_1)^{1-\rho} S_2(t_2)^{1-\rho}}{(S_1(t_1)^{-\sigma^2} + S_2(t_2)^{-\sigma^2} - 1)^{\frac{\rho}{\sigma^2}}}.$$

Consequently, the copula of the correlated gamma frailty model can be derived from the copula of the shared gamma frailty model without any interpretation related to frailty. The association function $\phi(t_1, t_2)$ in this case is of the form

$$\phi(t_1, t_2) = \frac{\sigma^2 \mu_1(t_1) \mu_2(t_2) S_1(t_1)^{-\sigma^2} S_2(t_2)^{-\sigma^2}}{(S_1(t_1)^{-\sigma^2} + S_2(t_2)^{-\sigma^2} - 1)^2}. \tag{6.9}$$

In the positive stable model, a similar extension can be performed starting from the copula of the shared positive frailty model (4.7):

$$\tilde{S}(t_1, t_2) = S_1(t_1)^{1-\rho} S_2(t_2)^{1-\rho} \exp\left[\rho\left((-\ln S_1(t_1))^{1/\gamma} + (-\ln S_2(t_2))^{1/\gamma}\right)^{\gamma}\right].$$

It should be noted that a correlated positive stable frailty model similar to the other correlated frailty models with explicit joint survival function does not exist, because the moments of the positive stable distribution are all infinite. Consequently, no correlation between the frailties in a cluster exist, which makes the interpretation of the parameter ρ more difficult. The association function becomes

$$\phi(t_1, t_2) = \frac{1 - \gamma}{\gamma} \mu_1(t_1) \mu_2(t_2) \left((-\ln S_1(t_1))^{\frac{1}{\gamma}} + (-\ln S_2(t_2))^{\frac{1}{\gamma}}\right)^{\gamma - 2}$$
$$\times (-\ln S_1(t_1))^{\frac{1}{\gamma} - 1} (-\ln S_2(t_2))^{\frac{1}{\gamma} - 1}.$$

The same extension holds also in the more general case of the compound Poisson model, including the gamma and the inverse Gaussian model as special cases. Starting with the copula of the shared compound Poisson frailty model (4.8), the copula of the correlated compound Poisson frailty model (5.14) is obtained by applying relation (6.6):

$$\tilde{S}(t_1, t_2) = S_1(t_1)^{1-\rho} S_2(t_2)^{1-\rho}$$
$$\times \exp\left[\frac{\rho(1 - \gamma)}{\gamma\sigma^2}\left(1 - \left((1 - \frac{\gamma\sigma^2}{1 - \gamma} \ln S_1(t_1))^{\frac{1}{\gamma}} + (1 - \frac{\gamma\sigma^2}{1 - \gamma} \ln S_2(t_2))^{\frac{1}{\gamma}} - 1\right)^{\gamma}\right)\right]$$

and association function

$$\phi(t_1, t_2)$$

$$= \sigma^2 \mu_1(t_1) \mu_2(t_2) \left(\left(1 - \frac{\gamma\sigma^2}{1-\gamma} \ln S_1(t_1)\right)^{\frac{1}{\gamma}} + \left(1 - \frac{\gamma\sigma^2}{1-\gamma} \ln S_2(t_2)\right)^{\frac{1}{\gamma}} - 1 \right)^{\gamma-2}$$

$$\times \left(1 - \frac{\gamma\sigma^2}{1-\gamma} \ln S_1(t_1)\right)^{\frac{1}{\gamma}-1} \left(1 - \frac{\gamma\sigma^2}{1-\gamma} \ln S_2(t_2)\right)^{\frac{1}{\gamma}-1}.$$

The following theorem extends the general copula model considered previously to the case of negative ρ, resulting in negative association between survival times in a cluster.

THEOREM 6.2

(Yashin and Iachine 1999a) Let the conditions of Theorem 6.1 hold. Then, for any ρ satisfying

$$\max_{t_1, t_2} \left(-\frac{\mu_1(t_1)\mu_2(t_2)}{\phi(t_1, t_2)} \right) < \rho < 0, \qquad (6.10)$$

the function $\tilde{S}(t_1, t_2)$ given by (6.6) determines a bivariate distribution of negatively correlated survival times.

Proof: Note that for any $\rho < 0$, we have

$$\big((\rho - 1)\mu_1(t_1) - \rho\mu_1(t_1, t_2)\big)\big((\rho - 1)\mu_2(t_2) - \rho\mu_2(t_1, t_2)\big) \geq \mu_1(t_1)\mu_2(t_2) \geq 0$$

because of $\mu_i(t_i) \geq \mu_i(t_1, t_2)$ due to $\phi(t_1, t_2) \geq 0$, and hence, (6.8) yields

$$\tilde{S}_{t_1 t_2}(t_1, t_2) \geq \tilde{S}(t_1, t_2)\big[\mu_1(t_1)\mu_2(t_2) + \rho\phi(t_1, t_2)\big]$$

Thus, $\tilde{S}_{t_1 t_2}(t_1, t_2)$ is nonnegative when ρ satisfies (6.10). The covariance of $\tilde{T}_1$, $\tilde{T}_2$ is

$$\mathbf{cov}(\tilde{T}_1, \tilde{T}_2) = \int_0^\infty \int_0^\infty \tilde{S}(u, v)\, du\, dv - \int_0^\infty \int_0^\infty S_1(u) S_2(v)\, du\, dv.$$

Using representation (6.6) for $\tilde{S}(t_1, t_2)$, we get

$$\mathbf{cov}(\tilde{T}_1, \tilde{T}_2) = \int_0^\infty \int_0^\infty S_1(u) S_2(v)(e^{\rho A(u,v)} - 1)\, du\, dv.$$

So, if $A(u, v) > 0$, then the sign of $\mathbf{cov}(\tilde{T}_1, \tilde{T}_2)$ coincides with the sign of ρ. This completes the proof. ∎

The extension of the copula model to negative values of ρ is important for several reasons. For example, negatively correlated lifespans are of interest in the situation of dependent competing risks such as competing causes of death in medical applications. Another aspect is testing of hypotheses. When ρ is considered as an association parameter (similar to the frailty model), researchers are frequently interested in testing the null hypothesis $H_0 : \rho = 0$ versus the alternative $H_A : \rho > 0$ about the independence of the lifetimes. By extending the model to $\rho < 0$, the point $\rho = 0$ becomes an internal point of the parameter space, and standard test theory for the likelihood ratio test can be applied, simplifying the analysis. In the following we consider condition (6.10) in more detail for the correlated gamma, positive stable, and the compound Poisson/PVF copulas. For the correlated gamma frailty copula model, relation (6.10) becomes

$$\max_{t_1,t_2} \left(- \frac{\mu_1(t_1)\mu_2(t_2)}{\phi(t_1,t_2)} \right) = \max_{t_1,t_2} \left(- \frac{\left(S_1(t_1)^{-\sigma^2} + S_2(t_2)^{-\sigma^2} - 1\right)^2}{\sigma^2 S_1(t_1)^{-\sigma^2} S_2(t_2)^{-\sigma^2}} \right) = \frac{-1}{\sigma^2}$$

by using (6.9). If σ^2 is smaller than one, the parameter ρ can take on all values between -1 and 1. In the correlated positive stable copula, it turns out that

$$\max_{t_1,t_2} \left(- \frac{\mu_1(t_1)\mu_2(t_2)}{\phi(t_1,t_2)} \right)$$
$$= \max_{t_1,t_2} \left(- \frac{\gamma\left(\left(-\ln S_1(t_1)\right)^{\frac{1}{\gamma}} + \left(-\ln S_2(t_2)\right)^{\frac{1}{\gamma}}\right)^{2-\gamma}}{(1-\gamma)\left(-\ln S_1(t_1)\right)^{\frac{1}{\gamma}-1}\left(-\ln S_2(t_2)\right)^{\frac{1}{\gamma}-1}} \right) = 0,$$

meaning that the correlated positive stable copula cannot be extended to negative values of ρ. In the general compound Poisson frailty model, it holds that

$$\max_{t_1,t_2} \left(- \frac{\mu_1(t_1)\mu_2(t_2)}{\phi(t_1,t_2)} \right)$$
$$= \max_{t_1,t_2} \left(- \frac{\left(\left(1 - \frac{\gamma\sigma^2}{1-\gamma}\ln S_1(t_1)\right)^{\frac{1}{\gamma}} + \left(1 - \frac{\gamma\sigma^2}{1-\gamma}\ln S_2(t_2)\right)^{\frac{1}{\gamma}} - 1\right)^{2-\gamma}}{\sigma^2\left(1 - \frac{\gamma\sigma^2}{1-\gamma}\ln S_1(t_1)\right)^{\frac{1}{\gamma}-1}\left(1 - \frac{\gamma\sigma^2}{1-\gamma}\ln S_2(t_2)\right)^{\frac{1}{\gamma}-1}} \right) = \frac{-1}{\sigma^2},$$

giving the same result as in the correlated gamma copula model.

6.4 Cross-Ratio Function

A measure of local dependence in dependent event times describing changes over time is the cross-ratio function introduced by Clayton (1978)

$$\theta(t_1, t_2) = \frac{\mu(t_1|T_2 = t_2)}{\mu(t_1|T_2 > t_2)}.$$

This expression has a nice interpretation. For twins considered as example through the last chapter, the ratio compares the hazard of the first partner to experience the event at time t_1, given that the second partner experiences the event at time t_2, to the hazard of the first partner at time t_1, given that the second partner experience the event later than time t_2. It is often helpful to write the cross-ratio function in terms of the survival function and their derivatives (Oakes 1989):

$$\theta(t_1, t_2) = \frac{S(t_1, t_2)S_{t_1 t_2}(t_1, t_2)}{S_{t_1}(t_1, t_2)S_{t_2}(t_1, t_2)}. \tag{6.11}$$

It should be noted that the cross-ratio function in the shared frailty model depends on t_1 and t_2 only through the joint survival function $S(t_1, t_2)$ because it is an Archimedean copula (Duchateau and Janssen 2008). The copula of the correlated gamma frailty model is not an Archimedean copula and their cross-ratio function can therefore not be represented as a function of $S(t_1, t_2)$. In the following we calculate the cross-ratio for the correlated gamma copula. The derivatives needed are provided in Appendix A.2. First we consider the numerator.

$$
\begin{aligned}
&S(t_1, t_2)S_{t_1 t_2}(t_1, t_2) \\
&= S(t_1)^{1-\rho}S(t_2)^{1-\rho}(S(t_1)^{-\sigma^2} + S(t_2)^{-\sigma^2} - 1)^{-\frac{\rho}{\sigma^2}} \\
&\quad \times S(t_1)^{-\rho}f(t_1)S(t_2)^{-\rho}f(t_2)(S(t_1)^{-\sigma^2} + S(t_2)^{-\sigma^2} - 1)^{-\frac{\rho}{\sigma^2}-2} \\
&\quad \times \left((1-\rho)^2(S(t_1)^{-\sigma^2} + S(t_2)^{-\sigma^2} - 1)^2 \right. \\
&\quad + (1-\rho)\rho S(t_2)^{-\sigma^2}(S(t_1)^{-\sigma^2} + S(t_2)^{-\sigma^2} - 1) \\
&\quad + (1-\rho)\rho S(t_1)^{-\sigma^2}(S(t_1)^{-\sigma^2} + S(t_2)^{-\sigma^2} - 1) + \rho(\rho+\sigma^2)S(t_1)^{-\sigma^2}S(t_2)^{-\sigma^2}\Big) \\
&= S(t_1)^{1-\rho}S(t_2)^{1-\rho}(S(t_1)^{-\sigma^2} + S(t_2)^{-\sigma^2} - 1)^{-\frac{\rho}{\sigma^2}} \\
&\quad \times S(t_1)^{-\rho}f(t_1)S(t_2)^{-\rho}f(t_2)(S(t_1)^{-\sigma^2} + S(t_2)^{-\sigma^2} - 1)^{-\frac{\rho}{\sigma^2}-2} \\
&\quad \times \left(\big((1-\rho)(S(t_1)^{-\sigma^2} + S(t_2)^{-\sigma^2} - 1) + \rho S(t_1)^{-\sigma^2}\big)\right. \\
&\quad \times \big((1-\rho)(S(t_1)^{-\sigma^2} + S(t_2)^{-\sigma^2} - 1) + \rho S(t_2)^{-\sigma^2}\big) + \rho\sigma^2 S(t_1)^{-\sigma^2}S(t_2)^{-\sigma^2}\Big).
\end{aligned}
$$

The denominator of the cross-ratio function is given by

$$
\begin{aligned}
S_{t_1}(t_1, t_2)S_{t_2}(t_1, t_2) &= S(t_1)^{-\rho}f(t_1)S(t_2)^{1-\rho}(S(t_1)^{-\sigma^2} + S(t_2)^{-\sigma^2} - 1)^{-\frac{\rho}{\sigma^2}-1} \\
&\times \big(- S(t_1)^{-\sigma^2} - (1-\rho)S(t_2)^{-\sigma^2} + (1-\rho) \big) \\
&\times S(t_1)^{1-\rho}S(t_2)^{-\rho}f(t_2)(S(t_1)^{-\sigma^2} + S(t_2)^{-\sigma^2} - 1)^{-\frac{\rho}{\sigma^2}-1} \\
&\times \big(- (1-\rho)S(t_1)^{-\sigma^2} - S(t_2)^{-\sigma^2} + (1-\rho) \big) \\
&= S(t_1)^{-\rho}f(t_1)S(t_2)^{1-\rho}(S(t_1)^{-\sigma^2} + S(t_2)^{-\sigma^2} - 1)^{-\frac{\rho}{\sigma^2}-1} \\
&\times S(t_1)^{1-\rho}S(t_2)^{-\rho}f(t_2)(S(t_1)^{-\sigma^2} + S(t_2)^{-\sigma^2} - 1)^{-\frac{\rho}{\sigma^2}-1} \\
&\times \big((1-\rho)(S(t_1)^{-\sigma^2} + S(t_2)^{-\sigma^2} - 1) + \rho S(t_1)^{-\sigma^2}\big) \\
&\times \big((1-\rho)(S(t_1)^{-\sigma^2} + S(t_2)^{-\sigma^2} - 1) + \rho S(t_2)^{-\sigma^2}\big).
\end{aligned}
$$

Using the preceding expressions the cross-ratio function (6.11) of the correlated gamma copula can be obtained as

$$
\theta(t_1, t_2) =
$$

$$
1 + \frac{\rho\sigma^2 S(t_1)^{-\sigma^2} S(t_2)^{-\sigma^2}}{\big((1-\rho)(S(t_2)^{-\sigma^2} - 1) + S(t_1)^{-\sigma^2}\big)\big((1-\rho)(S(t_1)^{-\sigma^2} - 1) + S(t_2)^{-\sigma^2}\big)}.
$$

In the following we consider some interesting special cases. At the beginning of the follow-up for both individuals, the cross-ratio function simplifies to the expression $\theta(0, 0) = 1 + \rho\sigma^2$. In the case of the shared gamma copula it holds $\rho = 1$, and we obtain the well-known time-independent cross-ratio function $\theta(t_1, t_2) = 1 + \sigma^2$ (compare with relation (6.3)). If times converge to infinity, it holds that

$$
\lim_{t_1 \to \infty} \theta(t_1, t_2) = \lim_{t_2 \to \infty} \theta(t_1, t_2) = 1
$$

and

$$
\lim_{t_1, t_2 \to \infty} \theta(t_1, t_2) = 1 + \frac{\rho\sigma^2}{(2-\rho)^2}.
$$

For $\rho = 0$, the two lifetimes are independent, indicated by $\theta(t_1, t_2) = 1$. The cross-ratio function of the correlated compound Poisson copula can be obtained in a similar way (the derivation is not shown here) by using the shorthands $a(t_1) = 1 - \frac{\gamma\sigma^2}{1-\gamma} \ln S(t_1)$ and $a(t_2) = 1 - \frac{\gamma\sigma^2}{1-\gamma} \ln S(t_2)$:

$$\theta(t_1, t_2) =$$

$$1 + \frac{\rho \sigma^2 a(t_1)^{1/\gamma - 1}(a(t_1)^{1/\gamma} + a(t_2)^{1/\gamma} - 1)^\gamma}{(1 - \rho)(a(t_1)^{1/\gamma} + a(t_2)^{1/\gamma} - 1) + \rho a(t_1)^{1/\gamma - 1}(a(t_1)^{1/\gamma} + a(t_2)^{1/\gamma} - 1)^\gamma}$$

$$\times \frac{a(t_2)^{1/\gamma - 1}}{(1 - \rho)(a(t_1)^{1/\gamma} + a(t_2)^{1/\gamma} - 1) + \rho a(t_2)^{1/\gamma - 1}(a(t_1)^{1/\gamma} + a(t_2)^{1/\gamma} - 1)^\gamma}.$$

With the shared compound Poisson copula obtained by $\rho = 1$, this expression simplifies to

$$\theta(t_1, t_2) = 1 + \frac{\sigma^2}{(a(t_1)^{1/\gamma} + a(t_2)^{1/\gamma} - 1)^\gamma}$$

(see Duchateau and Janssen 2008). The gamma model is obtained as limiting case for $\gamma \to 0$. It turns out that $a_j^{1/\gamma - 1} \to S(t_j)^{-\sigma^2}$ and $a_j^{1/\gamma} \to S(t_j)^{-\sigma^2}$ ($j = 1, 2$). Furthermore, it holds $(a(t_1)^{1/\gamma} + a(t_2)^{1/\gamma} - 1)^\gamma \to 1$. Consequently,

$$\theta(t_1, t_2)$$

$$= 1 + \frac{\rho \sigma^2 a(t_1)^{1/\gamma - 1}(a(t_1)^{1/\gamma} + a(t_2)^{1/\gamma} - 1)^\gamma}{(1 - \rho)(a(t_1)^{1/\gamma} + a(t_2)^{1/\gamma} - 1) + \rho a(t_1)^{1/\gamma - 1}(a(t_1)^{1/\gamma} + a(t_2)^{1/\gamma} - 1)^\gamma}$$

$$\times \frac{a(t_2)^{1/\gamma - 1}}{(1 - \rho)(a(t_1)^{1/\gamma} + a(t_2)^{1/\gamma} - 1) + \rho a(t_2)^{1/\gamma - 1}(a(t_1)^{1/\gamma} + a(t_2)^{1/\gamma} - 1)^\gamma}$$

$$\to 1 + \frac{\rho \sigma^2 S(t_1)^{-\sigma^2}}{(1 - \rho)(S(t_1)^{-\sigma^2} + S(t_2)^{-\sigma^2} - 1) + \rho S(t_1)^{-\sigma^2}}$$

$$\times \frac{S(t_2)^{-\sigma^2}}{(1 - \rho)(S(t_1)^{-\sigma^2} + S(t_2)^{-\sigma^2} - 1) + \rho S(t_2)^{-\sigma^2}}$$

$$= 1 + \frac{\rho \sigma^2 S(t_1)^{-\sigma^2} S(t_2)^{-\sigma^2}}{\left((1 - \rho)(S(t_2)^{-\sigma^2} - 1) + S(t_1)^{-\sigma^2}\right)\left((1 - \rho)(S(t_1)^{-\sigma^2} - 1) + S(t_2)^{-\sigma^2}\right)}$$

The cross-ratio function at the beginning of the follow-up for both individuals is $\theta(0, 0) = 1 + \rho \sigma^2$. In the case $\rho = 0$, the two lifetimes are independent.

Chapter 7

Different Aspects of Frailty Modeling

This chapter presents a nonsystematic collection of problems related to very different types of mainly nonstandard frailty models in various applications not covered in the preceding chapters. Most of the problems are not treated in detail here; they are just mentioned and shortly discussed. Additionally, references are given for further reading.

7.1 Dependence and Interaction between Frailty and Observed Covariates

Nearly all contributions and applications on frailty models in a regression setting like (3.2) consider the unobserved frailty variable Z as independent of the observed explanatory variables $\mathbf{X}$. This assumption is usually made only for mathematical convenience. Of course, in some cases this independence assumption could be inappropriate. In the case of competing risk models, di Serio (1997) analyzed this question to explain the effect of unexpected protectivity. This problem occurs when a covariate shows a protective impact not expected from a medical point of view. A simulation study was conducted by di Serio (1997) in a two competing risks scenario with two frailties. Each frailty is related to one of the competing events. It turns out that dependence between the two frailties alone does not cause false protectivity; conversely, false protectivity may occur according to the magnitude and the sign of the dependence between frailty and the observed covariate. Here, dependence between the two frailties implies dependence of the two competing event times, resulting in a univariate lifetime model with dependence between lifetimes and censoring times. The problem is that an assumption about the distribution of frailty is not enough since what we need are actually nontestable assumptions about the direction and the intensity of the dependence between frailty and the observable covariates, which makes the data analysis quite arbitrary. Thus, survival models where the observed covariates depend on unobserved random effects may not be identifiable from univariate survival data without additional assumptions.

It turns out that such models can be identified from bivariate (multivariate) data when they are embedded into a frailty model by using the relation

$$\sigma(X) = \sigma e^{\gamma X},$$

where γ is a parameter to be estimated, and σ^2 denotes the variance of the frailty Z. Thus, the distribution of Z (or more specifically, its variance) depends on the observed covariate values X. An example of such models in the multivariate case can be found in Wassell and Moeschberger (1993), who have studied the impact of interventions in the Framingham Heart Study by introducing their concept of modified gamma frailty. Yashin et al. (1999b) have investigated the heritability of susceptibility to death after accounting for the dependence between frailty and observed covariates (BMI and smoking) in Danish twins. Noh et al. (2006) suggested the notion of dispersed frailty for such kind of models and applied them to the well-known kidney infection data from McGilchrist and Aisbett (1991) to verify the hypothesis of heterogeneity in frailty distribution in the study population.

Several authors have considered the problem of unobserved heterogeneity caused by omitted covariates in randomized clinical trials. However, usually no interaction between the omitted covariate and the binary treatment variable is allowed. Exceptions are the papers by Li et al. (2002) and Xu (2004).

Li et al. (2002) considered asymptotic relative efficiency and power of the log-rank test in models with an interaction between normally distributed random effects W_i and a binary covariate X_i (for example, representing the treatment effect in a randomized trial) in a univariate model:

$$\mu(t|X_i, W_i) = \mu_0(t)e^{\beta X_i + W_i + \alpha W_i X_i}. \tag{7.1}$$

The interaction of the frailty term with observed covariates is incorporated on the same scale as the fixed effects. This model is flexible in the sense that the test on interaction can be based on the parameter α, whereas the test on unobserved heterogeneity is based on the variance parameter of the random effects.

Xu (2004) discussed a multivariate survival model with normal distributed random effects. As an example, for a multicenter trial, if a binary covariate X_{ij} indicates one of two treatment assignments for individual j in center i, the following model can be used to capture center-specific treatment effects:

$$\mu(t|X_{ij}, W_i) = \mu_0(t)e^{\beta X_{ij} + W_i X_{ij}}, \tag{7.2}$$

with W_i denoting the additional random treatment effects specific to the ith center, assumed to follow a normal distribution with zero expectation and some unknown variance. The proposed MCEM algorithm allows estimating the random effects, which could be, for example, used to rank the centers with respect to their treatment success.

Some research efforts have been undertaken to study extensions of the shared frailty approach to more general models allowing, for example, for interaction between treatment and center in a multicenter clinical trial (Yamaguchi and Ohashi 1999, Vaida and Xu 2000, Legrand et al. 2005, 2006, Massonnet et al. 2008) or interaction between treatment and study in a meta-analysis with event time outcome (Rondeau et al. 2008). The hazard function in this model is

$$\mu(t|\mathbf{X}_{ij}, \mathbf{W}_i) = \mu_0(t)e^{\boldsymbol{\beta}'\mathbf{X}_{ij}+W_{0i}+W_{1i}X_{ij1}}, \tag{7.3}$$

with $\mathbf{W}_i' = (W_{0i}, W_{1i})$, where W_{0i} denotes the shared random effect and $W_{1i}X_{ij1}$ the random interaction term with covariate X_{ij1}, which could be, for example, a binary treatment variable. Here, the covariate X_{ij1} is usually a component of the vector $\mathbf{X}_{ij}$. The random effects W_{0i} and W_{1i} are assumed to follow a bivariate Gaussian distribution with

$$\begin{pmatrix} W_{0i} \\ W_{1i} \end{pmatrix} \sim \mathrm{N}\left(\begin{pmatrix} 0 \\ 0 \end{pmatrix}, \begin{pmatrix} \sigma_0^2 & \rho\sigma_0\sigma_1 \\ \rho\sigma_0\sigma_1 & \sigma_1^2 \end{pmatrix} \right).$$

There are two sources of heterogeneity between clusters included in the model. First, heterogeneity between clusters may arises from the treatment itself, meaning the treatment is stronger in some clusters than in others. Such treatment by center interaction may reflect unobserved differences in patient characteristics and in implementation of the study protocol. This is accounted for by the random interaction between treatment and cluster. Second, the variation in outcomes between clusters may be attributed to differences in the baseline hazards reflecting, for example, differences in medical practices or in patient populations. Such kind of heterogeneity can be accounted for by the shared frailty term in the random effects model. A similar model based on the AFT approach can be found in Komárek et al. (2007).

This model was considered with independent random effects by several authors. It can be estimated by using an extension of the REML approach suggested by McGilchrist (1993) to accommodate for two random effects (Yamaguchi and Ohashi 1999). Vaida and Xu (2000) used a Monte Carlo EM algorithm with MCMC sampling in the E step. Legrand et al. (2005, 2006) proposed a Bayesian approach.

Ripatti and Palmgren (2000) used the penalized partial likelihood approach combined with a Laplace approximation in a model with dependent random effects. Massonnet et al. (2008) applied a transformation technique to estimate the parameters in this model. Rondeau et al. (2008) suggested a penalized marginal likelihood method, resulting in smoothed estimates of the hazard function. Allowing for a possible correlation between the two random effects, the heterogeneity of the baseline hazard between clusters may depend on the heterogeneity of the treatment effect. This seems to be reasonable because the treatment effect is usually expected to be larger in clusters with high baseline hazard, and vice versa.

7.2 Cox Model with General Gaussian Random Effects

A very general and flexible survival model with Gaussian random effects is considered by Vaida and Xu (2000), and Ripatti and Palmgren (2000). The model is given in terms of the conditional hazard

$$\mu(t|\mathbf{X}_{ij}, \mathbf{W}_i) = \mu_0(t)e^{\boldsymbol{\beta}'\mathbf{X}_{ij}+\mathbf{Y}'_{ij}\mathbf{W}_i}, \tag{7.4}$$

where $\mathbf{X}_{ij}$ and $\mathbf{Y}_{ij}$ denote the covariate vectors for the fixed and random effects. $\mathbf{W}_i$ is the random effect from the ith cluster. The random effects are assumed to follow a Gaussian distribution with expectation vector zero and some covariance matrix. Vaida and Xu (2000) considered the case of diagonal covariance matrices, resulting in independent random effects. In (7.4) $\mathbf{Y}_{ij}$ is often a subset of $\mathbf{X}_{ij}$, apart from possibly an "1" which represents the cluster effect on the baseline. For a better understanding, assume for a moment that $\mathbf{Y}'_{ij} = (1, \mathbf{X}_{ij})$ and $\mathbf{W}'_i = (W_{0i}, \mathbf{W}_{1i})$. Each component of $\mathbf{W}_{1i}$ represents the interaction between the cluster and the respective covariate, while the corresponding element of the parameter vector $\boldsymbol{\beta}$ represents the main effect of the covariate. W_{0i} is the random effect shared by all individuals in the ith cluster. Vaida and Xu (2000) obtain maximum likelihood estimates of the regression parameters, the variances of the random effects, and the baseline hazard function via a modified EM algorithm. In the E step, MCMC methods are used for the calculation of conditional expectations of functions of the random effects. Ripatti and Palmgren (2000) used Laplace approximation of the likelihood function in combination with a penalized partial likelihood approach, where the marginal distribution of the random effects determines the penalty term.

The flexibility of the above model is demonstrated best by discussing some of its interesting submodels. The univariate model by Li et al. (2002) given in (7.1) with parameter specification $\alpha = 1$ is a special case of this model with cluster size one, $\mathbf{Y}'_{ij} = (1, X_i)$, $\mathbf{W}'_i = (W_i, W_i)$, and $\mathbf{X}_{ij} = X_i$ as a binary covariate. The univariate log-normal frailty model with general covariates is obtained with cluster size one, $\mathbf{Y}_{ij} = 1$, and a one-dimensional random effect W_i. Furthermore, the model considered by Xu (2004) and specified in (7.2) is a special case with $\mathbf{Y}_{ij} = X_{ij}$, $\mathbf{W}_i$ as a one-dimensional random effect, and X_{ij} as a binary variable. The above model simplifies to the shared log-normal frailty model with $Y_{ij} = 1$ and a one-dimensional random effect $\mathbf{W}_i$. Furthermore, the interaction model (7.3) considered in the last section is a submodel via $\mathbf{Y}'_{ij} = (1, X_{ij1})$ and $\mathbf{W}'_i = (W_{0i}, W_{1i})$.

In the following section, nested (hierarchical) frailty models are considered. It is necessary to note that nested frailty models in general are not included in model class (7.4).

7.3 Nested Frailty Models

The shared frailty model is often used to model clustered survival data when the compound symmetry assumption seems appropriate. Multilevel clustered failure time data arise when the clustering of data occurs at more than one level. In studies about the relationship between environmental factors such as air pollution and mortality, for example, individuals are grouped in cities, and furthermore, in subclusters like districts. The hypothesis of independent observations is questionable in this setting, so a flexible survival model with two nested random effects at city and district level seems appropriate. Other fields of application are multicenter studies with recurrent events, where center is one cluster level and patients form the nested subclusters. Ignoring the additional subgroups may invalidate the results of data analysis. Thus, nested frailty models are of interest in problems in which data are naturally clustered at different hierarchical levels (e.g., families in different cities), or generated by a hierarchical sampling design (e.g., districts in cities). Sastry (1997) suggested a nested frailty model with two hierarchical levels

$$\mu(t|\mathbf{X}_{ijk}, Z_i, Z_{ij}) = Z_i Z_{ij} \mu_0(t) e^{\boldsymbol{\beta}' \mathbf{X}_{ijk}}, \tag{7.5}$$

where $\mathbf{X}_{ijk}$ denotes the covariate vector of the kth individual in the jth subcluster belonging to the ith cluster. Frailty Z_i denotes the cluster-specific random effect, and Z_{ij} is the subcluster-specific random effect. Both Z_i and Z_{ij} are independent gamma-distributed random variables with mean one and variances σ_1^2 and σ_2^2, respectively.

Nested frailty models account for the hierarchical clustering by including cluster-level-specific random effects. However, the extension of the estimation procedures of the shared frailty model to the case of two or more frailty terms is difficult. Sastry (1997) first adapted the EM algorithm to the nested frailty model. Manda (2001) used Bayesian methods in a nested gamma frailty model with piecewise constant baseline hazard. Rondeau et al. (2006) applied a semiparametric maximum penalized likelihood estimation procedure to model (7.5), which provides as a by-product a smooth estimator of the hazard function.

More complicated nested frailty models allowing for dependence between the cluster and subcluster-specific frailties are considered by Ma et al. (2003) using a Poisson modeling approach, and by Shih and Lu (2009). Yau (2001) suggested a nested log-normal frailty model of the type

$$\mu(t|\mathbf{X}_{ijk}, W_i, W_{ij}) = \mu_0(t) e^{\boldsymbol{\beta}' \mathbf{X}_{ijk} + W_i + W_{ij}} \tag{7.6}$$

with similar notation as above. W_i, W_{ij} are independent normally distributed random effects with mean zero and variances s_1^2 and s_2^2, respectively.

7.4   Recurrent Event Time Data

Up to now, in all cases were parallel event times considered. However, one important field for application of frailty models is the analysis of recurrent event time data. A common feature of recurrent event time data is that the events are naturally ordered and occur in a certain sequence over time. Reviews of models for recurrence data appeared recently in Cook und Lawless (2007) and Finkelstein (2008) with links to the field of reliability. However, there is a growing interest in models for recurrence data in other fields also. Medical examples of such data include cancer recurrences, asthma attacks, infections, admissions to hospital, and headaches. To analyze such type of data, many researchers estimate and compare event rates using the chi-square test or event times until the occurrence of the first event, or the overall event time using the Cox model. Such conventional methods are inefficient because they use only parts of the available information in the data. If data have repeated events with censored event times in longitudinal studies, complex analytic approaches are needed to obtain accurate estimates and efficient inferences. These models allow the use of all available information to accurately estimate the relative risk of recurrence. We will not go into much detail, but would like to mention the most common approaches. Therneau and Grambsch (2000) distinguishes three categories: independent increment, marginal, and conditional models. In all models, observations from one individual are grouped to one cluster. The main difference between models is the definition of risk sets and stratification of the baseline hazard function.

Andersen et al. (1982) proposed a model assuming independent increments. Here, individuals are assumed to be under risk for all their events until censoring. The baseline hazard is not stratified. This means that the risk of an event is unaffected by the occurrence of any previous event. The numbers of events in disjoint time interval are independent. For a parametric baseline hazard, this model is equivalent to the nonhomogeneous Poisson process. As an alternative, the gap times between events can be considered. Assuming that these times are independent and identically distributed, and the baseline hazard is parametric, the model reduces to a renewal process with covariates.

The well-known marginal model was introduced by Wei et al. (1989). All individuals are assumed to be under risk for a future event until the occurrence of this event or censoring. The baseline hazards may be stratified with respect to the event number. To account for correlation between the observed events, the variance is adjusted without explicitly modeling the correlation. As with the analysis of longitudinal data, regression parameters are estimated from generalized estimating equations, and the corresponding variance–covariance estimators are corrected properly to account for the dependence structure. An excellent review of the robust and well-developed marginal approach is given in Lin (1994).

The model introduced by Prentice et al. (1981) measures the conditional risk of experiencing an event. An individual is only at risk for an event from the occurrence of the previous event until the occurrence of this event or censoring. Therefore, an event-specific baseline hazard is assumed. In general, the model by Prentice et al. (1981) is approximating the real situation best.

In the models by Prentice et al. (1981) and Wei et al. (1989), in-subject correlation is accounted for through stratification of the baseline hazard. In the Andersen–Gill model, independent increments are assumed. All models can be expanded to allow for between-subject correlation. As proposed by McGilchrist (1991), a subject-specific frailty term can be used in the hazard. For all observations belonging to one subject, the same frailty term is used. The frailty variables of different subjects are independent realizations of a common frailty distribution.

Duchateau et al. (2003) applied different parametric and nonparametric models, both with and without frailty, to recurrent asthma events from an asthma prevention trial in young children. One problem, however, is the decision about the time scale to use. In the gap-time approach, only the time until the occurrence of the last event is considered. An alternative time scale is total time, measuring the time from the beginning of follow-up, disregarding other events having occurred meanwhile.

Frailty models specially designed for recurrence data are considered in detail by Aalen et al. (1995), McGilchrist and Yau (1996), Yau and McGilchrist (1998), and Manda and Meyer (2005). An overview in the field is given in Duchateau et al. (2003) and Lim et al. (2007).

The observation of recurrent event times could usually be terminated by loss to follow-up, end of study, or a terminal event such as death. In the analysis of recurrent even times discussed above, the assumption of noninformative censoring of the recurrent event process by death is made, which can be violated. For example, the recurrence of serious events, such as tumors or opportunistic infections, is often associated with an increased risk of death. To circumvent this problem, joint frailty models provide a useful alternative. Here, the recurrent event hazard and the death hazard are modeled separately but share some random effect, causing dependence between the recurrent event times and the lifetime. The model can be specified by the hazard functions

$$\mu_1(t|\mathbf{X}_{i1}, Z_i) = Z_i \mu_{01}(t) e^{\boldsymbol{\beta}_1' \mathbf{X}_{i1}} \tag{7.7}$$

$$\mu_2(t|\mathbf{X}_{i2}, Z_i) = Z_i^\gamma \mu_{02}(t) e^{\boldsymbol{\beta}_2' \mathbf{X}_{i2}}, \tag{7.8}$$

where μ_1 denotes the hazard of the recurrent events and μ_2 is the hazard of the terminal event. When $\gamma = 0$, then μ_2 does not depend on the frailty and is independent of the recurrent event times. If the frailty distribution is degenerated, there is no unobserved heterogeneity in the data, and the recurrent event times become independent. Liu et al. (2004) and Rondeau et al. (2007) assume a gamma distribution of the frailty.

7.5 Tests for Heterogeneity

In the practical application of methods from survival analysis, the researcher is usually confronted with the question of whether unobserved heterogeneity is present in the data or not. For this problem a number of tests of heterogeneity have been proposed during the last 15 years. The relevant testing problem for the null hypothesis of no unobserved heterogeneity is $H_0 : \sigma^2 = 0$ versus $H_A : \sigma^2 > 0$, where σ^2 denotes the frailty variance (unobserved heterogeneity). For ease of presentation, the case of infinite moments of the frailty distribution (positive stable distribution) is excluded here. In this situation, a one-sided testing hypothesis is natural. The main problem is that the heterogeneity parameter lays on the boundary of its parameter space under H_0, and the classical likelihood ratio asymptotic distribution theory is no longer valid. It turns out that, in many cases, the likelihood ratio statistic has an asymptotic distribution under the null hypothesis, which is an equal mixture of a point mass at zero and a chi-square distribution with one degree of freedom, often denoted by $0.5\,\chi_0^2 + 0.5\,\chi_1^2$. Rigourously established limiting distributions of the likelihood ratio test statistic are provided by Maller and Zhou (2003) and Claeskens et al. (2008). Other generally more applied results about tests for heterogeneity in survival data can be found in Oakes (1982), Blossfeld and Hamerle (1989, 1992), Hamerle (1992), Commenges and Andersen (1995), Gray (1995), Commenges and Jacqmin-Gadda (1997), Verweij et al. (1998), Bordes and Commenges (2001), Dunson and Chen (2004), and Dominicus et al. (2006).

Andersen et al. (1999) used the test suggested by Commenges and Andersen (1995) and found advantages of the mixed model when compared with the fixed-effects model, especially in the case where it is known to which subgroup the individuals belong if the number of subgroups in the total population is large and the number of individuals in each subgroup is only moderate. They applied the test to a multicenter clinical trial with survival outcome.

A test procedure for proportional hazards in the presence of unobserved heterogeneity is suggested by McCall (1994). Kimber and Zhu (1999) consider the situation where the conditional lifetimes are Weibull, and frailty follows a (shared) positive stable model. For this very specific situation, simple tests for frailty are proposed. Kimber (1996) already considered the case of gamma-distributed frailty and Weibull baseline.

A pseudo likelihood ratio test is proposed by Glidden (2000) and Andersen (2005) to test the assumption regarding heterogeneity distribution. In PVF frailty models, the gamma frailty model and the positive stable frailty model are at the boundary of the parameter space. Therefore, as discussed in Andersen (2005), the classical likelihood ratio test is not valid. Andersen (2005) gives the asymptotic distribution for the pseudo likelihood ratio test (but without rigorous proof).

7.6 Log-Rank Test in Frailty Models

In analyzing time-to-event data of two (or more) groups with the log-rank test, a proportional hazards model is usually assumed. Nevertheless, this hypothesis is no longer valid in the case of unobserved covariates. Omission of a balanced covariate from a proportional hazards model generally leads to a model with nonproportional hazards. As a consequence, the simple log-rank test is no longer optimal. A general treatment of this problem is given in Oakes and Jeong (1998). The authors establish connections between theories of weighted log-rank tests and of frailty models, and analyze parametric as well as nonparametric models. Furthermore, the authors consider different frailty distributions: positive stable, inverse Gaussian, gamma, and two-point distribution and the models are extended to include random censoring. The optimal limiting weight function is

$$w(t) = 1 + M_0(t)\left(\frac{\mathbf{L}''(M_0(t))}{\mathbf{L}'(M_0(t))} - \frac{\mathbf{L}'(M_0(t))}{\mathbf{L}(M_0(t))}\right),$$

where $\mathbf{L}'$ and $\mathbf{L}''$ are the first and second derivative of the Laplace transform $\mathbf{L}$ of the frailty distribution. For example, in the gamma frailty model, Oakes and Jeong (1998) derived the expression

$$w(t) = (1 + \sigma^2 M_0(t))^{-1}$$

(corrected for an error in their formula and translated to our notation). The asymptotic relative efficiency of the simple log-rank test and of the optimally weighted log-rank test relative to the adjusted test that would be used if the covariate values were known are given in terms of the Laplace transform of the frailty distributions. These frailties represent the effect of the missing covariates. Two main conclusions are derived by Oakes and Jeong (1998) from their analysis. First, the loss of efficiency from omitting a covariate is generally more important than the additional loss due to the misspecification of the resulting nonproportional hazards model. Furthermore, the loss of efficiency increases in general with higher variance of the frailty distribution. However, binary frailty distributions can provide exceptions to this rule, reflecting the fact that, for a very extreme frailty distribution, one can identify the values of the frailties from the ordering of the failures; the individuals who experience the event of interest first are almost certain to have the higher (of the only two possible) values of frailty. Consequently, the knowledge of the values of the frailties (which means the values of missing covariates) becomes less important. Second, censoring tends to remove the late events and, consequently, reduces the loss of efficiency in the simple log-rank test compared to the adjusted log-rank test. The above results depend on the knowledge of the usually unknown frailty variance σ^2; consequently, their practical applicability is limited.

Jeong (2003) extends the foregoing results to visualize and quantify the loss of efficiency of the log-rank test when a dependence structure between survival and censoring times is being ignored. The assumed dependence structure is based on a correlated gamma frailty model (Section 5.2). In the given situation the loss of efficiency is minimal under the proportional hazards model, even when the correlation between potential survival and censoring times is strong, unless the dependent censoring causes a severe nonproportionality.

Broët et al. (1999) suggest a more practical approach for taking into account unobserved covariates in a weighted log-rank test. The construction of the test is based on a gamma distribution of the frailty. For the frailty parameter σ^2, a range is assumed. Simulations investigate the power of the test for different frailty distributions.

Rank tests for clustered event time data when dependent subunits are randomized are considered by Jeong and Jung (2006).

Li et al. (2002) arrive at the conclusion that the log-rank test is nearly fully efficient relative to the optimally weighted log-rank test if the unobserved heterogeneity does not interact with the binary treatment variable. This is not the case if frailty interacts with treatment. Such situation could happen, for example, if unobserved heterogeneity is caused by genetic factors, which interact with treatment.

7.7 Time-Dependent Frailty Models

Standard frailty models assume that the individual frailty Z is determined at time zero (begin of follow-up) and follows the individual throughout the rest of the life, resulting in the individual's susceptibility (frailty) later in life being perfectly correlated with that at the beginning. It is clearly of interest to overcome this restrictive assumption of fixed frailty in order to develop more flexible models. However, it turns out that this is a difficult problem.

There exist different approaches dealing with time-dependent frailty by considering the individual hazard as a stochastic process. This provides individual flexibility. However, since what is observable is the average hazard function, the problem is to find models that show a tractable mathematical connection between the individual hazard function and the average one. One attempt to tackle this problem was suggested by Yashin and Manton (1997), defining the hazard function as a diffusion process by means of a stochastic differential equation. By using Ornstein–Uhlenbeck-type processes, such kind of models reflect the fact that many biological parameters tend to stabilize around certain values, which is called *homeostasis*. The quadratic hazard frailty model in Section 3.9 is a special case of this model with fixed frailty.

In a second approach, McGilchrist and Yau (1996), and Yau and McGilchrist (1998), focus on recurrent event time data. Often interrecurrence times close to each other on the time scale are highly associated, while times that are further apart from each other on the time scale are less correlated. To model such kinds of serial dependence, a dynamic frailty model can be constructed by assuming that the frailties of subsequent time intervals follow an autoregressive process of order one, denoted by AR(1). Yau and McGilchrist (1998) adopted AR(1) frailty models to analyze chronic granulomatous disease data. A similar but simpler idea without using an AR(1) process was suggested by Wintrebert et al. (2004). A Bayesian approach to the problem can be found in the paper by Manda and Meyer (2005).

The third approach is based on Lévy processes (Gjessing et al. 2003, Aalen et al. 2008). Like diffusion processes, hazard functions driven by Lévy processes also yield some degree of tractability. It is possible to get explicit formulas for the relationship between conditional and unconditional hazard, and the frailty and hazard of survivors may be estimated. A basic difference between this and the first approach is the jump nature of the Lévy processes. However, it could well be imagined that the individual hazard may increase in jumps, for example, with the onset of an acute disease. The model is an extension of Lévy frailty models with fixed frailty in Aalen and Hjort (2002), discussed in Section 3.10.

Example 7.1

Gamma processes: Let the value of the process at time point u be gamma distributed with shape parameter ku and scale parameter λ. Then it holds that

$$\mathbf{L}(s; u) = \left(1 + \frac{s}{\lambda}\right)^{-ku} = e^{-ku\left(\ln(\lambda+s) - \ln \lambda\right)}, \qquad k, \lambda > 0,$$

with $\psi(s) = k\left(\ln(\lambda + s) - \ln \lambda\right)$ as characteristic exponent (Section 3.6). ∎

Example 7.2

Standard compound Poisson processes: A Poisson process of rate ρ is running on time scale u, and to each jump there is a gamma random variable, independent of the past, with shape parameter k and scale parameter λ. The compound Poisson process is the sum of the gamma variables up to time u. The Laplace transform of the random value of the process at time u is given by

$$\mathbf{L}(s; u) = e^{-u\frac{k}{\gamma}\left((\lambda+s)^{\gamma} - \lambda^{\gamma}\right)}, \qquad \gamma < 0.$$

Hence, the characteristic exponent is given by $\psi(s) = \frac{k}{\gamma}\left((\lambda + s)^{\gamma} - \lambda^{\gamma}\right)$. ∎

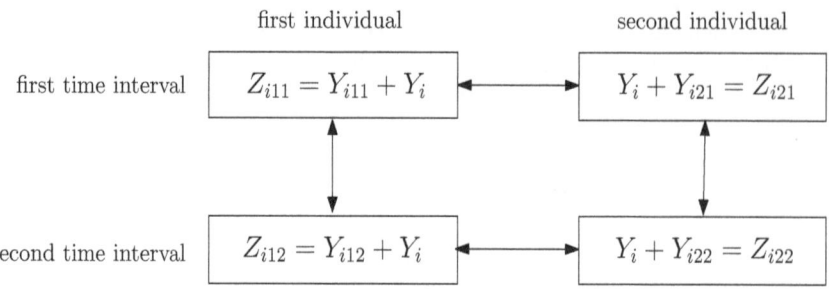

Figure 7.1: Time-varying frailties of two relatives from family i in two time intervals in the Paik model.

Example 7.3

Stable processes: The Laplace transform of a stable distributed random variable takes the form $\mathbf{L}(s; u) = e^{-u\frac{k}{\gamma}s^\gamma}$. Hence, $\psi(s) = \frac{k}{\gamma}s^\gamma$. ∎

Example 7.4

PVF processes: The power variance function distributions constitute a general class of distributions. A class of Lévy processes may be defined from the PVF distributions by $\psi(s) = \frac{k}{\gamma}\left((\lambda + s)^\gamma - \lambda^\gamma\right)$ $(\gamma > 0)$. The special case $\gamma = 0$ is defined by continuity and gives the gamma process. For $\gamma < 0$, the model yields the standard compound Poisson process. ∎

Paik et al. (1994) suggest another extension of the correlated gamma frailty model. They consider the case of clustered individuals but with varying frailties over time. For this purpose, the time scale is divided into intervals. The approach uses a decomposition of the frailty in each interval into a shared and a unique part, for example, $Z_{ijl} = Y_i + Y_{ijl}$ with independent random variables $Y_i \sim \Gamma(k_1, \lambda_1)$ and $Y_{ijl} \sim \Gamma(k_2, \lambda_2)$. In the correlated gamma frailty model, the assumption $\lambda_1 = \lambda_2$ is essential because it yields the gamma distribution of Z_1 and Z_2. Paik et al. (1994) allow the λ's to differ which, on the one hand, complicates the computation of the likelihood function, but on the other hand, it generates a more flexible model. In both models the expectation of the frailties is restricted to one. The main feature of the model in Paik et al. (1994) is to allow the frailty (and, consequently, the dependence function) to vary over time intervals. Restricting the model to two related individuals with two recurrent observation times each gives the structure of frailties shown in Figure 7.1.

Note that Paik et al. (1994) considered a noncompeting risk situation, which means it is assumed that all lifetimes are observable (with independent censoring). Different extensions of the Paik model are discussed in Wintrebert et al. (2004) and Wintrebert (2007).

7.8 Identifiability of Frailty Models

One of the aims of frailty modeling is to study the properties of the hazard function and the frailty distribution in real-life applications. Such analysis is possible if the frailty distribution, as well as the hazard function, are identifiable from the survival data. There is a substantial literature on the identification of frailty models. Especially in the econometric literature (where these models are named *mixed proportional hazards models*), the problem of identifiability is considered in detail for univariate as well as multivariate models.

7.8.1 Univariate frailty models

It is useful to consider the frailty model in a more general form based on the general proportional hazards model (2.9):

$$\mu(t|\mathbf{X}, Z) = Z\mu_0(t)h(\mathbf{X}).$$

It is possible to consider this model in a completely nonparametric form, for example, without any distributional assumptions about the cumulative baseline hazard M_0, the form of the function h, and the distribution of the frailty term Z (for example, given by their distribution function F_Z). We would like to point out that this situation is more general than the situation considered in the present monograph, where usually the function h is specified by $h(\mathbf{X}) = e^{\boldsymbol{\beta}'\mathbf{X}}$ and distributional assumptions are made about the frailty distribution. So the literature about identifiability of frailty models is (at least partially) concerned with nonparametric identifiability. It is useful to determine identifiability as a property of the mapping from the three determinants (M_0, h, F_Z), given their domain, to the data. The frailty model is now specified by the unique mapping from the domain to the data. The model is identifiable if this mapping has an inverse, meaning for given data there exists a unique set of functions (M_0, h, F_Z) in the domain that is able to generate these data. We will not go into much detail here, but refer the reader interested in identifiability results to Elbers and Ridder (1982), who were the first to prove nonparametric identifiability of frailty models. Their proof is not constructive. Constructive identification proofs are more attractive because they express the underlying functions (M_0, h, F_Z) directly in terms of observable quantities and therefore suggest an estimation method. Constructive proofs are provided by Heckman and Singer (1984b), Melino and Sueyoshi (1990), Ridder (1990), Heckman (1991), Heckman and Taber (1994), Kortram et al. (1995), and Horowitz (1999) under different model assumptions. For an overview, see van den Berg (2001). The most important assumption here is $\mathbf{E}Z < \infty$. In the case of nonidentifiability, the adoption of a model that is observationally equivalent to (but different from) the true model leads to biased parameter estimates. This is a difficult problem because it is usually hard to make justified assumptions about the frailty distribution based on the observed survival data.

The fundamental identification problem was addressed by Ridder (1990) in detail. He showed that, for every frailty model with $\mathbf{E}Z < \infty$, there exists an observational equivalent model with $\mathbf{E}Z = \infty$. Therefore, the assumption $\mathbf{E}Z < \infty$ imposes identifiability on a class of models that are not identifiable. The identifiability of the frailty distribution is a consequence of the nonproportionality of the unconditional hazards (Hougaard 1991, van den Berg 1992, Keiding 1998). Heckman and Taber (1994) and Kortram et al. (1995) show that the mapping from the data generating process to the data is not continuous, which results in the problem that two different frailty models can generate very similar data. Furthermore, convergence rates are sometimes very small, for example, convergence rates for the estimation of the baseline hazard λ and regression parameters β can be at most almost equal to $n^{-2/5}$ under some regularity assumptions. For the estimation of the frailty distribution, the rate of convergence is extremely small with $(\log n)^{-2}$ (Horowitz 1999). Consequently, based on sample sizes occurring in practical applications, the estimation in this nonparametric univariate frailty model is often very unstable, and interpretations based on such results should be performed with extreme caution.

One solution to the foregoing identifiability problem is to impose parametric assumptions about the frailty distribution as done in the present monograph. Let us now return to this situation, and let $S(t)$ represent some survival function. It turns out that $S(t)$ can always be represented as a marginal survival function in some model with unobserved frailty Z and cumulative baseline hazard $M_0(t)$. In other words, univariate frailty models are not identifiable if only the marginal distribution of the failure times (without any observed covariates) are known. Lancaster and Nickell (1980) discussed this identifiability problem in detail. Indeed, let $\mathbf{L}$ be the Laplace transform of some arbitrary distribution of the nonnegative random variable Z, and let $\mathbf{L}^{-1}$ be the inverse function of $\mathbf{L}$. For any $0 \leq t < \infty$, the cumulative hazard is defined as

$$M(t) = \mathbf{L}^{-1}(S(t)).$$

To prove that $M(t)$ is a cumulative hazard function of a survival distribution, it is sufficient to show that $M(t)$ is a nondecreasing function. This follows from the fact that both $S(t)$ and $\mathbf{L}^{-1}(t)$ are nonincreasing functions of t. Thus, for any given survival function $S(t)$ and probability distribution on the positive half-line (given by Laplace transform $\mathbf{L}$), one can construct a frailty model with marginal survival function $S(t)$. The nonidentifiability aspect of specific distributions of frailty was discussed by Heckman and Singer (1982a, 1984a) and Hoem (1990), among others. Elbers and Ridder (1982) show that if the frailty distribution has a finite mean, then the presence of covariates makes the univariate proportional hazards frailty model identifiable. Other conditions are given by Heckman and Honoré (1989). These findings stimulated the use of frailty models with observed covariates (regression models) in the analysis of univariate survival data (Andersen et al. 1993).

In the more general case of a frailty cure model (modeling a cure fraction and unobserved heterogeneity together), it holds that

$$S^*(t|\mathbf{X}_1, \mathbf{X}_2) = 1 - \phi(\mathbf{X}_2) + \phi(\mathbf{X}_2)\mathbf{L}(M_0(t)e^{\beta'\mathbf{X}_1}). \tag{7.9}$$

Peng and Zhang (2008b) establish mild conditions that imply identifiability of the model. Here, $\mathbf{L}$ again denotes the Laplace transform of a frailty variable. Two kinds of covariates are considered: $\mathbf{X}_2$ influences the probability to be cured, whereas $\mathbf{X}_1$ influences the event time in susceptible individuals. The identifiability of the frailty model is obtained as a special case but with a much simpler proof compared to the one in Elbers and Ridder (1982). The above frailty cure model with covariates in the cure fraction and the survival function of the noncured population is identifiable if the cure fraction $\phi(\mathbf{X}_2)$ is nonconstant and some technical assumptions such a finite mean of the frailty distribution are fulfilled. It turns out that the case of identical covariates $\mathbf{X}_1 = \mathbf{X}_2$ needs additional assumptions and is therefore treated separately by Peng and Zhang (2008b).

7.8.2 Multivariate frailty models

Bivariate (as well as multivariate) data present an opportunity to identify both the frailty distribution as well as the baseline hazard under much weaker assumptions than in the univariate case. For example, all shared frailty models are identifiable from bivariate data without additional information such as observed covariates or parametric assumptions about the baseline hazard as shown by Honoré (1993). Furthermore, the baseline hazard may depend on observed covariates $\mathbf{X}$ in an unspecified way, and frailty Z and covariates $\mathbf{X}$ may be dependent. It turns out that the identifiability property holds for a broader class of frailty models, including correlated frailty models. Furthermore, the condition of a finite mean required for identifiability in a univariate frailty model with covariates by Elbers and Ridder (1982) is not needed in this case. For more details of this situation, see Yashin and Iachine (1999b). Identifiability aspects of the correlated frailty model were analyzed in more detail by Iachine and Yashin (1998), and were further extended by Iachine (2004), with the latter paper discussing an interesting counterexample based on the positive stable frailty model.

Nielsen et al. (1992, end of Section 4) mentioned in the shared gamma frailty model the need for a positive probability of at least two failures per cluster to ensure identifiability.

7.9 Applications of Frailty Models

This section provides a collection of examples from the literature dealing with interesting frailty models usually not covered by the approaches considered in the foregoing chapters. The main emphasis is to give an overview of the variety of applications of frailty models in the solution of different statistical problems. The presentation of the material here is kept very short, and the reader is referred to related publications.

A model combining relative survival and frailty is given in Goeman et al. (2004). The authors look at the excess hazard for a specific disease when a concurrent disease is present. The main idea of this model is a hazard function of the form

$$\mu(t|Z) = \mu_0(t) + Z[\mu_1(t) + \mu_2(t)].$$

Here, μ_0 is a background hazard function from the risk of death by other causes assumed to be known (the general population mortality statistics if the disease under study contributes only a small part to overall mortality), μ_1 describes the excess hazard of the concurrent disease (assumed to be known from the literature), and μ_2 is the excess hazard caused by the primary disease. Results are shown to be independent of the chosen frailty distribution if heterogeneity is small. The model is applied to data on patients with head/neck tumors using information on previous tumors.

Zahl (1997) considers a similar problem by applying different versions of the shared and correlated gamma frailty model to cause-specific mortality data in Norway in order to model the excess hazard of cancer mortality. The study has the drawback that, because of a small number of cases, a reasonable estimation of the parameters was not possible. Nevertheless, the paper demonstrates the advantage of correlated frailty models in cause-specific mortality data (competing risks).

O'Quigley and Stare (2002) discuss some of the fundamental concepts of univariate and shared frailty models. The authors claimed that univariate frailty models are of limited practical value. Any frailty model $S(t|\mathbf{X}, Z)$ is equivalent to a usually nonproportional hazards model $S^*(t|\mathbf{X})$, in which the individual effects disappear:

$$S^*(t|\mathbf{X}) = \int_0^\infty S(t|\mathbf{X}, z) \, f_Z(z) \, dz$$

which would correspond to a homogeneous population. Keeping this in mind, any assertion about unobserved heterogeneity must be entirely arbitrary. The assertion is fully determined by an arbitrary model choice. The statistician who chooses $S(t|\mathbf{X}, Z)$ will conclude that heterogeneity is clearly evident. The statistician who decides for $S^*(t|\mathbf{X})$ will come to the opposite conclusion.

Consequently, both conclusions are arbitrary; the model we choose determines our conclusion. The data themselves will not allow us to decide which model is the true one. Decisions about the two situations cannot be made by looking at the data without making further strong, parametric assumptions about the baseline hazard or the frailty distribution. A test for the presence of frailties is equivalent to a test of fit against time-varying covariate effects. Unobserved heterogeneity cannot be distinguished from homogeneity under a nonproportional hazards model. Consequently, O'Quigley and Stare (2002) conclude that univariate frailty models cannot be used to incorporate the effects of unobserved covariates without additional information.

In contradiction to the univariate case, the authors state that, in the multi-variate case, frailty models can be used to advantage; especially for moderate to large numbers of small families (up to five members), the efficiency gains of frailty models could be important. For the analysis of data on large families, the authors recommend the use of stratified proportional hazards models. This is possible under the assumption of shared frailties in families, which implies proportional hazards even when the frailty is unknown.

Warwick et al. (2003) used a modified gamma frailty model with piecewise constant baseline hazards to model time-dependent effects on survival in breast cancer. It was shown that the effects of tumor size, lymph node status, and histologic grade are important predictors still after 20 years of follow-up, but the effects of these risk factors progressively diminish with time from prognosis. Frailty models are one possibility to allow for such kind of attenuation of prognostic effects.

Dos Santos et al. (1995) applied different shared frailty models with Weibull baseline hazard to the recurrence of breast cancer. The data set contains 917 women treated for breast cancer between 1980 and 1985 at the Christie Hospital in Manchester (U.K.) and their subsequent monitoring until 1991. The authors used two explanatory variables: age and stage of the disease at the initial treatment. The outcome of interest is the duration to recurrence after treatment. In modeling repeated durations, the covariate state (a factor with tree levels) was included. Death from other causes was treated as right censoring and therefore assumed to be noninformative. Four parametric models are considered in the analysis: a Cox model and three frailty models with gamma, log-normal, and four-point frailty. There is a considerable increase in the log-likelihood when a frailty term is included in the model. Although formal likelihood ratio tests are not appropriate, the discrete four-point frailty model shows a better fit to the data compared to the gamma and log-normal frailty models, respectively.

Guo and Rodriguez (1992) and Guo (1993) applied a shared frailty model with observed covariates to child survival data in Guatemala, using gamma and binary frailty distributions and piecewise constant hazards. The authors compare their results with an analysis based on a proportional hazards model with piecewise constant hazard function. In all three models, the estimates of the observed covariates effects are remarkably stable.

Moreno (1994) analyzed the influence of frailty distribution on the association between survival times under gamma, inverse Gaussian, discrete k-point, and Poisson distributions. He shows that the pattern and strength of this association depends on the specification of the frailty distribution.

Banerjee et al. (2003) applied a spatially correlated frailty model to infant mortality data in Minnesota. Each county in Minnesota forms a cluster, with common frailty for all observations in a cluster (shared frailty model). Additionally, the frailties of different clusters are not independent as in the classical frailty models. A correlation matrix for the frailties is used to model spatial correlations between clusters (correlated frailty model). Other spatial frailty models are investigated, for example, by Banerjee and Carlin (2003) and Jin and Carlin (2005).

In dental research, researchers are often faced to the problem of clustered event times. However, applications of frailty models to patient-oriented dental research are sparse. Kalwitzki et al. (2002) considered times until occurrence of caries. Sealant retention was analyzed by Morgan et al. (2002) using a Poisson frailty model. Chuang et al. (2005) and Chuang and Cai (2006) evaluated lifetimes of dental implants. Wong et al. (2006) applied a multi-level log-normal frailty model to lifetimes of treatment restorations of carious lesions of Chinese school children.

More general censoring and truncation patterns in univariate frailty models than left truncation and right censoring, as considered in the present book, are treated by Huber-Carol and Vonta (2004).

7.10   Software for Frailty Models

The applicability of newly developed statistical methods depend strongly on their availability in common statistical packages. The proportional hazards model is provided by all standard statistical packages, and the regression parameters in this model can be estimated consistently by maximization of a partial likelihood function (Cox 1975) that does not depend on the baseline hazard. The baseline hazard can be estimated nonparametrically. This is one of the great advantages of the proportional hazards model, but it does not carry over to frailty models. Here, more sophisticated estimation procedures are needed. Unfortunately frailty models are not standard tools provided by large standard packages such as SPSS and SAS as a standard routine. There exists different procedures freely available, such as COXPH, COXME, PHMM, FRAILTYPACK, SPGAM, or SPNL3. This makes it difficult to find the appropriate tool for the specific problem considered. Advantages and limitations of the procedures are discussed, and a short overview of the software for different frailty models is given in this section.

7.10.1 R packages

R is a free software environment for statistical computing and graphics. It runs on a wide variety of UNIX platforms, Windows, and MacOS and has become more and more attractive to statisticians as well for nonstatisticians. The software can be assessed on http://cran.R-project.org.

FRAILTYPACK: This package by Rondeau and González (2005) was mainly extended by Rondeau et al. (2010). It fits semiparametric gamma frailty models. It also provides parameter estimation in more complex settings such as the interaction model (7.3) with two dependent Gaussian random effects. Also, the nested frailty model (7.5) with two gamma-distributed frailties can be fitted. Furthermore, the joint modeling of recurrent events and a terminal event by a shared gamma frailty (7.7-7.8) is implemented in the package. It accommodates left-truncated and right-censored data. Stratified analysis with two strata is possible. FRAILTYPACK uses the penalization of the hazard function described by (3.34), applying the robust Marquardt algorithm, which is a combination between a Newton–Raphson and a steepest-descent algorithm. As a consequence of this estimation procedure, a smooth estimate of the hazard function is provided.

COXME: The procedure COXME was created by Therneau and works with the penalized partial likelihood algorithm. It provides estimation in the general Cox proportional hazards model with Gaussian random effects described by model (7.4). Furthermore, COXME is able to handle nested frailty models (7.5). The package was originally a function in the kinship package in recognition of the fact that it was primarily targeted toward genetic problems. COXME was also distributed as part of the base survival package in S plus. The current version from 2009 is more broad in its capabilities. It turns out to be useful to modify the convergence criteria eps from 10^{-6} to 10^{-9} and the maximum iteration number for the partial likelihood procedure iter.max from 20 to 40. This increases the precision of the estimation procedure to a reasonable size but at the cost of computer time.

SURVIVAL: This package was also written by Therneau for survival data. One function of the package is COXPH. It fits the proportional hazards model and is able to deal with time-dependent covariates and strata, multiple events per subject, and other extensions. One of these extensions include univariate and shared frailty models. The syntax is similar to that of the COXME procedure. The frailty distributions gamma, log-t, and log-normal are supported (Therneau et al. 2003). Similar to the COXME procedure, modification of the parameters eps and iter.max is recommended.

PHMM: This package steams from Donohue and Ronghui in 2009/2010. It fits the proportional hazards model incorporating Gaussian random effects given in (7.4). The estimation procedure is based on the EM algorithm using Markov Chain Monte Carlo methods in the E step. The software provides no convergence criterion; the number of iterations has to be fixed.

To make R and SAS procedures comparable, the option ties = "breslow" for the handling of ties should be used in all R procedures. Furthermore, despite the wide range of models covered, the R packages do not provide standard errors of the random effects variance estimates, which is a major drawback. An exception is the recent version of FRAILTYPACK.

7.10.2 SAS packages

In SAS there are only a few macros dealing with frailty models. It is important to note that the SAS macros provide standard errors of the frailty variance estimates in contrast to most of the R procedures.

GAMFRAIL: This macro by Klein uses the EM algorithm (Klein 1992) to fit semiparametric gamma frailty models and can be downloaded from http://www.mcw.edu/biostatistics/Research/Software.htm. It suffers from a very slow estimation procedure. The handling of the macro is not very user-friendly; for example, the data need to be arranged in a fixed order.

PS-FRAIL: This macro steams from Shu and Klein (1999) and can be obtained from http://www.mcw.edu/biostatistics/Research/Software.htm. It provides estimation of the semiparametric positive stable frailty model.

SPGAM: This macro implements the ML-EM algorithm for the semiparametric shared gamma frailty models, described by Vu (2003). The newer version allows for left censoring in the data. Additionally, there exists a version for estimation in the parametric shared gamma frailty model, which is called PGAM. The macros are available on http://lib.stat.cmu.edu.

SPNL: This is a macro to fit the semiparametric shared log-normal frailty models with left censoring, using the ML-EM algorithm described in Vu (2004). The syntax is similar to the SPGAM macro; just the argument N is added. N denotes the integer that controls the precision of the integrals involved inside the macro. It is available on http://lib.stat.cmu.edu.

A macro providing a score test for unobserved heterogeneity in event times is available on http://www.mcw.edu/biostatistics/Research/Software.htm.

7.10.3 STATA package

STATA is so far the only large commercial statistical package that supports frailty analysis. It is able to handle gamma and log-normal frailty models. However, analysis is restricted to parametric models. The package provides exponential, Weibull, Gompertz, log-normal, log-logistic, and generalized gamma distribution of the baseline hazard function.

Appendix A

Appendix

The aim of this appendix is to give some statistical key results that are important for the field of frailty models. These results are more technical and, for that reason, moved to the appendix to allow a fluent reading of the main parts of the book. The next part deals with bivariate event-time data. The bivariate case is used here to illustrate the main ideas of correlated frailty models in this simple situation. It turns out that the likelihood of the survival data can be represented in terms of the survival function and its partial derivatives. A model specification in terms of the survival function eases the computational burden of handling censoring and truncation.

A.1 Bivariate Lifetime Models

In Section 2.2, the likelihood function for univariate right-censored and left-truncated data was already derived. The present section deals with right censoring and left truncation in bivariate failure data. For this purpose, let $(T_1, T_2, \Delta_1, \Delta_2)$ be the censored bivariate observations with $T_j = \min\{T_j^*, C_j\}$, $\Delta_j = 1(T_j^* \leq C_j)$, $(j = 1, 2)$ and denoting the bivariate survival function of (T_1^*, T_2^*) by $S(t_1^*, t_2^*)$. Furthermore, denote the density of (T_1^*, T_2^*) and (C_1, C_2), respectively, by $f(t_1^*, t_2^*)$ and $g(c_1, c_2)$. Assume that the lifetimes (T_1^*, T_2^*) and censoring times (C_1, C_2) are independent.

$$
\begin{aligned}
H(t_1, t_2, 1, 1) &= \mathbf{P}(T_1 > t_1, T_2 > t_2, \Delta_1 = 1, \Delta_2 = 1) \\
&= \mathbf{P}(T_1^* > t_1, T_2^* > t_2, T_1^* \leq C_1, T_2^* \leq C_2) \\
&= \iiiint\limits_{\{t_1^* > t_1, t_2^* > t_2, t_1^* \leq c_1, t_2^* \leq c_2\}} f(t_1^*, t_2^*) g(c_1, c_2) \, dt_1^* dt_2^* dc_1 dc_2 \\
&= \int_{t_2}^{\infty} \int_{t_1}^{\infty} f(t_1^*, t_2^*) \left(\int_{t_2^*}^{\infty} \int_{t_1^*}^{\infty} g(c_1, c_2) \, dc_1 dc_2 \right) dt_1^* dt_2^*
\end{aligned}
$$

Consequently, the subdensity for noncensored pairs of lifetimes is

$$
h(t_1, t_2, 1, 1) = H_{t_1, t_2}(t_1, t_2, 1, 1) = f(t_1, t_2) \int_{t_2}^{\infty} \int_{t_1}^{\infty} g(c_1, c_2) \, dc_1 dc_2.
$$

The calculation of the other subdensities is analogous:

$$
\begin{aligned}
H(t_1, t_2, 1, 0) &= \mathbf{P}(T_1 > t_1, T_2 > t_2, \Delta_1 = 1, \Delta_2 = 0) \\
&= \mathbf{P}(T_1^* > t_1, C_2 > t_2, T_1^* \le C_1, T_2^* > C_2) \\
&= \iiiint\limits_{\{t_1^* > t_1, c_2 > t_2, t_1^* \le c_1, t_2^* > c_2\}} f(t_1^*, t_2^*) g(c_1, c_2) \, dt_1^* dt_2^* dc_1 dc_2 \\
&= \int_{t_2}^{\infty} \int_{t_1}^{\infty} \left(\int_{c_2}^{\infty} f(t_1^*, t_2^*) \, dt_2^* \int_{t_1^*}^{\infty} g(c_1, c_2) \, dc_1 \right) dt_1^* dc_2.
\end{aligned}
$$

Because of $-S_{t_1}(t_1, t_2) = \int_{t_2}^{\infty} f(t_1, t_2^*) \, dt_2^*$ it holds that

$$
h(t_1, t_2, 1, 0) = H_{t_1, t_2}(t_1, t_2, 1, 0) = -S_{t_1}(t_1, t_2) \int_{t_1}^{\infty} g(c_1, t_2) \, dc_1.
$$

$$
\begin{aligned}
H(t_1, t_2, 0, 1) &= \mathbf{P}(T_1 > t_1, T_2 > t_2, \Delta_1 = 0, \Delta_2 = 1) \\
&= \mathbf{P}(C_1 > t_1, T_2^* > t_2, T_1^* > C_1, T_2^* \le C_2) \\
&= \iiiint\limits_{\{c_1 > t_1, t_2^* > t_2, t_1^* > c_1, t_2^* \le c_2\}} f(t_1^*, t_2^*) g(c_1, c_2) \, dt_1^* dt_2^* dc_1 dc_2 \\
&= \int_{t_2}^{\infty} \int_{t_1}^{\infty} \left(\int_{c_1}^{\infty} f(t_1^*, t_2^*) \, dt_1^* \int_{t_2^*}^{\infty} g(c_1, c_2) \, dc_2 \right) dc_1 dt_2^*.
\end{aligned}
$$

Hence,

$$
h(t_1, t_2, 0, 1) = H_{t_1, t_2}(t_1, t_2, 0, 1) = -S_{t_2}(t_1, t_2) \int_{t_2}^{\infty} g(t_1, c_2) \, dc_2.
$$

$$
\begin{aligned}
H(t_1, t_2, 0, 0) &= \mathbf{P}(T_1 > t_1, T_2 > t_2, \Delta_1 = 0, \Delta_2 = 0) \\
&= \mathbf{P}(C_1 > t_1, C_2 > t_2, T_1^* > C_1, T_2^* > C_2) \\
&= \iiiint\limits_{\{c_1 > t_1, c_2 > t_2, t_1^* > c_1, t_2^* > c_2\}} f(t_1^*, t_2^*) g(c_1, c_2) \, dt_1^* dt_2^* dc_1 dc_2 \\
&= \int_{t_2}^{\infty} \int_{t_1}^{\infty} \left(\int_{c_2}^{\infty} \int_{c_1}^{\infty} f(t_1^*, t_2^*) \, dt_1^* dt_2^* \right) g(c_1, c_2) \, dc_1 dc_2.
\end{aligned}
$$

Consequently,

$$
h(t_1, t_2, 0, 0) = H_{t_1, t_2}(t_1, t_2, 0, 1) = S(t_1, t_2) g(t_1, t_2).
$$

Hence, the likelihood function under independent and noninformative right censoring can be expressed in terms of the bivariate survival function by

$$
S_{t_1 t_2}(t_1, t_2)^{\delta_1 \delta_2} S_{t_1}(t_1, t_2)^{\delta_1 (1 - \delta_2)} S_{t_2}(t_1, t_2)^{(1 - \delta_1)\delta_2} S(t_1, t_2)^{(1 - \delta_1)(1 - \delta_2)}. \quad \text{(A.1)}
$$

Now the case of nonrandom left truncation will be considered. Observations are made conditional on the fact that both survival times are larger than the respective truncation times:

$$
\mathbf{P}(T_1^+ > t_1, T_2^+ > t_2, \Delta_1 = \delta_1, \Delta_2 = \delta_2)
$$
$$
= \mathbf{P}(T_1 > t_1, T_2 > t_2, \Delta_1 = \delta_1, \Delta_2 = \delta_2 | T_1 > t_1^+, T_2 > t_2^+)
$$
$$
= \frac{\mathbf{P}(T_1 > t_1, T_2 > t_2, \Delta_1 = \delta_1, \Delta_2 = \delta_2)}{\mathbf{P}(T_1 > t_1^+, T_2 > t_2^+)}.
$$

Finally, with a sample of n pairs, we obtain the likelihood

$$
\prod_{i=1}^{n} S_{t_{i1} t_{i2}}(t_{i1}, t_{i2})^{\delta_{i1} \delta_{i2}} S_{t_{i1}}(t_{i1}, t_{i2})^{\delta_{i1}(1-\delta_{i2})} S_{t_{i2}}(t_{i1}, t_{i2})^{(1-\delta_{i1})\delta_{i2}} \tag{A.2}
$$
$$
\times S(t_{i1}, t_{i2})^{(1-\delta_{i1})(1-\delta_{i2})} S(t_{i1}^+, t_{i2}^+)^{-1}.
$$

A.2 Correlated Gamma Frailty Model

From the previous section it follows that the likelihood of bivariate event-time data depends mainly on the derivatives from the survival function. Here, in this section, these derivatives for the correlated gamma frailty model are calculated, forming the basis for parameter estimation in this model. The main ideas from the bivariate correlated gamma frailty model are used later on for other correlated frailty models, for example, the correlated compound Poisson frailty model, in the next section. The survival function in the bivariate correlated gamma frailty model is given by (5.6):

$$
S(t_1, t_2) = S_1(t_1)^{1 - \frac{\sigma_1}{\sigma_2} \rho} S_2(t_2)^{1 - \frac{\sigma_2}{\sigma_1} \rho} (S_1(t_1)^{-\sigma_1^2} + S_2(t_2)^{-\sigma_2^2} - 1)^{-\frac{\rho}{\sigma_1 \sigma_2}}.
$$

Hence, the densities are of the form

$$
S_{t_1}(t_1, t_2) =
$$
$$
- (1 - \frac{\sigma_1}{\sigma_2} \rho) S_1(t_1)^{-\frac{\sigma_1}{\sigma_2} \rho} f_1(t_1) S_2(t_2)^{1 - \frac{\sigma_2}{\sigma_1} \rho} (S_1(t_1)^{-\sigma_1^2} + S_2(t_2)^{-\sigma_2^2} - 1)^{-\frac{\rho}{\sigma_1 \sigma_2}}
$$
$$
- \frac{\sigma_1}{\sigma_2} \rho S_1(t_1)^{-\frac{\sigma_1}{\sigma_2} \rho - \sigma_1^2} f_1(t_1) S_2(t_2)^{1 - \frac{\sigma_2}{\sigma_1} \rho} (S_1(t_1)^{-\sigma_1^2} + S_2(t_2)^{-\sigma_2^2} - 1)^{-\frac{\rho}{\sigma_1 \sigma_2} - 1}
$$
$$
= S_1(t_1)^{-\frac{\sigma_1}{\sigma_2} \rho} f_1(t_1) S_2(t_2)^{1 - \frac{\sigma_2}{\sigma_1} \rho} (S_1(t_1)^{-\sigma_1^2} + S_2(t_2)^{-\sigma_2^2} - 1)^{-\frac{\rho}{\sigma_1 \sigma_2} - 1}
$$
$$
\times \left(- S_1(t_1)^{-\sigma_1^2} - (1 - \frac{\sigma_1}{\sigma_2} \rho) S_2(t_2)^{-\sigma_2^2} + (1 - \frac{\sigma_1}{\sigma_2} \rho) \right),
$$

$$S_{t_2}(t_1, t_2) =$$
$$- S_1(t_1)^{1-\frac{\sigma_1}{\sigma_2}\rho}(1 - \frac{\sigma_2}{\sigma_1}\rho)S_2(t_2)^{-\frac{\sigma_2}{\sigma_1}\rho}f_2(t_2)(S_1(t_1)^{-\sigma_1^2} + S_2(t_2)^{-\sigma_2^2} - 1)^{-\frac{\rho}{\sigma_1\sigma_2}}$$
$$- S_1(t_1)^{1-\frac{\sigma_1}{\sigma_2}\rho}\frac{\sigma_2}{\sigma_1}\rho S_2(t_2)^{-\frac{\sigma_2}{\sigma_1}\rho-\sigma_2^2}f_2(t_2)(S_1(t_1)^{-\sigma_1^2} + S_2(t_2)^{-\sigma_2^2} - 1)^{-\frac{\rho}{\sigma_1\sigma_2}-1}$$
$$= S_1(t_1)^{1-\frac{\sigma_1}{\sigma_2}\rho}S_2(t_2)^{-\frac{\sigma_2}{\sigma_1}\rho}f_2(t_2)(S_1(t_1)^{-\sigma_1^2} + S_2(t_2)^{-\sigma_2^2} - 1)^{-\frac{\rho}{\sigma_1\sigma_2}-1}$$
$$\times \left(- (1 - \frac{\sigma_2}{\sigma_1}\rho)S_1(t_1)^{-\sigma_1^2} - S_2(t_2)^{-\sigma_2^2} + (1 - \frac{\sigma_2}{\sigma_1}\rho)\right),$$

and finally, the second derivative

$$S_{t_1 t_2}(t_1, t_2)$$
$$= (1 - \frac{\sigma_1}{\sigma_2}\rho)(1 - \frac{\sigma_2}{\sigma_1}\rho)S_1(t_1)^{-\frac{\sigma_1}{\sigma_2}\rho}f_1(t_1)S_2(t_2)^{-\frac{\sigma_2}{\sigma_1}\rho}f_2(t_2)$$
$$\times (S_1(t_1)^{-\sigma_1^2} + S_2(t_2)^{-\sigma_2^2} - 1)^{-\frac{\rho}{\sigma_1\sigma_2}}$$
$$+ (1 - \frac{\sigma_1}{\sigma_2}\rho)\frac{\sigma_2}{\sigma_1}\rho S_1(t_1)^{-\frac{\sigma_1}{\sigma_2}\rho}f_1(t_1)S_2(t_2)^{-\frac{\sigma_2}{\sigma_1}\rho-\sigma_2^2}f_2(t_2)$$
$$\times (S_1(t_1)^{-\sigma_1^2} + S_2(t_2)^{-\sigma_2^2} - 1)^{-\frac{\rho}{\sigma_1\sigma_2}-1}$$
$$+ (1 - \frac{\sigma_2}{\sigma_1}\rho)\frac{\sigma_1}{\sigma_2}\rho S_1(t_1)^{-\frac{\sigma_1}{\sigma_2}\rho-\sigma_1^2}f_1(t_1)S_2(t_2)^{-\frac{\sigma_2}{\sigma_1}\rho}f_2(t_2)$$
$$\times (S_1(t_1)^{-\sigma_1^2} + S_2(t_2)^{-\sigma_2^2} - 1)^{-\frac{\rho}{\sigma_1\sigma_2}-1}$$
$$+ \rho(\rho + \sigma_1\sigma_2)S_1(t_1)^{-\frac{\sigma_1}{\sigma_2}\rho-\sigma_1^2}f_1(t_1)S_2(t_2)^{-\frac{\sigma_2}{\sigma_1}\rho-\sigma_2^2}f_2(t_2)$$
$$\times (S_1(t_1)^{-\sigma_1^2} + S_2(t_2)^{-\sigma_2^2} - 1)^{-\frac{\rho}{\sigma_1\sigma_2}-2}$$
$$= S_1(t_1)^{-\frac{\sigma_1}{\sigma_2}\rho}f_1(t_1)S_2(t_2)^{-\frac{\sigma_2}{\sigma_1}\rho}f_2(t_2)(S_1(t_1)^{-\sigma_1^2} + S_2(t_2)^{-\sigma_2^2} - 1)^{-\frac{\rho}{\sigma_1\sigma_2}-2}$$
$$\times \left((1 - \frac{\sigma_1}{\sigma_2}\rho)(1 - \frac{\sigma_2}{\sigma_1}\rho)(S_1(t_1)^{-\sigma_1^2} + S_2(t_2)^{-\sigma_2^2} - 1)^2\right.$$
$$+ (1 - \frac{\sigma_1}{\sigma_2}\rho)\frac{\sigma_2}{\sigma_1}\rho S_2(t_2)^{-\sigma_2^2}(S_1(t_1)^{-\sigma_1^2} + S_2(t_2)^{-\sigma_2^2} - 1)$$
$$+ (1 - \frac{\sigma_2}{\sigma_1}\rho)\frac{\sigma_1}{\sigma_2}\rho S_1(t_1)^{-\sigma_1^2}(S_1(t_1)^{-\sigma_1^2} + S_2(t_2)^{-\sigma_2^2} - 1)$$
$$+ \rho(\rho + \sigma_1\sigma_2)S_1(t_1)^{-\sigma_1^2}S_2(t_2)^{-\sigma_2^2}\right).$$

Plugging these expressions into formula (A.2) gives the likelihood function of the correlated gamma frailty model. It is easy to see that, even in the simple bivariate case, the likelihood becomes formidable because of the necessary derivatives. The problem increases with larger cluster size. Furthermore, the maximum likelihood method is only applicable in the parametric case with full specification of the baseline hazard function. Therefore, more sophisticated strategies for parameter estimation are necessary, especially in the case of cluster size larger than two.

A.3 Correlated Compound Poisson Frailty Model

The correlated compound Poisson frailty model is a natural extension of the correlated gamma frailty model. Similar to the gamma model, we start with the bivariate marginal survival function, which is given for the compound Poisson frailty model by (5.14):

$$S(t_1, t_2) = S(t_1)^{1-\rho} S(t_2)^{1-\rho}$$
$$\times \exp\left(\frac{\rho(1-\gamma)}{\gamma\sigma^2}\left[1 - \left((1 - \frac{\gamma\sigma^2}{1-\gamma}\ln S(t_1))^{\frac{1}{\gamma}} + (1 - \frac{\gamma\sigma^2}{1-\gamma}\ln S(t_2))^{\frac{1}{\gamma}} - 1)^\gamma\right]\right).$$

The derivatives with respect to the first and second event time can be easily calculated by

$$S_{t_1}(t_1, t_2) =$$
$$- (1-\rho)f(t_1)S(t_1)^{-\rho}S(t_2)^{1-\rho}$$
$$\times \exp\left(\frac{\rho(1-\gamma)}{\gamma\sigma^2}\left[1 - \left((1 - \frac{\gamma\sigma^2}{1-\gamma}\ln S(t_1))^{\frac{1}{\gamma}} + (1 - \frac{\gamma\sigma^2}{1-\gamma}\ln S(t_2))^{\frac{1}{\gamma}} - 1)^\gamma\right]\right)$$
$$- \rho f(t_1)S(t_1)^{-\rho}S(t_2)^{1-\rho}(1 - \frac{\gamma\sigma^2}{1-\gamma}\ln S(t_1))^{\frac{1}{\gamma}-1}$$
$$\times \exp\left(\frac{\rho(1-\gamma)}{\gamma\sigma^2}\left[1 - \left((1 - \frac{\gamma\sigma^2}{1-\gamma}\ln S(t_1))^{\frac{1}{\gamma}} + (1 - \frac{\gamma\sigma^2}{1-\gamma}\ln S(t_2))^{\frac{1}{\gamma}} - 1)^\gamma\right]\right)$$
$$\times \left((1 - \frac{\gamma\sigma^2}{1-\gamma}\ln S(t_1))^{\frac{1}{\gamma}} + (1 - \frac{\gamma\sigma^2}{1-\gamma}\ln S(t_2))^{\frac{1}{\gamma}} - 1\right)^{\gamma-1}$$

and

$$S_{t_2}(t_1, t_2) =$$
$$- (1-\rho)f(t_2)S(t_1)^{1-\rho}S(t_2)^{-\rho}$$
$$\times \exp\left(\frac{\rho(1-\gamma)}{\gamma\sigma^2}\left[1 - \left((1 - \frac{\gamma\sigma^2}{1-\gamma}\ln S(t_1))^{\frac{1}{\gamma}} + (1 - \frac{\gamma\sigma^2}{1-\gamma}\ln S(t_2))^{\frac{1}{\gamma}} - 1)^\gamma\right]\right)$$
$$- \rho f(t_2)S(t_1)^{1-\rho}S(t_2)^{-\rho}(1 - \frac{\gamma\sigma^2}{1-\gamma}\ln S(t_2))^{\frac{1}{\gamma}-1}$$
$$\times \exp\left(\frac{\rho(1-\gamma)}{\gamma\sigma^2}\left[1 - \left((1 - \frac{\gamma\sigma^2}{1-\gamma}\ln S(t_1))^{\frac{1}{\gamma}} + (1 - \frac{\gamma\sigma^2}{1-\gamma}\ln S(t_2))^{\frac{1}{\gamma}} - 1)^\gamma\right]\right)$$
$$\times \left((1 - \frac{\gamma\sigma^2}{1-\gamma}\ln S(t_1))^{\frac{1}{\gamma}} + (1 - \frac{\gamma\sigma^2}{1-\gamma}\ln S(t_2))^{\frac{1}{\gamma}} - 1\right)^{\gamma-1}.$$

The derivative with respect to both event times is given by

$$S_{t_1 t_2}(t_1, t_2) =$$
$$(1-\rho)^2 f(t_1) S(t_1)^{-\rho} f(t_2) S(t_2)^{-\rho}$$
$$\times \exp\left(\frac{\rho(1-\gamma)}{\gamma\sigma^2}\left[1 - ((1 - \frac{\gamma\sigma^2}{1-\gamma}\ln S(t_1))^{\frac{1}{\gamma}} + (1 - \frac{\gamma\sigma^2}{1-\gamma}\ln S(t_2))^{\frac{1}{\gamma}} - 1)^{\gamma}\right]\right)$$
$$+ \rho(1-\rho) f(t_1) S(t_1)^{-\rho} f(t_2) S(t_2)^{-\rho}(1 - \frac{\gamma\sigma^2}{1-\gamma}\ln S(t_1))^{\frac{1}{\gamma}-1}$$
$$\times \exp\left(\frac{\rho(1-\gamma)}{\gamma\sigma^2}\left[1 - ((1 - \frac{\gamma\sigma^2}{1-\gamma}\ln S(t_1))^{\frac{1}{\gamma}} + (1 - \frac{\gamma\sigma^2}{1-\gamma}\ln S(t_2))^{\frac{1}{\gamma}} - 1)^{\gamma}\right]\right)$$
$$\times ((1 - \frac{\gamma\sigma^2}{1-\gamma}\ln S(t_1))^{\frac{1}{\gamma}} + (1 - \frac{\gamma\sigma^2}{1-\gamma}\ln S(t_2))^{\frac{1}{\gamma}} - 1)^{\gamma-1}$$
$$+ \rho(1-\rho) f(t_1) S(t_1)^{-\rho} f(t_2) S(t_2)^{-\rho}(1 - \frac{\gamma\sigma^2}{1-\gamma}\ln S(t_2))^{\frac{1}{\gamma}-1}$$
$$\times \exp\left(\frac{\rho(1-\gamma)}{\gamma\sigma^2}\left[1 - ((1 - \frac{\gamma\sigma^2}{1-\gamma}\ln S(t_1))^{\frac{1}{\gamma}} + (1 - \frac{\gamma\sigma^2}{1-\gamma}\ln S(t_2))^{\frac{1}{\gamma}} - 1)^{\gamma}\right]\right)$$
$$\times ((1 - \frac{\gamma\sigma^2}{1-\gamma}\ln S(t_1))^{\frac{1}{\gamma}} + (1 - \frac{\gamma\sigma^2}{1-\gamma}\ln S(t_2))^{\frac{1}{\gamma}} - 1)^{\gamma-1}$$
$$+ \rho^2 f(t_1) S(t_1)^{-\rho} f(t_2) S(t_2)^{-\rho}$$
$$\times \exp\left(\frac{\rho(1-\gamma)}{\gamma\sigma^2}\left[1 - ((1 - \frac{\gamma\sigma^2}{1-\gamma}\ln S(t_1))^{\frac{1}{\gamma}} + (1 - \frac{\gamma\sigma^2}{1-\gamma}\ln S(t_2))^{\frac{1}{\gamma}} - 1)^{\gamma}\right]\right)$$
$$\times ((1 - \frac{\gamma\sigma^2}{1-\gamma}\ln S(t_1))^{\frac{1}{\gamma}} + (1 - \frac{\gamma\sigma^2}{1-\gamma}\ln S(t_2))^{\frac{1}{\gamma}} - 1)^{2\gamma-2}$$
$$\times (1 - \frac{\gamma\sigma^2}{1-\gamma}\ln S(t_1))^{\frac{1}{\gamma}-1}(1 - \frac{\gamma\sigma^2}{1-\gamma}\ln S(t_2))^{\frac{1}{\gamma}-1}$$
$$+ \rho\sigma^2 f(t_1) S(t_1)^{-\rho} f(t_2) S(t_2)^{-\rho}$$
$$\times \exp\left(\frac{\rho(1-\gamma)}{\gamma\sigma^2}\left[1 - ((1 - \frac{\gamma\sigma^2}{1-\gamma}\ln S(t_1))^{\frac{1}{\gamma}} + (1 - \frac{\gamma\sigma^2}{1-\gamma}\ln S(t_2))^{\frac{1}{\gamma}} - 1)^{\gamma}\right]\right)$$
$$\times ((1 - \frac{\gamma\sigma^2}{1-\gamma}\ln S(t_1))^{\frac{1}{\gamma}} + (1 - \frac{\gamma\sigma^2}{1-\gamma}\ln S(t_2))^{\frac{1}{\gamma}} - 1)^{\gamma-2}$$
$$\times (1 - \frac{\gamma\sigma^2}{1-\gamma}\ln S(t_1))^{\frac{1}{\gamma}-1}(1 - \frac{\gamma\sigma^2}{1-\gamma}\ln S(t_2))^{\frac{1}{\gamma}-1}.$$

Substituting these expressions in (A.2) yields the likelihood function of the bivariate correlated compound Poisson frailty model. The model was used in Section 5.5 to analyze the ages at onset of breast cancer in Swedish female twin pairs. As discussed there in more detail, the correlated gamma and the correlated inverse Gaussian frailty model are special cases of the compound Poisson frailty model.

A.4 Correlated Quadratic Hazard Frailty Model

In the following, the unconditional bivariate survival function in the quadratic hazard frailty model (5.15) is derived by integrating the conditional survival function first with respect to the random effects using the same form of the two-dimensional normal density as in (5.16).

$$
\begin{aligned}
S(t_1, t_2) &= \mathbf{E}S(t_1, t_2 | W_1, W_2) \\
&= \frac{1}{2\pi s_1 s_2 \sqrt{1 - r^2}} \iint S(t_1, t_2 | w_1, w_2) \\
&\quad \times e^{\frac{-1}{1-r^2} \left(\frac{(w_1 - m_1)^2}{2s_1^2} - r\frac{(w_1 - m_1)(w_2 - m_2)}{s_1 s_2} + \frac{(w_2 - m_2)^2}{2s_2^2} \right)} \, dw_1 dw_2 \\
&= \frac{1}{2\pi s_1 s_2 \sqrt{1 - r^2}} \iint e^{-w_1^2 M_0(t_1)} e^{-w_2^2 M_0(t_2)} \\
&\quad \times e^{\frac{-1}{1-r^2} \left(\frac{(w_1 - m_1)^2}{2s_1^2} - r\frac{w_2 - m_2}{s_1 s_2} w_1 \right)} e^{\frac{-1}{1-r^2} \left(\frac{(w_2 - m_2)^2}{2s_2^2} + r\frac{w_2 - m_2}{s_1 s_2} m_1 \right)} \, dw_1 dw_2 \\
&= \frac{1}{\sqrt{2\pi} s_2} \int e^{-w_2^2 M_0(t_2)} I(w_2) e^{\frac{-1}{1-r^2} \left(\frac{(w_2 - m_2)^2}{2s_2^2} + r\frac{w_2 - m_2}{s_1 s_2} m_1 \right)} \, dw_2
\end{aligned}
$$

with

$$
I(w_2) = \frac{1}{\sqrt{2\pi} s_1 \sqrt{1 - r^2}} \int e^{-w_1^2 M_0(t_1)} e^{\frac{-1}{1-r^2} \left(\frac{(w_1 - m_1)^2}{2s_1^2} - r\frac{w_2 - m_2}{s_1 s_2} w_1 \right)} \, dw_1.
$$

In the next paragraph, we first calculate the integral $I(w_2)$:

$$
\begin{aligned}
&I(w_2) \\
&= \frac{1}{\sqrt{2\pi} s_1 \sqrt{1 - r^2}} \int e^{-w_1^2 M_0(t_1)} e^{\frac{-1}{1-r^2} \left(\frac{(w_1 - m_1)^2}{2s_1^2} - r\frac{w_2 - m_2}{s_1 s_2} w_1 \right)} \, dw_1 \\
&= \frac{1}{\sqrt{2\pi} s_1 \sqrt{1 - r^2}} \int e^{-\frac{(1 + 2s_1^2(1 - r^2) M_0(t_1)) s_2 w_1^2 - 2m_1 s_2 w_1 - 2r(w_2 - m_2) s_1 w_1 + m_1^2 s_2}{2s_1^2(1 - r^2) s_2}} \, dw_1 \\
&= \frac{\frac{1}{\sqrt{1 + 2s_1^2(1 - r^2) M_0(t_1)}}}{\frac{\sqrt{2\pi} s_1 \sqrt{1 - r^2}}{\sqrt{1 + 2s_1^2(1 - r^2) M_0(t_1)}}} \exp \left\{ \frac{\left(\frac{m_1 + r(w_2 - m_2)\frac{s_1}{s_2}}{1 + 2s_1^2(1 - r^2) M_0(t_1)} \right)^2 - \frac{m_1^2}{1 + 2s_1^2(1 - r^2) M_0(t_1)}}{2\frac{s_1^2(1 - r^2)}{1 + 2s_1^2(1 - r^2) M_0(t_1)}} \right\} \\
&\quad \times \int \exp \left\{ -\frac{w_1^2 - 2\frac{m_1 + r(w_2 - m_2)\frac{s_1}{s_2}}{1 + 2s_1^2(1 - r^2) M_0(t_1)} w_1 + \left(\frac{m_1 + r(w_2 - m_2)\frac{s_1}{s_2}}{1 + 2s_1^2(1 - r^2) M_0(t_1)} \right)^2}{2\frac{s_1^2(1 - r^2)}{1 + 2s_1^2(1 - r^2) M_0(t_1)}} \right\} dw_1
\end{aligned}
$$

Because of

$$\frac{1}{\frac{\sqrt{2\pi}s_1\sqrt{1-r^2}}{\sqrt{1+2s_1^2(1-r^2)M_0(t_1)}}} \int \exp\left\{-\frac{\left(w_1 - \frac{m_1+r(w_2-m_2)\frac{s_1}{s_2}}{1+2s_1^2(1-r^2)M_0(t_1)}\right)^2}{2\frac{s_1^2(1-r^2)}{1+2s_1^2(1-r^2)M_0(t_1)}}\right\}dw_1 = 1,$$

it holds that

$$I(w_2) = \frac{1}{\sqrt{1+2s_1^2(1-r^2)M_0(t_1)}}e^{\frac{-2s_1^2(1-r^2)M_0(t_1)m_1^2+2rm_1(w_2-m_2)\frac{s_1}{s_2}+r^2(w_2-m_2)^2\frac{s_1^2}{s_2^2}}{2s_1^2(1-r^2)(1+2s_1^2(1-r^2)M_0(t_1))}}$$

$$= \frac{1}{\sqrt{1+2s_1^2(1-r^2)M_0(t_1)}}e^{\frac{-M_0(t_1)m_1^2}{1+2s_1^2(1-r^2)M_0(t_1)}}e^{\frac{2rm_1(w_2-m_2)\frac{s_1}{s_2}+r^2(w_2-m_2)^2\frac{s_1^2}{s_2^2}}{2s_1^2(1-r^2)(1+2s_1^2(1-r^2)M_0(t_1))}}$$

$$= I_1 I_2 I_3(w_2).$$

Now it is necessary to integrate the conditional survival function with respect to the second random effect. Considering the foregoing three terms in more detail, it turns out that the first two terms I_1 and I_2 are independent of w_2. The third term $I_3(w_2)$ contains w_2 and has to be included in the integral with respect to w_2. Consequently, it holds that

$S(t_1, t_2)$

$$= \frac{I_1 I_2}{\sqrt{2\pi}s_2}\int e^{-w_2^2 M_0(t_2)}e^{\frac{-1}{1-r^2}\left(\frac{(w_2-m_2)^2}{2s_2^2}+r\frac{w_2-m_2}{s_1 s_2}m_1\right)}I_3(w_2)\,dw_2$$

$$= \frac{I_1 I_2}{\sqrt{2\pi}s_2}\int e^{-w_2^2 M_0(t_2)}e^{\frac{-1}{1-r^2}\left(\frac{(w_2-m_2)^2}{2s_2^2}+r\frac{w_2-m_2}{s_1 s_2}m_1\right)}$$

$$\times e^{\frac{2rm_1(w_2-m_2)\frac{s_1}{s_2}+r^2(w_2-m_2)^2\frac{s_1^2}{s_2^2}}{2s_1^2(1-r^2)(1+2s_1^2(1-r^2)M_0(t_1))}}\,dw_2$$

$$= \frac{I_1 I_2}{\sqrt{2\pi}s_2}\int e^{-w_2^2 M_0(t_2)}e^{-\frac{(w_2-m_2)^2 s_1^2(1+2s_1^2(1-r^2)M_0(t_1))}{2s_1^2(1-r^2)s_2^2(1+2s_1^2(1-r^2)M_0(t_1))}}$$

$$\times e^{-\frac{2rm_1 s_1 s_2(1+2s_1^2(1-r^2)M_0(t_1))(w_2-m_2)-2rm_1 s_1 s_2(w_2-m_2)-r^2(w_2-m_2)^2 s_1^2}{2s_1^2(1-r^2)s_2^2(1+2s_1^2(1-r^2)M_0(t_1))}}\,dw_2$$

$$= \frac{I_1 I_2}{\sqrt{2\pi}s_2}\int e^{-\frac{(1+2s_1^2 M_0(t_1))(w_2-m_2)^2+2s_2^2(1+2s_1^2(1-r^2)M_0(t_1))M_0(t_2)w_2^2}{2s_2^2(1+2s_1^2(1-r^2)M_0(t_1))}}$$

$$\times e^{-\frac{4rm_1 s_1 s_2 M_0(t_1)(w_2-m_2)}{2s_2^2(1+2s_1^2(1-r^2)M_0(t_1))}}\,dw_2$$

$$= \frac{I_1 I_2}{\sqrt{2\pi}s_2}\int e^{-\frac{(1+2s_1^2 M_0(t_1)+2s_2^2(1+2s_1^2(1-r^2)M_0(t_1))M_0(t_2))w_2^2}{2s_2^2(1+2s_1^2(1-r^2)M_0(t_1))}}$$

$$\times e^{-\frac{-2((1+2s_1^2 M_0(t_1))m_2-2rm_1 s_1 s_2 M_0(t_1))w_2}{2s_2^2(1+2s_1^2(1-r^2)M_0(t_1))}}\,dw_2\, e^{-\frac{(1+2s_1^2 M_0(t_1))m_2^2-4rm_1 m_2 s_1 s_2 M_0(t_1)}{2s_2^2(1+2s_1^2(1-r^2)M_0(t_1))}}.$$

Substituting the last factor by the shorthand

$$I_4 = e^{-\frac{(1+2s_1^2 M_0(t_1))m_2^2 - 4rm_1 m_2 s_1 s_2 M_0(t_1)}{2s_2^2(1+2s_1^2(1-r^2)M_0(t_1))}},$$

then

$$S(t_1, t_2)$$

$$= \frac{I_1 I_2 I_4}{\sqrt{2\pi}s_2} \int e^{-\frac{(1+2s_1^2 M_0(t_1)+2s_2^2(1+2s_1^2(1-r^2)M_0(t_1))M_0(t_2))w_2^2}{2s_2^2(1+2s_1^2(1-r^2)M_0(t_1))}} \, dw_2$$

$$\times e^{-\frac{-2((1+2s_1^2 M_0(t_1))m_2 - 2rm_1 s_1 s_2 M_0(t_1))w_2}{2s_2^2(1+2s_1^2(1-r^2)M_0(t_1))}} \, dw_2$$

$$= \frac{I_1 I_2 I_4}{\sqrt{2\pi}s_2} \int \exp\left\{ -\frac{w_2^2 - \frac{2((1+2s_1^2 M_0(t_1))m_2 - 2rm_1 s_1 s_2 M_0(t_1))w_2}{1+2s_1^2 M_0(t_1)+2s_2^2 M_0(t_2)+4s_1^2 s_2^2(1-r^2)M_0(t_1)M_0(t_2)}}{\frac{2s_2^2(1+2s_1^2(1-r^2)M_0(t_1))}{1+2s_1^2 M_0(t_1)+2s_2^2 M_0(t_2)+4s_1^2 s_2^2(1-r^2)M_0(t_1)M_0(t_2)}} \right\} \, dw_2$$

$$= I_1 I_2 I_4 \frac{\sqrt{1+2s_1^2(1-r^2)M_0(t_1)}}{\sqrt{1+2s_1^2 M_0(t_1)+2s_2^2 M_0(t_2)+4s_1^2 s_2^2(1-r^2)M_0(t_1)M_0(t_2)}}$$

$$\times \exp\left\{ -\frac{-\left(\frac{(1+2s_1^2 M_0(t_1))m_2 - 2rm_1 s_1 s_2 M_0(t_1)}{1+2s_1^2 M_0(t_1)+2s_2^2 M_0(t_2)+4s_1^2 s_2^2(1-r^2)M_0(t_1)M_0(t_2)}\right)^2}{\frac{2s_2^2(1+2s_1^2(1-r^2)M_0(t_1))}{1+2s_1^2 M_0(t_1)+2s_2^2 M_0(t_2)+4s_1^2 s_2^2(1-r^2)M_0(t_1)M_0(t_2)}} \right\}.$$

Here I_1 cancels out. Furthermore, we introduce

$$I_5 - \frac{1}{\sqrt{1+2s_1^2 M_0(t_1)+2s_2^2 M_0(t_2)+4s_1^2 s_2^2(1-r^2)M_0(t_1)M_0(t_2)}},$$

which implies that

$$S(t_1, t_2)$$

$$= I_2 I_5 e^{-\frac{((1+2s_1^2 M_0(t_1))m_2 - 2rm_1 s_1 s_2 M_0(t_1))^2}{2s_2^2(1+2s_1^2(1-r^2)M_0(t_1))(1+2s_1^2 M_0(t_1)+2s_2^2 M_0(t_2)+4s_1^2 s_2^2(1-r^2)M_0(t_1)M_0(t_2))}}$$

$$\times e^{-\frac{((1+2s_1^2 M_0(t_1))m_2^2 - 4rm_1 m_2 s_1 s_2 M_0(t_1))(1+2s_1^2 M_0(t_1)+2s_2^2 M_0(t_2)+4s_1^2 s_2^2(1-r^2)M_0(t_1)M_0(t_2))}{2s_2^2(1+2s_1^2(1-r^2)M_0(t_1))(1+2s_1^2 M_0(t_1)+2s_2^2 M_0(t_2)+4s_1^2 s_2^2(1-r^2)M_0(t_1)M_0(t_2))}}$$

$$= I_2 I_5 e^{-\frac{-2r^2 m_1^2 s_1^2 M_0^2(t_1)+m_2^2 M_0(t_2)(1+2s_1^2 M_0(t_1))(1+2s_1^2(1-r^2)M_0(t_1))}{(1+2s_1^2(1-r^2)M_0(t_1))(1+2s_1^2 M_0(t_1)+2s_2^2 M_0(t_2)+4s_1^2 s_2^2(1-r^2)M_0(t_1)M_0(t_2))}}$$

$$\times e^{-\frac{-4rm_1 m_2 s_1 s_2 M_0(t_1)M_0(t_2)(1+2s_1^2(1-r^2)M_0(t_1))}{(1+2s_1^2(1-r^2)M_0(t_1))(1+2s_1^2 M_0(t_1)+2s_2^2 M_0(t_2)+4s_1^2 s_2^2(1-r^2)M_0(t_1)M_0(t_2))}}.$$

Substituting the term I_2 back, it holds that

$$S(t_1, t_2)$$

$$= I_5 e^{-\frac{m_1^2 M_0(t_1)(1+2s_1^2 M_0(t_1)+2s_2^2 M_0(t_2)+4s_1^2 s_2^2(1-r^2)M_0(t_1)M_0(t_2))-2r^2 m_1^2 s_1^2 M_0^2(t_1)}{(1+2(1-r^2)s_1^2 M_0(t_1))(1+2s_1^2 M_0(t_1)+2s_2^2 M_0(t_2)+4s_1^2 s_2^2(1-r^2)M_0(t_1)M_0(t_2))}}$$

$$\times e^{-\frac{m_2^2 M_0(t_2)(1+2s_1^2 M_0(t_1))-4r m_1 m_2 s_1 s_2 M_0(t_1)M_0(t_2)}{1+2s_1^2 M_0(t_1)+2s_2^2 M_0(t_2)+4s_1^2 s_2^2(1-r^2)M_0(t_1)M_0(t_2)}}$$

$$= \frac{1}{\sqrt{1+2s_1^2 M_0(t_1)+2s_2^2 M_0(t_2)+4s_1^2 s_2^2(1-r^2)M_0(t_1)M_0(t_2)}}$$

$$\times e^{-\frac{m_2^2 M_0(t_2)(1+2s_1^2 M_0(t_1))-4r m_1 m_2 s_1 s_2 M_0(t_1)M_0(t_2)+m_1^2 M_0(t_1)(1+2s_2^2 M_0(t_2))}{(1+2s_1^2 M_0(t_1)+2s_2^2 M_0(t_2)+4s_1^2 s_2^2(1-r^2)M_0(t_1)M_0(t_2))}}.$$

In the case of independence $r = 0$, this results in

$$\frac{1}{\sqrt{1+2s_1^2 M_0(t_1)}} e^{\frac{-M_0(t_1)m_1^2}{1+2s_1^2 M_0(t_1)}} \frac{1}{\sqrt{1+2s_2^2 M_0(t_2)}} e^{\frac{-M_0(t_2)m_2^2}{1+2s_2^2 M_0(t_2)}}.$$

Now we are considering the case of $m_1 = m_2 = 0$ and $s_1^2 = s_2^2 = s^2$, but $r \neq 0$. For this special case, it is straightforward to derive the log-likelihood function, requiring the first and second derivatives of the unconditional survival function $S(t_1, t_2)$. Using the relation $S(t) = (1 + 2s^2 M_0(t))^{-1/2}$, the bivariate survival function becomes, in the copula form,

$$S(t_1, t_2) = \left(S(t_1)^{-2} S(t_2)^{-2} - r^2(S(t_1)^{-2} - 1)(S(t_2)^{-2} - 1)\right)^{-\frac{1}{2}}$$

$$S_{t_1}(t_1, t_2) = -\left(S(t_1)^{-2} S(t_2)^{-2} - r^2(S(t_1)^{-2} - 1)(S(t_2)^{-2} - 1)\right)^{-\frac{3}{2}}$$
$$\times f(t_1)S(t_1)^{-3}((1 - r^2)S(t_2)^{-2} + r^2)$$

$$S_{t_2}(t_1, t_2) = -\left(S(t_1)^{-2} S(t_2)^{-2} - r^2(S(t_1)^{-2} - 1)(S(t_2)^{-2} - 1)\right)^{-\frac{3}{2}}$$
$$\times f(t_2)S(t_2)^{-3}((1 - r^2)S(t_1)^{-2} + r^2).$$

For the second derivative, it holds that

$$S_{t_1 t_2}(t_1, t_2)$$

$$= 3\left(S(t_1)^{-2} S(t_2)^{-2} - r^2(S(t_1)^{-2} - 1)(S(t_2)^{-2} - 1)\right)^{-\frac{5}{2}}$$
$$\times f(t_1)S(t_1)^{-3} f(t_2)S(t_2)^{-3}((1 - r^2)S(t_1)^{-2} + r^2)((1 - r^2)S(t_2)^{-2} + r^2)$$
$$- 2(1 - r^2)\left(S(t_1)^{-2} S(t_2)^{-2} - r^2(S(t_1)^{-2} - 1)(S(t_2)^{-2} - 1)\right)^{-\frac{3}{2}}$$
$$\times f(t_1)S(t_1)^{-3} f(t_2)S(t_2)^{-3}$$

$$= \left(S(t_1)^{-2} S(t_2)^{-2} - r^2(S(t_1)^{-2} - 1)(S(t_2)^{-2} - 1)\right)^{-\frac{5}{2}} f(t_1)S(t_1)^{-3}$$
$$\times f(t_2)S(t_2)^{-3}\left(((1 - r^2)S(t_1)^{-2} + r^2)((1 - r^2)S(t_2)^{-2} + r^2) + 2r^2\right).$$

This expression can now be used in the bivariate likelihood function (A.2).

A.5 Dependent Competing Risks Model

Here a specific four-dimensional correlated gamma frailty model is derived to model dependent competing risks in twin survival data. The following relations are used in the calculations: Let $V_1, V_8 \sim \Gamma(k_1, \lambda_0)$, $V_2 \sim \Gamma(k_2, \lambda_1)$, $V_3 \sim \Gamma(k_3, \lambda_2)$, $V_4, V_7 \sim \Gamma(k_4, \lambda_2)$, $V_5, V_6 \sim \Gamma(k_5, \lambda_1)$ be independent gamma-distributed random variables with parameters $k_1 + k_2 + k_5 := \lambda_1 = \frac{1}{\sigma_1^2}$ and $k_1 + k_3 + k_4 := \lambda_2 = \frac{1}{\sigma_2^2}$. Hence, it holds that $\mathbf{E}Z_1 = \mathbf{E}Z_2 = \mathbf{E}Z_3 = \mathbf{E}Z_4 = 1$, $\mathbf{V}(Z_1) = \mathbf{V}(Z_3) = \frac{1}{k_1+k_2+k_5} = \sigma_1^2$, and $\mathbf{V}(Z_2) = \mathbf{V}(Z_4) = \frac{1}{k_1+k_3+k_4} = \sigma_2^2$. It holds that

$$\mathbf{cov}(Z_1, Z_3) = \mathbf{cov}(\frac{\lambda_0}{\lambda_1}V_1 + V_2 + V_5, V_2 + V_6 + \frac{\lambda_0}{\lambda_1}V_8) = \mathbf{V}(V_2) = \frac{k_2}{\lambda_1^2}.$$

Consequently, the correlation coefficient between Z_1 and Z_3 is

$$\rho_1 = \mathbf{corr}(Z_1, Z_3) = \frac{\mathbf{cov}(Z_1, Z_3)}{\sqrt{\mathbf{V}(Z_1)\mathbf{V}(Z_3)}} = \frac{k_2}{\lambda_1} = k_2\sigma_1^2. \tag{A.3}$$

Here, ρ_1 is the correlation between the frailties of twins with respect to the first risk. By similar calculations it is easy to obtain $\rho_2 = \mathbf{corr}(Z_2, Z_4) = k_3\sigma_2^2$, which describes the correlation between frailties of twin partners regarding the second competing risk. In the following we calculate the correlation coefficient $\rho = \mathbf{corr}(Z_1, Z_2) = \mathbf{corr}(Z_3, Z_4)$, describing the correlation between the frailty terms of the two competing risks. It holds that

$$\mathbf{cov}(Z_1, Z_2) = \mathbf{cov}(\frac{\lambda_0}{\lambda_1}V_1 + V_2 + V_5, \frac{\lambda_0}{\lambda_2}V_1 + V_3 + V_4) = \frac{\lambda_0^2}{\lambda_1\lambda_2}\mathbf{V}(V_1) = \frac{k_1}{\lambda_1\lambda_2}.$$

The correlation coefficient between Z_1 and Z_2 (and between Z_3 and Z_4) is given by

$$\rho = \mathbf{corr}(Z_1, Z_2) = \frac{\mathbf{cov}(Z_1, Z_2)}{\sqrt{\mathbf{V}(Z_1)\mathbf{V}(Z_2)}} = \frac{k_1}{\sqrt{\lambda_1\lambda_2}} = k_1\sigma_1\sigma_2. \tag{A.4}$$

Consequently, $k_1 + k_2 + k_5 = \frac{1}{\sigma_1^2}$, $k_1 + k_3 + k_4 = \frac{1}{\sigma_2^2}$, and relations (A.3) and (A.4) result in

$$k_5 = \frac{1}{\sigma_1^2} - k_2 - k_1 = \frac{1}{\sigma_1^2} - \frac{\rho_1}{\sigma_1^2} - \frac{\rho}{\sigma_1\sigma_2}$$

and

$$k_4 = \frac{1}{\sigma_2^2} - k_3 - k_4 = \frac{1}{\sigma_2^2} - \frac{\rho_2}{\sigma_2^2} - \frac{\rho}{\sigma_1\sigma_2}.$$

For gamma-distributed random variables $Y \sim \Gamma(k, \lambda)$, the Laplace transform is given by $\mathbf{E}e^{-sY} = (1+\frac{s}{\lambda})^{-k}$. Now we are in the state to derive the survival function in (5.25):

$$S(t_1, y_1, t_2, y_2)$$
$$= \mathbf{E}S_1(t_1)^{Z_1} S_2(y_1)^{Z_2} S_1(t_2)^{Z_3} S_2(y_2)^{Z_4}$$
$$= \mathbf{E}e^{-V_1(\frac{\lambda_0}{\lambda_1}M_{01}(t_1)+\frac{\lambda_0}{\lambda_2}M_{02}(y_1))}e^{-V_2(M_{01}(t_1)+M_{01}(t_2))}$$
$$\times e^{-V_3(M_{02}(y_1)+M_{02}(y_2))}e^{-V_8(\frac{\lambda_0}{\lambda_1}M_{01}(t_2)+\frac{\lambda_0}{\lambda_2}M_{02}(y_2))}$$
$$\times e^{-V_4 M_{02}(y_1)}e^{-V_5 M_{01}(t_1)}e^{-V_6 M_{01}(t_2)}e^{-V_7 M_{02}(y_2)}$$
$$= \left(1 + \frac{M_{01}(t_1)}{\lambda_1} + \frac{M_{02}(y_1)}{\lambda_2}\right)^{-k_1}\left(1 + \frac{M_{01}(t_1)}{\lambda_1} + \frac{M_{01}(t_2)}{\lambda_1}\right)^{-k_2}$$
$$\times \left(1 + \frac{M_{02}(y_1)}{\lambda_2} + \frac{M_{02}(y_2)}{\lambda_2}\right)^{-k_3}\left(1 + \frac{M_{01}(t_2)}{\lambda_1} + \frac{M_{02}(y_2)}{\lambda_2}\right)^{-k_1}$$
$$\times \left(1 + \frac{M_{02}(y_1)}{\lambda_2}\right)^{-k_4}\left(1 + \frac{M_{01}(t_1)}{\lambda_1}\right)^{-k_5}\left(1 + \frac{M_{01}(t_2)}{\lambda_1}\right)^{-k_5}\left(1 + \frac{M_{02}(y_2)}{\lambda_2}\right)^{-k_4}$$
$$= \left(S_1(t_1)^{-\sigma_1^2} + S_1(t_2)^{-\sigma_1^2} - 1\right)^{-\frac{\rho_1}{\sigma_1^2}}\left(S_2(y_1)^{-\sigma_2^2} + S_2(y_2)^{-\sigma_2^2} - 1\right)^{-\frac{\rho_2}{\sigma_2^2}}$$
$$\times \left(S_1(t_1)^{-\sigma_1^2} + S_2(y_1)^{-\sigma_2^2} - 1\right)^{-\frac{\rho}{\sigma_1\sigma_2}}\left(S_1(t_2)^{-\sigma_1^2} + S_2(y_2)^{-\sigma_2^2} - 1\right)^{-\frac{\rho}{\sigma_1\sigma_2}}$$
$$\times S_2(y_1)^{1-\rho_2-\frac{\sigma_2}{\sigma_1}\rho}S_1(t_1)^{1-\rho_1-\frac{\sigma_1}{\sigma_2}\rho}S_1(t_2)^{1-\rho_1-\frac{\sigma_1}{\sigma_2}\rho}S_2(y_2)^{1-\rho_2-\frac{\sigma_2}{\sigma_1}\rho}.$$

To derive the likelihood function of the bivariate dependent competing risk data, it is necessary to keep in mind that the above four-dimensional model is not fully observable. Only the minimum of the three competing risk times (t_j, y_j, c_j) is observable for twin j ($j = 1, 2$). Because of (5.23), the likelihood contribution of the truncated data takes the form

$$\Big(1(\delta_1 = 1, \delta_2 = 1)S_{t_1,t_2}(t_1, t_1, t_2, t_2)$$
$$+ 1(\delta_1 = 1, \delta_2 = 0)S_{t_1}(t_1, t_1, c_2, c_2)$$
$$+ 1(\delta_1 = 0, \delta_2 = 1)S_{t_2}(c_1, c_1, t_2, t_2)$$
$$+ 1(\delta_1 = 0, \delta_2 = 0)S(c_1, c_1, c_2, c_2)$$
$$+ 1(\delta_1 = -1, \delta_2 = -1)S_{y_1 y_2}(y_1, y_1, y_2, y_2)$$
$$+ 1(\delta_1 = -1, \delta_2 = 0)S_{y_1}(y_1, y_1, c_2, c_2)$$
$$+ 1(\delta_1 = 0, \delta_2 = -1)S_{y_2}(c_1, c_1, y_2, y_2)$$
$$+ 1(\delta_1 = 1, \delta_2 = -1)S_{t_1 y_2}(t_1, t_1, y_2, y_2)$$
$$+ 1(\delta_1 = -1, \delta_2 = 1)S_{y_1 t_2}(y_1, y_1, t_2, t_2)\Big)/S(t^+, t^+, t^+, t^+),$$

where t^+ denotes the truncation time. In the following the derivatives of the survival function needed for the likelihood expression are calculated.

$$S_{t_1}(t_1, y_1, t_2, y_2)$$

$$= -\rho_1(S_1(t_1)^{-\sigma_1^2} + S_1(y_1)^{-\sigma_1^2} - 1)^{-\frac{\rho_1}{\sigma_1^2}-1}(S_2(t_2)^{-\sigma_2^2} + S_2(y_2)^{-\sigma_2^2} - 1)^{-\frac{\rho_2}{\sigma_2^2}}$$

$$\times (S_1(t_1)^{-\sigma_1^2} + S_2(t_2)^{-\sigma_2^2} - 1)^{-\frac{\rho}{\sigma_1\sigma_2}}(S_1(y_1)^{-\sigma_1^2} + S_2(y_2)^{-\sigma_2^2} - 1)^{-\frac{\rho}{\sigma_1\sigma_2}}$$

$$\times S_1(t_1)^{1-\rho_1-\frac{\sigma_1}{\sigma_2}\rho-\sigma_1^2}\mu_1(t_1)S_1(y_1)^{1-\rho_1-\frac{\sigma_1}{\sigma_2}\rho}S_2(t_2)^{1-\rho_2-\frac{\sigma_2}{\sigma_1}\rho}S_2(y_2)^{1-\rho_2-\frac{\sigma_2}{\sigma_1}\rho}$$

$$- \frac{\sigma_1}{\sigma_2}\rho(S_1(t_1)^{-\sigma_1^2} + S_1(y_1)^{-\sigma_1^2} - 1)^{-\frac{\rho_1}{\sigma_1^2}}(S_2(t_2)^{-\sigma_2^2} + S_2(y_2)^{-\sigma_2^2} - 1)^{-\frac{\rho_2}{\sigma_2^2}}$$

$$\times (S_1(t_1)^{-\sigma_1^2} + S_2(t_2)^{-\sigma_2^2} - 1)^{-\frac{\rho}{\sigma_1\sigma_2}-1}(S_1(y_1)^{-\sigma_1^2} + S_2(y_2)^{-\sigma_2^2} - 1)^{-\frac{\rho}{\sigma_1\sigma_2}}$$

$$\times S_1(t_1)^{1-\rho_1-\frac{\sigma_1}{\sigma_2}\rho-\sigma_1^2}\mu_1(t_1)S_1(y_1)^{1-\rho_1-\frac{\sigma_1}{\sigma_2}\rho}S_2(t_2)^{1-\rho_2-\frac{\sigma_2}{\sigma_1}\rho}S_2(y_2)^{1-\rho_2-\frac{\sigma_2}{\sigma_1}\rho}$$

$$- (1-\rho_1-\frac{\sigma_1}{\sigma_2}\rho)\sigma_1^2(S_1(t_1)^{-\sigma_1^2} + S_1(y_1)^{-\sigma_1^2} - 1)^{-\frac{\rho_1}{\sigma_1^2}}$$

$$\times (S_2(t_2)^{-\sigma_2^2} + S_2(y_2)^{-\sigma_2^2} - 1)^{-\frac{\rho_2}{\sigma_2^2}}(S_1(t_1)^{-\sigma_1^2} + S_2(t_2)^{-\sigma_2^2} - 1)^{-\frac{\rho}{\sigma_1\sigma_2}}$$

$$\times (S_1(y_1)^{-\sigma_1^2} + S_2(y_2)^{-\sigma_2^2} - 1)^{-\frac{\rho}{\sigma_1\sigma_2}}$$

$$\times S_1(t_1)^{1-\rho_1-\frac{\sigma_1}{\sigma_2}\rho}\mu_1(t_1)S_1(y_1)^{1-\rho_1-\frac{\sigma_1}{\sigma_2}\rho}S_2(t_2)^{1-\rho_2-\frac{\sigma_2}{\sigma_1}\rho}S_2(y_2)^{1-\rho_2-\frac{\sigma_2}{\sigma_1}\rho}$$

$$S_{y_1}(t_1, y_1, t_2, y_2)$$

$$= -\rho_1(S_1(t_1)^{-\sigma_1^2} + S_1(y_1)^{-\sigma_1^2} - 1)^{-\frac{\rho_1}{\sigma_1^2}-1}(S_2(t_2)^{-\sigma_2^2} + S_2(y_2)^{-\sigma_2^2} - 1)^{-\frac{\rho_2}{\sigma_2^2}}$$

$$\times (S_1(t_1)^{-\sigma_1^2} + S_2(t_2)^{-\sigma_2^2} - 1)^{-\frac{\rho}{\sigma_1\sigma_2}}(S_1(y_1)^{-\sigma_1^2} + S_2(y_2)^{-\sigma_2^2} - 1)^{-\frac{\rho}{\sigma_1\sigma_2}}$$

$$\times S_1(t_1)^{1-\rho_1-\frac{\sigma_1}{\sigma_2}\rho}S_1(y_1)^{1-\rho_1-\frac{\sigma_1}{\sigma_2}\rho-\sigma_1^2}\mu_1(y_1)S_2(t_2)^{1-\rho_2-\frac{\sigma_2}{\sigma_1}\rho}S_2(y_2)^{1-\rho_2-\frac{\sigma_2}{\sigma_1}\rho}$$

$$- \frac{\sigma_1}{\sigma_2}\rho(S_1(t_1)^{-\sigma_1^2} + S_1(y_1)^{-\sigma_1^2} - 1)^{-\frac{\rho_1}{\sigma_1^2}}(S_2(t_2)^{-\sigma_2^2} + S_2(y_2)^{-\sigma_2^2} - 1)^{-\frac{\rho_2}{\sigma_2^2}}$$

$$\times (S_1(t_1)^{-\sigma_1^2} + S_2(t_2)^{-\sigma_2^2} - 1)^{-\frac{\rho}{\sigma_1\sigma_2}}(S_1(y_1)^{-\sigma_1^2} + S_2(y_2)^{-\sigma_2^2} - 1)^{-\frac{\rho}{\sigma_1\sigma_2}-1}$$

$$\times S_1(t_1)^{1-\rho_1-\frac{\sigma_1}{\sigma_2}\rho}S_1(y_1)^{1-\rho_1-\frac{\sigma_1}{\sigma_2}\rho-\sigma_1^2}\mu_1(y_1)S_2(t_2)^{1-\rho_2-\frac{\sigma_2}{\sigma_1}\rho}S_2(y_2)^{1-\rho_2-\frac{\sigma_2}{\sigma_1}\rho}$$

$$- (1-\rho_1-\frac{\sigma_1}{\sigma_2}\rho)\sigma_1^2(S_1(t_1)^{-\sigma_1^2} + S_1(y_1)^{-\sigma_1^2} - 1)^{-\frac{\rho_1}{\sigma_1^2}}$$

$$\times (S_2(t_2)^{-\sigma_2^2} + S_2(y_2)^{-\sigma_2^2} - 1)^{-\frac{\rho_2}{\sigma_2^2}}(S_1(t_1)^{-\sigma_1^2} + S_2(t_2)^{-\sigma_2^2} - 1)^{-\frac{\rho}{\sigma_1\sigma_2}}$$

$$\times (S_1(y_1)^{-\sigma_1^2} + S_2(y_2)^{-\sigma_2^2} - 1)^{-\frac{\rho}{\sigma_1\sigma_2}}$$

$$\times S_1(t_1)^{1-\rho_1-\frac{\sigma_1}{\sigma_2}\rho}S_1(y_1)^{1-\rho_1-\frac{\sigma_1}{\sigma_2}\rho}\mu_1(y_1)S_2(t_2)^{1-\rho_2-\frac{\sigma_2}{\sigma_1}\rho}S_2(y_2)^{1-\rho_2-\frac{\sigma_2}{\sigma_1}\rho}$$

$$S_{t_2}(t_1, y_1, t_2, y_2)$$

$$= -\rho_2 (S_1(t_1)^{-\sigma_1^2} + S_1(y_1)^{-\sigma_1^2} - 1)^{-\frac{\rho_1}{\sigma_1^2}} (S_2(t_2)^{-\sigma_2^2} + S_2(y_2)^{-\sigma_2^2} - 1)^{-\frac{\rho_2}{\sigma_2^2}-1}$$

$$\times (S_1(t_1)^{-\sigma_1^2} + S_2(t_2)^{-\sigma_2^2} - 1)^{-\frac{\rho}{\sigma_1\sigma_2}} (S_1(y_1)^{-\sigma_1^2} + S_2(y_2)^{-\sigma_2^2} - 1)^{-\frac{\rho}{\sigma_1\sigma_2}}$$

$$\times S_1(t_1)^{1-\rho_1-\frac{\sigma_1}{\sigma_2}\rho} S_1(y_1)^{1-\rho_1-\frac{\sigma_1}{\sigma_2}\rho} S_2(t_2)^{1-\rho_2-\frac{\sigma_2}{\sigma_1}\rho-\sigma_2^2} \mu_2(t_2) S_2(y_2)^{1-\rho_2-\frac{\sigma_2}{\sigma_1}\rho}$$

$$- \frac{\sigma_2}{\sigma_1}\rho (S_1(t_1)^{-\sigma_1^2} + S_1(y_1)^{-\sigma_1^2} - 1)^{-\frac{\rho_1}{\sigma_1^2}} (S_2(t_2)^{-\sigma_2^2} + S_2(y_2)^{-\sigma_2^2} - 1)^{-\frac{\rho_2}{\sigma_2^2}}$$

$$\times (S_1(t_1)^{-\sigma_1^2} + S_2(t_2)^{-\sigma_2^2} - 1)^{-\frac{\rho}{\sigma_1\sigma_2}-1} (S_1(y_1)^{-\sigma_1^2} + S_2(y_2)^{-\sigma_2^2} - 1)^{-\frac{\rho}{\sigma_1\sigma_2}}$$

$$\times S_1(t_1)^{1-\rho_1-\frac{\sigma_1}{\sigma_2}\rho} S_1(y_1)^{1-\rho_1-\frac{\sigma_1}{\sigma_2}\rho} S_2(t_2)^{1-\rho_2-\frac{\sigma_2}{\sigma_1}\rho-\sigma_2^2} \mu_2(t_2) S_2(y_2)^{1-\rho_2-\frac{\sigma_2}{\sigma_1}\rho}$$

$$- (1-\rho_2-\frac{\sigma_2}{\sigma_1}\rho)\sigma_2^2 (S_1(t_1)^{-\sigma_1^2} + S_1(y_1)^{-\sigma_1^2} - 1)^{-\frac{\rho_1}{\sigma_1^2}}$$

$$\times (S_2(t_2)^{-\sigma_2^2} + S_2(y_2)^{-\sigma_2^2} - 1)^{-\frac{\rho_2}{\sigma_2^2}} (S_1(t_1)^{-\sigma_1^2} + S_2(t_2)^{-\sigma_2^2} - 1)^{-\frac{\rho}{\sigma_1\sigma_2}}$$

$$\times (S_1(y_1)^{-\sigma_1^2} + S_2(y_2)^{-\sigma_2^2} - 1)^{-\frac{\rho}{\sigma_1\sigma_2}}$$

$$\times S_1(t_1)^{1-\rho_1-\frac{\sigma_1}{\sigma_2}\rho} S_1(y_1)^{1-\rho_1-\frac{\sigma_1}{\sigma_2}\rho} S_2(t_2)^{1-\rho_2-\frac{\sigma_2}{\sigma_1}\rho} \mu_2(t_2) S_2(y_2)^{1-\rho_2-\frac{\sigma_2}{\sigma_1}\rho}$$

$$S_{y_2}(t_1, y_1, t_2, y_2)$$

$$= -\rho_2 (S_1(t_1)^{-\sigma_1^2} + S_1(y_1)^{-\sigma_1^2} - 1)^{-\frac{\rho_1}{\sigma_1^2}} (S_2(t_2)^{-\sigma_2^2} + S_2(y_2)^{-\sigma_2^2} - 1)^{-\frac{\rho_2}{\sigma_2^2}-1}$$

$$\times (S_1(t_1)^{-\sigma_1^2} + S_2(t_2)^{-\sigma_2^2} - 1)^{-\frac{\rho}{\sigma_1\sigma_2}} (S_1(y_1)^{-\sigma_1^2} + S_2(y_2)^{-\sigma_2^2} - 1)^{-\frac{\rho}{\sigma_1\sigma_2}}$$

$$\times S_1(t_1)^{1-\rho_1-\frac{\sigma_1}{\sigma_2}\rho} S_1(y_1)^{1-\rho_1-\frac{\sigma_1}{\sigma_2}\rho} S_2(t_2)^{1-\rho_2-\frac{\sigma_2}{\sigma_1}\rho} S_2(y_2)^{1-\rho_2-\frac{\sigma_2}{\sigma_1}\rho-\sigma_2^2} \mu_2(y_2)$$

$$- \frac{\sigma_1}{\sigma_2}\rho (S_1(t_1)^{-\sigma_1^2} + S_1(y_1)^{-\sigma_1^2} - 1)^{-\frac{\rho_1}{\sigma_1^2}} (S_2(t_2)^{-\sigma_2^2} + S_2(y_2)^{-\sigma_2^2} - 1)^{-\frac{\rho_2}{\sigma_2^2}}$$

$$\times (S_1(t_1)^{-\sigma_1^2} + S_2(t_2)^{-\sigma_2^2} - 1)^{-\frac{\rho}{\sigma_1\sigma_2}} (S_1(y_1)^{-\sigma_1^2} + S_2(y_2)^{-\sigma_2^2} - 1)^{-\frac{\rho}{\sigma_1\sigma_2}-1}$$

$$\times S_1(t_1)^{1-\rho_1-\frac{\sigma_1}{\sigma_2}\rho} S_1(y_1)^{1-\rho_1-\frac{\sigma_1}{\sigma_2}\rho} S_2(t_2)^{1-\rho_2-\frac{\sigma_2}{\sigma_1}\rho} S_2(y_2)^{1-\rho_2-\frac{\sigma_2}{\sigma_1}\rho-\sigma_2^2} \mu_2(y_2)$$

$$- (1-\rho_2-\frac{\sigma_2}{\sigma_1}\rho)\sigma_2^2 (S_1(t_1)^{-\sigma_1^2} + S_1(y_1)^{-\sigma_1^2} - 1)^{-\frac{\rho_1}{\sigma_1^2}}$$

$$\times (S_2(t_2)^{-\sigma_2^2} + S_2(y_2)^{-\sigma_2^2} - 1)^{-\frac{\rho_2}{\sigma_2^2}} (S_1(t_1)^{-\sigma_1^2} + S_2(t_2)^{-\sigma_2^2} - 1)^{-\frac{\rho}{\sigma_1\sigma_2}}$$

$$\times (S_1(y_1)^{-\sigma_1^2} + S_2(y_2)^{-\sigma_2^2} - 1)^{-\frac{\rho}{\sigma_1\sigma_2}}$$

$$\times S_1(t_1)^{1-\rho_1-\frac{\sigma_1}{\sigma_2}\rho} S_1(y_1)^{1-\rho_1-\frac{\sigma_1}{\sigma_2}\rho} S_2(t_2)^{1-\rho_2-\frac{\sigma_2}{\sigma_1}\rho} S_2(y_2)^{1-\rho_2-\frac{\sigma_2}{\sigma_1}\rho} \mu_2(y_2)$$

$S_{t_1,y_1}(t_1, y_1, t_2, y_2)$

$= \mu_1(t_1)\mu_1(y_1)(S_1(t_1)^{-\sigma_1^2} + S_1(y_1)^{-\sigma_1^2} - 1)^{-\rho_1/\sigma_1^2-2}(S_2(t_2)^{-\sigma_2^2} + S_2(y_2)^{-\sigma_2^2} - 1)^{-\rho_2/\sigma_2^2}$

$\times (S_1(t_1)^{-\sigma_1^2} + S_2(t_2)^{-\sigma_2^2} - 1)^{-\rho/\sigma_1\sigma_2-1}(S_1(y_1)^{-\sigma_1^2} + S_2(y_2)^{-\sigma_2^2} - 1)^{-\rho/\sigma_1\sigma_2-1}$

$\times S_1(t_1)^{1-\rho_1-\frac{\sigma_1}{\sigma_2}\rho}S_1(y_1)^{1-\sigma_1-\frac{\sigma_1}{\sigma_2}\rho}S_2(t_2)^{1-\rho_2-\frac{\sigma_2}{\sigma_1}\rho}S_2(y_2)^{1-\rho_2-\frac{\sigma_2}{\sigma_1}\rho}$

$\times \left[\rho^2\frac{\sigma_1^2}{\sigma_2^2}S_1(t_1)^{-\sigma_1^2}S_1(y_1)^{-\sigma_1^2} + S_1(y_1)^{-\sigma_1^2} - 1\right)^2$

$+ \rho\rho_1\frac{\sigma_1}{\sigma_2}S_1(t_1)^{-\sigma_1^2}S_1(y_1)^{-\sigma_1^2}(S_1(t_1)^{-\sigma_1^2} + S_1(y_1)^{-\sigma_1^2} - 1)(S_1(t_1)^{-\sigma_1^2} + S_2(t_2)^{-\sigma_2^2} - 1)$

$+ \rho(1 - \rho_1 - \frac{\sigma_1}{\sigma_2}\rho)\frac{\sigma_1}{\sigma_2}S_1(y_1)^{-\sigma_1^2}(S_1(t_-)^{-\sigma_1^2} + S_1(y_1)^{-\sigma_1^2} - 1)^2(S_1(t_1)^{-\sigma_1^2} + S_2(t_2)^{-\sigma_2^2} - 1)$

$+ \rho\rho_1\frac{\sigma_1}{\sigma_2}S_1(t_1)^{-\sigma_1^2}S_1(y_1)^{-\sigma_1^2}(S_1(t_1)^{-\sigma_1^2} + S_1(y_1)^{-\sigma_1^2} - 1)(S_1(y_1)^{-\sigma_1^2} + S_2(y_2)^{-\sigma_2^2} - 1)$

$+ \rho(1 - \rho_1 - \frac{\sigma_1}{\sigma_2}\rho)\frac{\sigma_1}{\sigma_2}S_1(t_1)^{-\sigma_1^2}(S_1(t_1)^{-\sigma_1^2} + S_1(y_1)^{-\sigma_1^2} - 1)^2(S_1(y_1)^{-\sigma_1^2} + S_2(y_2)^{-\sigma_2^2} - 1)$

$+ \rho_1(\rho_1 + \sigma_1^2)S_1(t_1)^{-\sigma_1^2}S_1(y_1)^{-\sigma_1^2}(S_1(t_1)^{-\sigma_1^2} + S_2(t_2)^{-\sigma_2^2} - 1)(S_1(y_1)^{-\sigma_1^2} - 1)$

$+ \rho_1(1 - \rho_1 - \frac{\sigma_1}{\sigma_2}\rho)S_1(t_1)^{-\sigma_1^2}(S_1(t_1)^{-\sigma_1^2} + S_1(y_1)^{-\sigma_1^2} - 1)$

$\times (S_1(t_1)^{-\sigma_1^2} + S_2(t_2)^{-\sigma_2^2} - 1)(S_1(y_1)^{-\sigma_1^2} + S_2(y_2)^{-\sigma_2^2} - 1)$

$+ \rho_1(1 - \rho_1 - \frac{\sigma_1}{\sigma_2}\rho)S_1(y_1)^{-\sigma_1^2}(S_1(t_1)^{-\sigma_1^2} + S_1(y_1)^{-\sigma_1^2} - 1)$

$\times (S_1(t_1)^{-\sigma_1^2} + S_2(t_2)^{-\sigma_2^2} - 1)(S_1(y_1)^{-\sigma_1^2} + S_2(y_2)^{-\sigma_2^2} - 1)$

$+ (1 - \rho_1 - \frac{\sigma_1}{\sigma_2}\rho)^2(S_1(t_1)^{-\sigma_1^2} + S_1(y_1)^{-\sigma_1^2} - 1)^2(S_1(t_1)^{-\sigma_1^2} + S_2(t_2)^{-\sigma_2^2} - 1)(S_1(y_1)^{-\sigma_1^2} + S_2(y_2)^{-\sigma}$

$$S_{t_1,y_2}(t_1, y_1, t_2, y_2)$$

$$= \mu_1(t_1)\mu_2(y_2)(S_1(t_1)^{-\sigma_1^2} + S_1(y_1)^{-\sigma_1^2} - 1)^{-\rho_1/\sigma_1^2-1}(S_2(t_2)^{-\sigma_2^2} + S_2(y_2)^{-\sigma_2^2} - 1)^{-\rho_2/\sigma_2^2-1}$$

$$\times (S_1(t_1)^{-\sigma_1^2} + S_2(t_2)^{-\sigma_2^2} - 1)^{-\rho/\sigma_1\sigma_2-1}(S_1(y_1)^{-\sigma_1^2} + S_2(y_2)^{-\sigma_2^2} - 1)^{-\rho/\sigma_1\sigma_2-1}$$

$$\times S_1(t_1)^{1-\rho_1-\frac{\sigma_1}{\sigma_2}\rho}S_1(y_1)^{1-\rho_1-\frac{\sigma_1}{\sigma_2}\rho}S_2(t_2)^{1-\rho_2-\frac{\sigma_2}{\sigma_1}\rho}S_2(y_2)^{1-\rho_2-\frac{\sigma_2}{\sigma_1}\rho}$$

$$\times \left[\rho\rho_2\frac{\sigma_1}{\sigma_2}S_1(t_1)^{-\sigma_1^2}S_2(y_2)^{-\sigma_2^2}(S_1(t_1)^{-\sigma_1^2} + S_1(y_1)^{-\sigma_1^2} - 1)(S_1(y_1)^{-\sigma_1^2} + S_2(y_2)^{-\sigma_2^2} - 1) \right.$$

$$+ \rho_1\rho_2 S_1(t_1)^{-\sigma_1^2}S_2(y_2)^{-\sigma_2^2}(S_1(t_1)^{-\sigma_1^2} + S_2(t_2)^{-\sigma_2^2} - 1)(S_1(y_1)^{-\sigma_1^2} + S_2(y_2)^{-\sigma_2^2} - 1)$$

$$+ \rho_2(1 - \rho_1 - \frac{\sigma_1}{\sigma_2}\rho)S_2(y_2)^{-\sigma_2^2}(S_1(t_1)^{-\sigma_1^2} + S_1(y_1)^{-\sigma_1^2} - 1)(S_1(t_1)^{-\sigma_1^2} + S_2(t_2)^{-\sigma_2^2} - 1)(S_1(y_1)^{-\sigma_1^2} + S_2$$

$$+ \rho^2 S_1(t_1)^{-\sigma_1^2}S_2(y_2)^{-\sigma_2^2}(S_1(t_1)^{-\sigma_1^2} + S_1(y_1)^{-\sigma_1^2} - 1)(S_2(t_2)^{-\sigma_2^2} + S_2(y_2)^{-\sigma_2^2} - 1)$$

$$+ \rho\rho_1\frac{\sigma_2}{\sigma_1}S_1(t_1)^{-\sigma_1^2}S_2(y_2)^{-\sigma_2^2}(S_2(t_2)^{-\sigma_2^2} + S_2(y_2)^{-\sigma_2^2} - 1)(S_1(t_1)^{-\sigma_1^2} + S_2(t_2)^{-\sigma_2^2} - 1)$$

$$+ \rho(1 - \rho_2 - \frac{\sigma_2}{\sigma_1}\rho)\frac{\sigma_1}{\sigma_2}S_1(t_1)^{-\sigma_1^2}(S_1(t_1)^{-\sigma_1^2} + S_1(y_1)^{-\sigma_1^2} - 1)$$

$$\times (S_2(t_2)^{-\sigma_2^2} + S_2(y_2)^{-\sigma_2^2} - 1)(S_1(y_1)^{-\sigma_1^2} + S_2(y_2)^{-\sigma_2^2} - 1)$$

$$+ \rho(1 - \rho_1 - \frac{\sigma_1}{\sigma_2}\rho)\frac{\sigma_2}{\sigma_1}S_2(y_2)^{-\sigma_2^2}(S_1(t_1)^{-\sigma_1^2} + S_1(y_1)^{-\sigma_1^2} - 1)$$

$$\times (S_2(t_2)^{-\sigma_2^2} + S_2(y_2)^{-\sigma_2^2} - 1)(S_1(t_1)^{-\sigma_1^2} + S_2(t_2)^{-\sigma_2^2} - 1)$$

$$+ \rho_1(1 - \rho_2 - \frac{\sigma_2}{\sigma_1}\rho)S_1(t_1)^{-\sigma_1^2}(S_2(t_2)^{-\sigma_2^2} + S_2(y_2)^{-\sigma_2^2} - 1)$$

$$\times (S_1(t_1)^{-\sigma_1^2} + S_2(t_2)^{-\sigma_2^2} - 1)(S_1(y_1)^{-\sigma_1^2} + S_2(y_2)^{-\sigma_2^2} - 1)$$

$$+ (1 - \rho_1 - \frac{\sigma_1}{\sigma_2}\rho)(1 - \rho_2 - \frac{\sigma_2}{\sigma_1}\rho)(S_1(t_1)^{-\sigma_1^2} + S_1(y_1)^{-\sigma_1^2} - 1)(S_2(t_2)^{-\sigma_2^2} + S_2(y_2)^{-\sigma_2^2} - 1)$$

$$\left. \times (S_1(t_1)^{-\sigma_1^2} + S_2(t_2)^{-\sigma_2^2} - 1)(S_1(y_1)^{-\sigma_1^2} + S_2(y_2)^{-\sigma_2^2} - 1) \right]$$

$$t_{2},y_{1}(t_{1}, y_{1}, t_{2}, y_{2})$$

$$= \mu_2(t_2)\mu_1(y_1)(S_1(t_1)^{-\sigma_1^2} + S_1(y_-)^{-\sigma_1^2} - 1)^{-\rho_1/\sigma_1^2-1}(S_2(t_2)^{-\sigma_2^2} + S_2(y_2)^{-\sigma_2^2} - 1)^{-\rho_2/\sigma_2^2-1}$$

$$\times (S_1(t_1)^{-\sigma_1^2} + S_2(t_2)^{-\sigma_2^2} - 1)^{-\rho/\sigma_1\sigma_2-1}(S_1(y_1)^{-\sigma_1^2} + S_2(y_2)^{-\sigma_2^2} - 1)^{-\rho/\sigma_1\sigma_2-1}$$

$$\times S_1(t_1)^{1-\rho_1-\frac{\sigma_1}{\sigma_2}\rho}S_1(y_1)^{1-\rho_1-\frac{\sigma_1}{\sigma_2}\rho}S_2(t_2)^{1-\rho_2-\frac{\sigma_2}{\sigma_1}\rho}S_2(y_2)^{1-\rho_2-\frac{\sigma_2}{\sigma_1}\rho}$$

$$\times \left[\rho\rho_2\frac{\sigma_1}{\sigma_2}S_2(t_2)^{-\sigma_2^2}S_1(y_1)^{-\sigma_1^2}(S_1(t_1)^{-\sigma_1^2} + S_1(y_1)^{-\sigma_1^2} - 1)(S_1(t_1)^{-\sigma_1^2} + S_2(t_2)^{-\sigma_2^2} - 1)\right.$$

$$+ \rho_1\rho_2 S_2(t_2)^{-\sigma_2^2}S_1(y_1)^{-\sigma_1^2}(S_1(t_1)^{-\sigma_1^2} + S_2(t_2)^{-\sigma_2^2} - 1)(S_1(y_1)^{-\sigma_1^2} + S_2(y_2)^{-\sigma_2^2} - 1)$$

$$+ \rho_2(1 - \rho_1 - \frac{\sigma_1}{\sigma_2}\rho)S_2(t_2)^{-\sigma_2^2}(S_1(t_1)^{-\sigma_1^2} + S_1(y_1)^{-\sigma_1^2} - 1)$$

$$\times (S_1(t_1)^{-\sigma_1^2} + S_2(t_2)^{-\sigma_2^2} - 1)(S_1(y_1)^{-\sigma_1^2} + S_2(y_2)^{-\sigma_2^2} - 1)$$

$$+ \rho^2 S_2(t_2)^{-\sigma_2^2}S_1(y_1)^{-\sigma_1^2}(S_1(t_1)^{-\sigma_1^2} + S_1(y_1)^{-\sigma_1^2} - 1)(S_2(t_2)^{-\sigma_2^2} + S_2(y_2)^{-\sigma_2^2} - 1)$$

$$+ \rho(1 - \rho_2 - \frac{\sigma_2}{\sigma_1}\rho)\frac{\sigma_1}{\sigma_2}S_1(y_1)^{-\sigma_1^2}(S_1(t_1)^{-\sigma_1^2} - S_1(y_1)^{-\sigma_1^2} - 1)$$

$$\times (S_2(t_2)^{-\sigma_2^2} + S_2(y_2)^{-\sigma_2^2} - 1)$$

$$+ \rho\rho_1\frac{\sigma_2}{\sigma_1}S_2(t_2)^{-\sigma_2^2}S_1(y_1)^{-\sigma_1^2}(S_2(t_2)^{-\sigma_2^2} + S_2(y_2)^{-\sigma_2^2} - 1)(S_1(y_1)^{-\sigma_1^2} + S_2(y_2)^{-\sigma_2^2} - 1)$$

$$+ \rho(1 - \rho_1 - \frac{\sigma_1}{\sigma_2}\rho)\frac{\sigma_2}{\sigma_1}S_2(t_2)^{-\sigma_2^2}(S_1(t_1)^{-\sigma_1^2} - S_1(y_1)^{-\sigma_1^2} - 1)$$

$$\times (S_2(t_2)^{-\sigma_2^2} + S_2(y_2)^{-\sigma_2^2} - 1)(S_1(y_1)^{-\sigma_1^2} - S_2(y_2)^{-\sigma_2^2} - 1)$$

$$+ \rho_1(1 - \rho_2 - \frac{\sigma_2}{\sigma_1}\rho)S_1(y_1)^{-\sigma_1^2}(S_2(t_2)^{-\sigma_2^2} + S_2(y_2)^{-\sigma_2^2} - 1)(S_1(t_1)^{-\sigma_1^2} + S_2(t_2)^{-\sigma_2^2} - 1)(S_1(y_1)^{-\sigma_1^2} + S_2(y_2)^{-\sigma_2^2} - 1)$$

$$+ (1 - \rho_1 - \frac{\sigma_1}{\sigma_2}\rho)(1 - \rho_2 - \frac{\sigma_2}{\sigma_1}\rho)(S_1(t_1)^{-\sigma_1^2} + S_1(y_1)^{-\sigma_1^2} - 1)(S_2(t_2)^{-\sigma_2^2} + S_2(y_2)^{-\sigma_2^2} - 1)(S_1(y_1)^{-\sigma_1^2} + S_2($$

$$\left.\times (S_1(t_1)^{-\sigma_1^2} + S_2(t_2)^{-\sigma_2^2} - 1)(S_1(y_1)^{-\sigma_1^2} + S_2(y_2)^{-\sigma_2^2} - 1)\right]$$

$$S_{t_2,y_2}(t_1,y_1,t_2,y_2)$$

$$= \mu_2(t_2)\mu_2(y_2)(S_1(t_1)^{-\sigma_1^2} + S_1(y_1)^{-\sigma_1^2} - 1)^{-\rho_1/\sigma_1^2} S_2(t_2)^{-\sigma_2^2} + S_2(y_2)^{-\sigma_2^2} - 1)^{-\rho_2/\sigma_2^2 - 2}$$

$$\times (S_1(t_1)^{-\sigma_1^2} + S_2(t_2)^{-\sigma_2^2} - 1)^{-\rho/\sigma_1\sigma_2 - 1}(S_1(y_1)^{-\sigma_1^2} + S_2(y_2)^{-\sigma_2^2} - 1)^{-\rho/\sigma_1\sigma_2 - 1}$$

$$\times S_1(t_1)^{1-\rho_1-\frac{\sigma_1}{\sigma_2}\rho} S_1(y_1)^{1-\rho_1-\frac{\sigma_2}{\sigma_1}\rho} S_2(t_2)^{1-\rho_2-\frac{\sigma_2}{\sigma_1}\rho} S_2(y_2)^{1-\rho_2-\frac{\sigma_2}{\sigma_1}\rho}$$

$$\times \left[\rho^2 \frac{\sigma_2^2}{\sigma_1^2} S_2(t_2)^{-\sigma_2^2} S_2(y_2)^{-\sigma_2^2} (S_2(t_2)^{-\sigma_2^2} + S_2(y_2)^{-\sigma_2^2} - 1)^2 \right.$$

$$+ \rho\rho_2 \frac{\sigma_2}{\sigma_1} S_2(t_2)^{-\sigma_2^2} S_2(y_2)^{-\sigma_2^2} (S_2(t_2)^{-\sigma_2^2} + S_2(y_2)^{-\sigma_2^2} - 1)(S_1(t_1)^{-\sigma_1^2} + S_2(t_2)^{-\sigma_2^2} - 1)$$

$$+ \rho(1 - \rho_2 - \frac{\sigma_2}{\sigma_1}\rho) \frac{\sigma_2}{\sigma_1} S_2(y_2)^{-\sigma_2^2} S_2(t_2)^{-\sigma_2^2} (S_2(y_2)^{-\sigma_2^2} + S_2(y_2)^{-\sigma_2^2} - 1)^2 (S_1(t_1)^{-\sigma_1^2} + S_2(t_2)^{-\sigma_2^2} - 1)$$

$$+ \rho\rho_2 \frac{\sigma_2}{\sigma_1} S_2(t_2)^{-\sigma_2^2} S_2(y_2)^{-\sigma_2^2} (S_2(t_2)^{-\sigma_2^2} + S_2(y_2)^{-\sigma_2^2} - 1)(S_1(y_1)^{-\sigma_1^2} + S_2(y_2)^{-\sigma_2^2} - 1)$$

$$+ \rho(1 - \rho_2 - \frac{\sigma_2}{\sigma_1}\rho) \frac{\sigma_2}{\sigma_1} S_2(t_2)^{-\sigma_2^2} S_2(t_2)^{-\sigma_2^2} (S_2(t_2)^{-\sigma_2^2} + S_2(y_2)^{-\sigma_2^2} - 1)^2 (S_1(y_1)^{-\sigma_1^2} + S_2(y_2)^{-\sigma_2^2} - 1)$$

$$+ \rho_2(\sigma_2^2 + \rho_2) S_2(t_2)^{-\sigma_2^2} S_2(y_2)^{-\sigma_2^2} (S_1(t_1)^{-\sigma_1^2} + S_2(t_2)^{-\sigma_2^2} - 1)(S_1(y_1)^{-\sigma_1^2} + S_2(y_2)^{-\sigma_2^2} - 1)$$

$$+ \rho_2(1 - \rho_2 - \frac{\sigma_2}{\sigma_1}\rho) S_2(t_2)^{-\sigma_2^2} S_2(t_2)^{-\sigma_2^2} (S_2(t_2)^{-\sigma_2^2} + S_2(y_2)^{-\sigma_2^2} - 1)$$

$$\times (S_1(t_1)^{-\sigma_1^2} + S_2(t_2)^{-\sigma_2^2} - 1)(S_1(y_1)^{-\sigma_1^2} + S_2(y_2)^{-\sigma_2^2} - 1)$$

$$+ \rho_2(1 - \rho_2 - \frac{\sigma_2}{\sigma_1}\rho) S_2(y_2)^{-\sigma_2^2} S_2(t_2)^{-\sigma_2^2} (S_2(t_2)^{-\sigma_2^2} + S_2(y_2)^{-\sigma_2^2} - 1)$$

$$\times (S_1(t_1)^{-\sigma_1^2} + S_2(t_2)^{-\sigma_2^2} - 1)(S_1(y_1)^{-\sigma_1^2} + S_2(y_2)^{-\sigma_2^2} - 1)$$

$$+ (1 - \rho_2 - \frac{\sigma_2}{\sigma_1}\rho)^2 (S_2(t_2)^{-\sigma_2^2} + S_2(y_2)^{-\sigma_2^2} - 1)^2 (S_1(t_1)^{-\sigma_1^2} + S_2(t_2)^{-\sigma_2^2} - 1)(S_1(y_1)^{-\sigma_1^2} + S_2(y_2)^{-\sigma}$$

A.6 Quantitative Genetics

One aim of genetic analysis is to determine whether and to which extent genetic variation may account for the variation of a specific phenotype (e.g., lifetime, susceptibility to disease). To address this question, measurements of the phenotype must be combined with genetic information. In studies of related individuals (families, twins, litter, etc.), genetic information is usually available as pedigree. Based on methods of quantitative genetics developed by Falconer (1990) and Neale and Cardon (1992), the relative role of genetic factors is determined by estimating heritability.

Twin studies are one of the most widely used methods for quantifying the influence of genetic and environmental factors on specific diseases. The classic twin method, attributed to Francis Galton (1887), argues that, whereas in MZ twins the differences in a pair must be due to environmental differences, for DZ twins it includes effects associated with their genetic difference. Through making a critical assumption that differences with respect to environmental factors between identical pairs are of the same (average) strength as those between DZ twins (equal environment assumption), inference can be made about the influence of genetic factors simply by comparing MZ and DZ pair correlations. In the case of binary traits (where the disease is either present or not), concordance analysis provides a powerful and widely accepted method in genetic epidemiology. Concordance rates are easy to calculate and allow for a clear interpretation (McGue 1993, Gatz et al. 2000). In many practical applications, time-to-event data (time of onset of disease, age at death) are available, but usually in a censored form. Censoring of bivariate observations can be a complex problem, as either or both individuals of a pair may be subject to censoring, and the censoring times need not be the same for both individuals. Furthermore, observed covariates are available in many cases. Unfortunately, it is difficult to manage censored lifetime data and covariates within the context of concordance analysis. A large part of the motivation for the methodology of this paragraph is exploring the potential for censored data and the inclusion of measured covariates.

Typical models of quantitative genetics can be incorporated with ease into the correlated frailty model described earlier. Models of quantitative genetics (Falconer 1990) are based on the decomposition of a phenotypic trait in a sum of different components, that are assumed to be independent. Using this approach, it is possible to estimate the proportion of the total variability of the phenotype that is related to genetic factors. In particular, a heritability estimate can be calculated for human longevity by identifying the phenotype with the lifespan variable (McGue et al. 1993). Usually, heritability is defined as the percentage of variation of the trait explained by the variation of genetic factors.

Yashin and Iachine (1995a) suggested an approach based on the frailty Z instead of the lifespan T. It is interesting to find out the relative importance of genes and the environment in determining individual susceptibility toward mortality (overall or cause specific). An advantage of this approach is that, through the additive decomposition of the frailty term into a genetic and an environmental component, one can obtain a competing risk structure for the respective survival model. In other words, observed mortality is represented as a sum of two terms: one depends on genetic, and the other on environmental, parameters, both estimated from bivariate data. In more detail, let the frailty be represented by

$$Z = genes + environment = A + D + I + C + E, \qquad (A.5)$$

where A represents additive genetic effects, D corresponds to genetic effects caused by dominance, I denotes epistatic genetic effects, and C and E stand for shared and nonshared environmental effects, respectively. All factors are assumed to be independent. The associated variance proportions of the components are defined as follows:

$$a^2 = \frac{V(A)}{V(Z)}, \ d^2 = \frac{V(D)}{V(Z)}, \ i^2 = \frac{V(I)}{V(Z)}, \ c^2 = \frac{V(C)}{V(Z)}, \ e^2 = \frac{V(E)}{V(Z)}.$$

The additive decomposition of the frailty variance and the correlation between co-twins' frailty hold that

$$1 = a^2 + d^2 + i^2 + c^2 + e^2 \qquad (A.6)$$

$$\rho = \rho_1 a^2 + \rho_2 d^2 + \rho_3 i^2 + \rho_4 c^2 + \rho_5 e^2, \qquad (A.7)$$

where lowercase letters a^2, d^2, i^2, c^2, e^2 indicate the proportions of the total variance σ^2 associated with the correspondent components of frailty, and ρ_i ($i = 1, ..., 5$) are correlations between respective components within a twin pair. In this case, broad sense heritability can be expressed as

$$H^2 = a^2 + d^2 + i^2,$$

where the term a^2 denotes small sense heritability. Standard assumptions of quantitative genetics models specify different values of ρ_i ($i = 1, ..., 5$) for monozygotic and dizygotic twins. In the case of monozygotic twins $\rho_i = 1$ ($i = 1, ..., 4$) and $\rho_5 = 0$, while for dizygotic twins $\rho_1 = 0.5$, $\rho_2 = 0.25$, $\rho_3 = m$, $\rho_4 = 1$, $\rho_5 = 0$, and $0 \leq m \leq 0.25$ is an unknown parameter. Not all parameters of the genetic decomposition of frailty can be estimated simultaneously, even under the assumption of no epistasis ($i^2 = 0$). In this case, it is only possible to conclude that the true heritability H^2 is in the interval (Iachine 2002)

$$\frac{4}{3}(\rho_{MZ} - \rho_{DZ}) \leq H^2 \leq \min\{\rho_{MZ}, 2(\rho_{MZ} - \rho_{DZ})\}.$$

The width of the interval is at most $\rho_{MZ} - \rho_{DZ}$, which represents the potential error in heritability estimation using only the correlation coefficients of MZ and DZ twins. The model in fact reduces to three equations (two relations (A.7) for monozygotic and dizygotic twins each, and one constraint (A.6)), allowing estimation of no more than three parameters at the same time. One possibility is to consider an ACE (additive genetic – common environment – uncommon environment) model. In this case, equations (A.6) and (A.7) lead to

$$
\begin{aligned}
1 &= a^2 + c^2 + e^2 \\
\rho_{MZ} &= a^2 + c^2 \\
\rho_{DZ} &= 0.5a^2 + c^2.
\end{aligned}
\tag{A.8}
$$

This system can be integrated into the correlated frailty model giving place to a reparameterization of the original model. The only difference is that, if we are interested in estimating the parameters of a genetic model, data for monozygotic and dizygotic twins have to be analyzed simultaneously and a likelihood function for combined data has to be drawn. Equally, other genetic models can be obtained combining no more than three components of frailty.

It is necessary to note that heritability estimation requires assumptions that are often difficult to verify in practice. For example, the trait must be represented as an additive combination of uncorrelated environmental and genetic factors, and the variances of phenotypic traits associated with related individuals must be the same. The classical twin method is based on the assumption that MZ and DZ twins have the same correlation with respect to environmental factors (equal environment assumption). This assumption is necessary for the identifiability of heritability, that is, so as to be able to interpret the difference in concordance between MZ and DZ twins as being explained in full by their difference in genetic concordance. However, without doubt, the assumption is also sometimes questionable: MZ twins are generally treated the same by their parents to a much greater extent than DZ twins. This implies an overestimation of heritability, especially for behavioral traits.

This does not decrease the statistical attractiveness of this direction of research. However, the interpretation of heritability estimates must be used with care as pointed out by Feldman and Lewontin (1975).

After the age of six, death rates for Danish twins born between 1870 and 1900 are almost the same as those for the same cohorts of the Danish population. The distributions of age at death for monozygotic twins are close to those of dizygotic twins for both sexes (Christensen et al. 1995). Recent papers dealing with twin cohorts born during the period 1870 – 1930 found similar mortality patterns for Danish twins and the general Danish population with respect to CHD (Wienke et al. 2001, Christensen et al. 2001). This similarity suggests that it is possible to generalize genetic results from survival analysis of twins to the total population with respect to mortality due to CHD.

References

Aalen, O.O. (1978) Nonparametric inference for a family of counting processes. *Annals of Statistics* 6, 701–726.

Aalen, O.O. (1987) Two examples of modelling heterogeneity in survival analysis. *Scandinavian Journal of Statistics* 14, 19–25.

Aalen, O.O. (1988) Heterogeneity in survival analysis. *Statistics in Medicine* 7, 1121–1137.

Aalen, O.O. (1992) Modelling heterogeneity in survival analysis by the compound Poisson distribution. *Annals of Applied Probability* 4, 951–972.

Aalen, O.O., Bjertness, E., Sønju, T. (1995) Analysis of dependent survival data applied to lifetimes of amalgam fillings. *Statistics in Medicine* 14, 1819–1829.

Aalen, O.O., Tretli, S. (1999) Analyzing incidence of testis cancer by means of a frailty model. *Cancer Causes and Control* 10, 285–292.

Aalen, O., Hjort, N.L. (2002) Frailty models that yield proportional hazards. *Statistics & Probability Letters* 58, 335–342.

Aalen, O.O., Borgan, O., Gjessing, H.K. (2008) *Survival and Event History Analysis: A Process Point of View.* Springer, Berlin.

Abbring, J., van den Berg, G.J. (2003) The identifiability of the mixed proportional hazards competing risks model. *Journal of the Royal Statistical Society (B)* 65, 701–710.

Abbring, J., van den Berg, G.J. (2007) The unobserved heterogeneity distribution in duration analysis. *Biometrika* 94, 87–99.

Akaike, H. (1974) A new look at the statistical model identification. *IEEE Transactions on Automatic Control* 19, 716–723.

Andersen, E.W. (2005) Two-stage estimation in copula models used in family studies. *Lifetime Data Analysis* 11, 333–350.

Andersen, P.K., Gill, R.D. (1982) Cox's regression model for counting processes: a large sample study. *Annals of Statistics* 10, 1100–1120.

Andersen, P.K., Borgan, O., Gill, R.D., Keiding, N. (1993) *Statistical Models based on Counting Processes.* Springer, New York.

Andersen, P.K., Klein, J.P., Zhang, M.-J. (1999) Testing for centre effects in multi-centre survival studies: a Monte Carlo comparison of fixed and random effects tests. *Statistics in Medicine* 18, 1489–1500.

Anderson, J.E., Louis, T.A. (1995) Survival analysis using a scale change random effects model. *Journal of the American Statistical Association* 90, 669–679.

Anderson, J.E., Louis, T.A., Holm, N.V., Harvald, B. (1992) Time dependent association measures for bivariate survival distributions. *Journal of the American Statistical Association* 87, 641–650.

Balakrishnan, N., Peng, Y. (2006) Generalized gamma frailty model. *Statistics in Medicine* 25, 2797–2816.

Bandeen-Roche, K.J., Liang, K-Y. (1996) Modelling failure-time associations in data with multiple levels of clustering. *Biometrika* 83, 29–39.

Bandyopadhyay, D., Basu, A. (1990) On a generalization of a model by Lindley and Singpurwalla. *Advances in Applied Probability* 22, 498–500.

Banerjee, S., Wall, M.M., Carlin, B.P. (2003) Frailty modeling for spatially correlated survival data, with application to infant mortality in Minnesota. *Biostatistics* 4, 123–142.

Banerjee, S., Carlin, B.P. (2003) Semiparametric spatio-temporal frailty modeling. *Environmetrics* 14, 523–535.

Barker, P., Henderson, R. (2004) Modelling converging hazards in survival analysis. *Lifetime Data Analysis* 10, 263–281.

Barker, P., Henderson, R. (2005) Small sample bias in the gamma frailty model for univariate survival. *Lifetime Data Analysis* 11, 265–284.

Beard, R.E. (1959) Note on some mathematical mortality models. In: *The Lifespan of Animals.* G.E.W. Wolstenholme, M.O'Conner (eds.), Ciba Foundation Colloquium on Ageing, Little, Brown, Boston, 302–311.

Bellamy, S., Li, Y., Ryan, L., Lipsitz, S., Canner, M., Wright, R. (2004) Analysis of clustered and interval censored data from a community-based study in asthma. *Statistics in Medicine* 23, 3607–3621.

Berkson, J., Gage, R. (1952) Survival curve for cancer patients following treatment. *Journal of the American Statistical Association* 47, 501–515.

Berry, G. (2007) Relative risk and acceleration in lung cancer. *Statistics in Medicine* 26, 3511–3517.

Bertoin, J. (1996) *Lévy Processes.* Cambridge University Press, Cambridge.

Besag, J., Green, P. (1993) Spatial statistics and Bayesian computation. *Journal of the Royal Statistical Society (B)* 55, 25–37.

Beutels, M., van Damme, P., Aelvoet, W., Desmyter, J., Dondeyne, F., Goilav, C., Mak, R, Muylle, L, Pierard, D, Stroobant, A, van Loock, F., Waumans, P., Vranckx, R. (1997) Prevalence of hepatitis A, B and C in the Flemish population. *European Journal of Epidemiology* 13, 275–80.

Blumen, I., Kogan, M., McCarthy, P.J. (1955) *The Industrial Mobility of Labor as a Probability Process.* Cornell University Press, New York.

Blossfeld, H.P., Hamerle, A. (1989) Unobserved heterogeneity in hazard rate models – a test and an illustration from a study of career mobility. *Quality & Quantity* 23, 129–141.

Blossfeld, H.P., Hamerle, A. (1992) Unobserved heterogeneity in event history models. *Quality & Quantity* 26, 157–168.

Boag, J.W. (1949) Maximum likelihood estimates of the proportion of patients cured by cancer therapy. *Journal of the Royal Statistical Society (B)* 11, 15–44.

Bollmann, A., Blankenburg, T., Haerting, J., Kuss, O., Schütte, W., Dunst, J., Neef, H. (2004) Survival of patients in clinical stages I-IIIb of non-small-cell lung cancer treated with radiation therapy alone. Results of a population-based study in Southern Saxony-Anhalt. *Strahlentherapie & Onkologie* 180, 488 - 496.

Bolstad, W.M., Manda, S.O. (2001) Investigating child mortality in Malawi using family and community random effects: a Bayesian analysis. *Journal of the American Statistical Association* 96, 12–19.

Bordes, L., Commenges, D. (2001) Asymptotics for homogeneity tests based on a multivariate random effects proportional hazards model. *Journal of Multivariate Analysis* 78, 83–102.

Bouchard, C. (1994) Genetics of obesity: overview and research directions. In: *The Genetics of Obesity.* C. Bouchard (ed.), CRC Press, Boca Raton, FL, pp. 223–233.

Box, G. (1976) Science and Statistics. *Journal of the American Statistical Association* 71, 791–802.

Breslow, N. (1974) Covariance analysis of censored survival data. *Biometrics* 30, 89–99.

Breslow, N., Crowley, J. (1974) A large sample study of the life table and product limit estimates under random censorship. *Annals of Statistics* 2, 437–453.

Bretagnolle, J., Huber-Carol, C. (1988) Effects of omitting covariates in Cox's model for survival data. *Scandinavian Journal of Statistics* 15, 125–138.

Broët, P., Moreau, T., Lellouch, J., Asselain, B. (1999) Unobserved covariates in the two-sample comparison of survival times: a maxmin efficiency robust test. *Statistics in Medicine* 18, 1791–1800.

Brooks, S.P., Gelman A. (1998) Alternative methods for monitoring convergence of iterative simulations. *Journal of Computational and Graphical Statistics* 7, 434–455.

Cai, J., Prentice, R.L. (1995) Estimating equations for hazard ratio parameters based on correlated failure time data. *Biometrika* 82, 151–164.

Carling, K., Jacobson, T. (1995) Modeling unemployment duration in a dependent competing risks framework: identification and estimation. *Lifetime Data Analysis* 1, 111 - 122

Caroni, C., Crowder, M., Kimber, A. (2010) Proportional hazards models with discrete frailty. *Lifetime Data Analysis* 16, 374–384.

Carvalho, M., Henderson, R., Shimakura, S., Sousa, I.P.S.C. (2003) Survival of hemodialysis patients: modeling differences in risk of dialysis centers. *International Journal for Quality in Health Care* 15, 189–196.

Cederlöf, R., Friberg, L., Jonsson, E., Kaij, L. (1961) Studies on similarity diagnosis in twins with the aid of mailed questionnaires. *Acta Genetica* 11, 338–362.

Chamberlain, G. (1992) Heterogeneity, omitted variable bias, and duration dependence. In: *Longitudinal Analysis of Labour Market Data*. J. Heckman, B. Singer (eds.) Cambridge University Press, pp. 3–38.

Chang, S.-H. (2004) Estimating marginal effects in accelerated failure time models for serial sojourn times among repeated events. *Lifetime Data Analysis* 10, 175–190.

Chang, I.-S., Wen, C.-C., Wu, Y.-J. (2007) A profile likelihood theory for the correlated gamma-frailty model with current status family data. *Statistica Sinica 17*, 1023–1046.

Chatterjee, N., Shih, J. (2001) A bivariate cure-mixture approach for modeling familial association in diseases. *Biometrics* 57, 779–786.

Chen, M.-C., Bandeen-Roche, K. (2005) A diagnostic for association in bivariate survival models. *Lifetime Data Analysis* 11, 245–264.

Christensen, K., Vaupel, J., Holm, N., Yashin, A. (1995) Mortality among twins after age 6: fetal origins hypothesis versus twin method. *British Medical Journal* 310, 432–436.

Christensen, K., Wienke, A., Skytthe, A., Holm, N., Vaupel, J., Yashin, A. (2001) Cardiovascular mortality in twins and fetal origins hypothesis. *Twin Research* 4, 344–349.

Chuang, S.K., Cai, T., Douglass, C.W., Wei, L.J., Dodson, T.B. (2005) Frailty approach for the analysis of clustered failure time observations in dental research. *Journal of Dental Research* 84, 54–58.

Chuang, S.K., Cai, T. (2006) Predicting clustered dental implant survival using frailty methods. *Journal of Dental Research* 85, 1147–1151.

Claeskens, G., Nguti, R., Janssen, P. (2008) One-sided tests in shared frailty models. *Test* 17, 69–82.

Clayton, D.G. (1978) A model for association in bivariate life tables and its application in epidemiological studies of familial tendency in chronic disease incidence. *Biometrika* 65, 141–151.

Clayton, D., Cuzick, J. (1985a) The semi-parametric Pareto model for regression analysis of survival times. *Proceedings of the 45th Session of the International Statistical Institute* 23, 1–18.

Clayton, D., Cuzick, J. (1985b) Multivariate generalizations of the proportional hazards model. *Journal of the Royal Statistical Society (A)* 148, 82–117.

Clayton, D., Kaldor, J.M. (1985) Heterogeneity models as an alternative to proportional hazards in cohort studies. *Bulletin of the International Statistical Institute* 51, 1–16.

Clayton, D. (1991) A Monte Carlo method for Bayesian inference in frailty models. *Biometrics* 47, 467–485.

Collett, D. (2003) *Modelling Survival Data in Medical Research.* Chapman & Hall/CRC, London.

Commenges, D., Andersen P.K. (1995) Score test of homogeneity for survival data. *Lifetime Data Analysis* 1, 145–160.

Commenges, D., Jacmin-Gadda, H. (1997) Generalized score test of homogeneity based on correlated random effects models. *Journal of the Royal Statistical Society (B)* 59, 157–171.

Congdon, P. (1995) Modelling frailty in area mortality. *Statistics in Medicine* 14, 1859–1874.

Cook, R., Ng, E., Mukherjee, J., Vaughan, D. (1999) Two-state mixed renewal processes for chronic disease. *Statistics in Medicine* 18, 175–188.

Cook, R.J., Lawless, J.F. (2007) *The Statistical Analysis of Recurrent Events.* Springer, Berlin.

Cox, D.R. (1959) Analysis of exponentially distributed life-times with two types of failure. *Journal of the Royal Statistical Society (B)* 21, 411–421.

Cox, D.R. (1972) Regression models and life-tables. *Journal of the Royal Statistical Society (B)* 34, 187–220.

Cox, D.R. (1975) Partial likelihood. *Biometrika* 62, 269–276.

Cox, D.R., Oakes, D. (1984) *Analysis of Survival Data.* Chapman & Hall, London.

Crowder, M. (1989) A multivariate distribution with Weibull connections. *Journal of the Royal Statistical Society (B)* 51, 93–107.

Cui, S., Sun, Y. (2004) Checking for the gamma frailty distribution under the marginal proportional hazards frailty model. *Statistica Sinica* 14, 249–267.

Davis, H.T., Feldstein, M. (1979) The generalized Pareto law as a model for progressively censored survival data. *Biometrika* 66, 299–306.

de Faire, U., Friberg, L., Lundman, T. (1975) Concordance for mortality with special reference to ischaemic heart and cerebrovascular disease: a study on the Swedish Twin Registry. *Preventive Medicine* 4, 509–517.

Dempster, A.P., Laird, N.M., Rubin, D.B. (1977) Maximum likelihood from incomplete data via the EM algorithm. *Journal of the Royal Statistical Society (B)* 39, 1–38.

Diamond, I.D., McDonald, J.W., Shah, I.H. (1986) Proportional hazards models for current status data - application to the study of differentials in age at weaning in Pakistan. *Demography* 23, 607–620.

di Serio, C. (1997) The protective impact of a covariate on competing failures with an example from bone marrow transplantation. *Lifetime Data Analysis* 3, 99–122.

Dominicus, A., Skrondal, A., Gjessing, H., Pedersen, N, Palmgren, J. (2006) Likelihood ratio tests in behavioral genetics: problems and solutions. *Behavior Genetics* 36, 331–340.

dos Santos, D., Davies, R, Francis, B. (1995) Nonparametric hazard versus nonparametric frailty distribution in modelling recurrence of breast cancer. *Journal of Statistical Planning and Inference* 47, 111–127.

Drapeau, M.D., Gassa, E.K., Simisona, M.D., Muellera, L.D., Rosea, M.R. (2000) Testing the heterogeneity theory of late-life mortality plateaus by using cohorts of Drosophila melanogaster. *Experimental Gerontology* 35, 71–84.

Drzewiecki, K.T., Ladefoged, C., Christensen, H.E. (1980a) Biopsy and prognosis for cutaneous malignant melanomas in clinical stage I. *Scandinavian Journal of Plastic and Reconstructive Surgery and Hand Surgery* 14, 141–144.

Drzewiecki, K.T., Christensen, H.E., Ladefoged, C., Poulsen, H. (1980b) Clinical course of cutaneous malignant melanoma related to histopathological criteria of primary tumour. *Scandinavian Journal of Plastic and Reconstructive Surgery and Hand Surgery* 14, 229–234.

Duchateau, L., Janssen, P., Lindsey, P., Legrand, C., Nguti, R., Sylvester, R. (2002) The shared frailty model and the power for heterogeneity tests in multicenter trials. *Computational Statistics & Data Analysis* 40, 603–20.

Duchateau, L., Janssen, P., Kezic, I., Fortpied, C. (2003) Evolution of recurrent asthma event rate over time in frailty models. *Journal of the Royal Statistical Society (B)* 52, 355–363.

Duchateau, L., Janssen, P. (2004) Penalized partial likelihood for frailties and smoothing splines in time to first insemination models for dairy cows. *Biometrics* 60, 608–614.

Duchateau, L., Janssen, P. (2008) *The Frailty Model.* Springer, New York.

Dunson, D.B., Chen, Z. (2004) Selecting factors predictive of heterogeneity in multivariate event time data. *Biometrics* 60, 352–358.

Economou, P., Caroni, C. (2005) Graphical tests for the assumption of gamma and inverse Gaussian frailty distributions. *Lifetime Data Analysis* 11, 565–582.

Economou, P., Caroni, C. (2008) Graphical tests for the frailty distribution in the shared frailty model. *Communications in Statistics - Simulations and Computation* 37, 978–992.

Efron, B. (1967) The two sample problem with censored data. *Proceedings of the 5th Berkeley Symposium on Mathematical Statistics and Probability*, pp. 831–853. University California Press

Efron, B. (1977) The efficiency of Cox's likelihood function for censored data. *Journal of the American Statistical Association* 72, 557–565.

Elbers, C., Ridder, G. (1982) True and spurious duration dependence: the identifiability of the proportional hazard model. *Review of Economic Studies* XLIX, 403–409.

Ellermann, R., Sullo, P., Tien, J.M. (1992) An alternative approach to modeling recidivism using quantile residual life functions. *Operations Research* 40, 485–504.

Emoto, S., Matthews, P. (1990) A Weibull model for dependent censoring. *Annals of Statistics* 18, 1556–1577.

Falconer, D.S. (1990) *Introduction to Quantitative Genetics*. Longman Group, New York.

Farewell, V.T. (1977) A model for a binary variable with time-censored observations. *Biometrika* 64, 43–46.

Farewell, V.T., Math, B., Math, M. (1977) The combined effect of breast cancer risk factors. *Cancer* 40, 931–936.

Farewell, V.T. (1982) The use of mixture models for the analysis of survival data with long-term survivors. *Biometrics* 38, 1041–1046.

Farrington, C., Kanaan, M., Gay, N. (2001) Estimation of the basic reproduction number for infectious diseases from age-stratified serological survey data. *Applied Statistics* 50, 251–292.

Feldman, M., Lewontin, R. (1975) The heritability hang-up. *Science* 190, 1163–1168.

Feller, W. (1971) *An Introduction to Probability Theory and its Applications*. John Wiley and Sons, New York.

Feuer, E.J., Wun, L.-M., Boring, C.C., Flanders, W.D., Timmel, M.J., Tong, T. (1993) The lifetime risk of developing breast cancer. *Journal of the National Cancer Institute* 85, 892–897.

Fine, J., Jiang, H. (2000) On association in a copula with time transformations. *Biometrika* 87, 559–571.

Fine, J., Glidden, D., Lee, K. (2003) A simple estimator for a shared frailty regression model. *Journal of the Royal Statistical Society (B)* 65, 317–29.

Finkelstein, M. (2008) *Failure Rate Modeling for Reliability and Risk*. Springer, New York.

Fisher R.A. (1958) Cancer and smoking. *Nature* 182, 596.

Fleming, T., Harrington, D. (1991) *Counting Processes and Survival Analysis*. Wiley & Sons, Chichester.

Flinn, C., Heckman, J. (1982) New methods for analyzing structural models of labor force dynamics. *Journal of Econometrics* 18, 115–168.

Gail, M.H., Wieand, S., Piantadosi, S. (1984) Biased estimates of treatment effect in randomized experiments with nonlinear regressions and omitted covariates. *Biometrika* 71, 431–444.

Galton, F. (1887) *Natural Inheritance.* Macmillan, London.

Gatz, M., Pedersen, N.L., Crowe, M., Fiske, A. (2000) Defining discordance in twin studies of risk and protective factors for late life disorders. *Twin Research* 3, 159–164.

Gelman, A., Rubin, D.B. (1992) Inference from iterative simulation using multiple sequences. *Statistical Science* 7, 457–511.

Geman, S., Geman, D. (1984) Stochastic relaxation, Gibbs distributions, and the Bayesian restauration of images. *IEEE Transactions on Pattern Analysis and Machine Intelligence* 6, 721–741.

Genest, C., MacKay, J. (1986) The joy of copulas: bivariate distributions with uniform marginals. *The American Statistician* 40, 280–283.

Giard, N. (2001) *A Four-Dimensional Correlated Frailty Model.* GCA-Verlag, Herdecke (Ph.D thesis).

Giard, N., Lichtenstein, P., Yashin, A. (2002) *A multistate model for genetic analysis of the ageing process.* Statistics in Medicine 21, 2511–2526.

Gilks, W.R., Richardson, S., Spiegelhalter, D.G. (1996) *Markov Chain Monte Carlo in Practice.* Chapman and Hall, London.

Gjessing, H.K., Aalen, O.O., Hjort, N.L. (2003) Frailty models based on Lévy processes. *Advances in Applied Probability* 35, 532–550.

Glidden, D.V. (1999) Checking the adequacy of the gamma frailty model for multivariate failure times. *Biometrika* 86, 381–393.

Glidden, D.V. (2000) A two-stage estimator of the dependence parameter for the Clayton–Oakes model. *Lifetime Data Analysis* 6, 141–156.

Glidden, D.V. (2007) Pairwise dependence diagnostics for clustered failure time data. *Biometrika* 94, 371–385.

Goeman, J.J., Le Cessie, S., Baatenburg de Jong, R.J., van de Geer, S.A. (2004) Predicting survival using disease history: a model combining relative survival and frailty. *Statistica Neerlandica* 58, 21–34.

Goethals, K., Janssen, P., Duchateau, L. (2008) Frailty models and copulas: similarities and differences. *Journal of Applied Statistics* 35, 1071–1079.

Gompertz, B. (1825) On the nature of the function expressive of the law of human mortality, and on a new mode of determining the value of life contingencies. *Philosophical Transactions of the Royal Society of London* 115, 513–585.

Gordon, S.C. (2000) A frailty model of negatively dependent competing risks. Unpublished Draft.

Gorfine, M., Zucker, D., Hsu, L. (2006) Prospective survival analysis with a general semiparametric shared frailty model: a pseudo full likelihood approach. *Biometrika* 93, 735–741.

Gray, R.J. (1995) Tests for variation over groups in survival data. *Journal of the American Statistical Association* 90, 198–203.

Greenwood, M., Yule, G.U. (1920) An inquiry into the nature of frequency distributions representative of multiple happenings with particular reference to the occurrence of multiple attacks of disease or of repeated accidents. *Journal of the Royal Statistical Society* 83, 255–279.

Greenwood, M. (1926) The natural duration of cancer. Reports on Public Health and Medical Subjects. *Her Majesty's Stationery Office* 33, 1–26.

Guo, G., Rodriguez, G. (1992) Estimating a multivariate proportional hazards model for clustered data using the EM algorithm, with an application to child survival in Guatemala. *Journal of the American Statistical Association* 87, 969–976.

Guo, G. (1993) Use of sibling data to estimate family mortality effects in Guatemala. *Demography* 30, 15–32.

Gupta, P. L., Gupta, R.D. (1990) A bivariate random environmental stress model. *Advances in Applied Probability* 22, 501–503.

Gupta, R. C., Gupta, R.D. (2009) General frailty model and stochastic orderings. *Journal of Statistical Planning and Inference* 139, 3277–3287.

Gustafson, P. (1997) Large hierarchical Baysian analysis of multivariate survival data. *Biometrics* 53, 230–242.

Hamerle, A. (1992) A test for detecting overdispersion in multiple spell failure time models. *Biometrical Journal* 34, 81–90.

Hanagal, D. (2009) Weibull extension of bivariate exponential regression model with different frailty distributions. *Statistical Papers* 50, 29–49.

Hanagal, D. (2010) Modeling heterogeneity for bivariate survival data by the compound Poisson distribution. *Model Assisted Statistics and Applications* 5, 1–9.

Hastings, W.K. (1970) Monte Carlo sampling methods using Markov Chains and their applications. *Biometrika* 57, 97–109.

Harvald, B., Hauge, M. (1970) Coronary occlusion in twins. *Acta Geneticae Medicae et Gemellologiae* 19, 248–250.

Hauge, M. (1981) The Danish twin register. In: *Prospective Longitudinal Research.* S. Mednich, A. Baert, B. Bachmann (eds.), Oxford Medical Publisher, Oxford, pp. 217–222.

Haukka, J., Suvisaari, J., Lönnqvist, J. (2003) Increasing age does not decrease risk of schizophrenia up to age 40. *Schizophrenia Research* 61, 105–110.

Heath, A., Madden, P. (1995) Genetic influences on smoking behavior. In: *Behavior: Genetic Approaches in Behavioral Medicine.* J.R. Turner, L.R. Cardon, J.K. Hewitt (eds.), Plenum Press, New York, 45–63.

Heckman, J.J., Honoré B.E. (1989) The identifiability of the competing risks model. *Biometrika* 76, 325–330.

Heckman, J.J., Singer, B. (1982a) The identification problem in econometric models for duration data. In: *Advances in Econometrics.* W. Hildenbrandt (ed.), Cambridge University Press, Cambridge, pp. 39–77.

Heckman, J.J., Singer, B. (1982b) Population heterogeneity in demographic models. In: *Multidimensional Mathematical Demography.* K. Land, A. Rogers (eds.), Academic Press, New York.

Heckman, J.J., Singer, B. (1984a) A method for minimizing the impact of distributional assumptions in econometric models for duration data. *Econometrica* 52, 271–320.

Heckman, J.J., Singer, B. (1984b) The identifiability of the proportional hazard model. *Review of Economic Studies* 51, 231–241.

Heckman, J.J., Walker J.R. (1990) Estimating fecundability from data on waiting-times to 1st conception. *Journal of the American Statistical Association* 85, 283–294.

Heckman, J.J. (1991) Identifying the hand of the past: distinguishing state dependence from heterogeneity. *American Economic Review* 81, 71–79.

Heckman, J.J., Taber, C.R. (1994) Econometric mixture models and more general models for unobservables in duration analysis. *Statistical Methods in Medical Research* 3, 279–302.

Henderson, R., Oman, P. (1999) Effect of frailty on marginal regression estimates in survival analysis. *Journal of the Royal Statistical Society (B)* 61, 367–379.

Henderson, R., Shimakura, S. (2003) A serially correlated gamma frailty model for longitudinal count data. *Biometrika* 90, 355–366.

Hens, N., Wienke, A., Aerts, M., Molenberghs, G. (2009) The correlated and shared gamma frailty model for bivariate current status data: an illustration for cross sectional serological data. *Statistics in Medicine* 28, 2785–2800.

Henschel, V., Engel, J., Hölzel, D., Mansmann, U. (2009) A semiparametric Bayesian proportional hazards model for interval censored data with frailty effects. *BMC Medical Research Methodology* 9, article 9.

Herskind, A.M., McGue, M., Iachine, I.A., Holm, N., Sørensen, T.I.A., Harvald, B., Vaupel, J.W. (1996a) Untangling genetic influences on smoking, body mass index and longevity: a multivariate study of 2464 Danish twins followed for 28 years. *Human Genetics* 98, 467–475.

Herskind, A.M., McGue, M., Sørensen, T.I.A., Harvald, B. (1996b) Sex and age specific assessment of genetic and environmental influences on body mass index in twins. *International Journal of Obesity* 20, 106–113.

Hoem, J.M. (1990) Identifiability in hazard models with unobserved heterogeneity: the compatibility of two apparently contradictionary results. *Theoretical Population Biology* 37, 124–128.

Holm, N.V. (1983) *The use of twin studies to investigate causes of diseases with complex etiology with a focus on cancer.* Ph.D. thesis (in Danish), Odense University, Odense.

Honoré, B. (1993) Identification results for duration models with multiple spells. *Review of Economic Studies* 60, 241–246.

Hopper, J.L. (1993) Variance components for statistical genetics: applications in medical research to characteristics related to human diseases and health. *Statistical Methods in Medical Research* 2, 199–223.

Horowitz, J.L. (1999) Semiparametric estimation of a proportional hazard model with unobserved heterogeneity. *Econometrica* 67, 1001–1028.

Hougaard, P. (1984) Life table methods for heterogeneous populations. *Biometrika* 71, 75–83.

Hougaard, P. (1986a) Survival models for heterogeneous populations derived from stable distributions. *Biometrika* 73, 387–396.

Hougaard, P. (1986b) A class of multivariate failure time distributions. *Biometrika* 73, 671–678.

Hougaard, P. (1987) Modeling multivariate survival. *Scandinavian Journal of Statistics* 14, 291–304.

Hougaard, P. (1991) Modeling heterogeneity in survival data. *Journal of Applied Probability* 28, 695–701.

Hougaard, P., Harvald, B., Holm, N.V. (1992) Measuring the similarities between the lifetimes of adult Danish twins born 1881 – 1930. *Journal of the American Statistical Association* 87, 17–24.

Hougaard, P., Myglegaard, P., Borch-Johnsen, K. (1994) Heterogeneity models of disease susceptibility, with application to diabetic nephropathy. *Biometrics* 50, 1178–1188.

Hougaard, P. (1995) Frailty models for survival data. *Lifetime Data Analysis* 1, 255–273.

Hougaard, P. (1999) Fundamentals of survival data. *Biometrics* 55, 13–22.

Hougaard, P. (2000) *Analysis of Multivariate Survival Data.* Springer, New York.

Huang, X., Wolfe, R.A. (2002) A frailty model for informative censoring. *Biometrics* 58, 510–520.

Huang, X., Wolfe, R.A., Hu, C. (2004) A test for informative censoring in clustered survival data. *Statistics in Medicine* 23, 2089–2107.

Huber-Carol, C., Vonta, I. (2004) Frailty models for arbitrarily censored and truncated data. *Lifetime Data Analysis* 10, 369–388.

Hutchinson, T.P., Lai, C.D. (1991) *The Engineering Statistician's Guide to Continuous Bivariate Distributions.* Rumsby, Adelaide.

Iachine, I.A. (1995) Parameter Estimation in the Bivariate Correlated Frailty Model with observed Covariates via the EM-Algorithm. Research Report, Population Studies of Ageing 16, Odense University.

Iachine, I.A. (2002) The Use of Twin and Family Survival Data in the Population Studies of Aging: Statistical Methods Based on Multivariate Survival Models. Ph.D. Thesis. Monograph 8, Department of Statistics and Demography, University of Southern Denmark.

Iachine, I. (2004) Identifiability of Bivariate Frailty Models. Preprint 5, Department of Statistics, University of Southern Denmark, Odense.

Iachine, I., Holm, N., Harris, J., Begun, A., Iachina, M., Laitinen, M., Kaprio, J., Yashin, A. (1998) How heritable is individual susceptibility to death? The results of an analysis of survival data on Danish, Swedish and Finnish twins. *Twin Research* 1, 196–205.

Iachine, I.A., Yashin, A.I. (1998) Identifiability of Bivariate Frailty Models based on Additive Independent Components. Research Report 8, Department of Statistics and Demography, University of Southern Denmark, Odense.

Ibrahim, J.G., Chen, M.-H., Sinha, D. (2001) *Bayesian Survival Analysis*. Springer, New York.

Izumi, S., Ohtaki, M. (2004) Aspects of the Armitage-Doll gamma frailty model for cancer incidence data. *Environmetrics* 15, 209–218.

Jeong, J. (2003) Efficiency of log-rank tests under dependent censoring. *Communications in Statistics, Theory and Methods* 32, 1197–1211.

Jeong, J., Jung, S., Wieand, S. (2003) A parametric model for long-term follow-up data from phase III breast cancer clinical trials. *Statistics in Medicine* 22, 339–352.

Jeong, J., Jung, S. (2006) Rank tests for clustered survival data when dependent subunits are randomized. *Statistics in Medicine* 25, 361–373.

Jin, X., Carlin, B. (2005) Multivariate parametric spatiotemporal models for county level breast cancer survival data. *Lifetime Data Analysis* 11, 5-27

Joe, H. (1993) Parametric families of multivariate distributions with given margins. *Journal of Multivariate Analysis* 46, 262–282.

Jones, B.L. (1998) A model for analyzing the impact of selective lapsation on mortality. *North American Actuarial Journal* 2, 79–86.

Jonker, M., Bhulai, S., Boomsma, D., Ligthart, R., Posthuma, D., van der Vaart, A. (2009) Gamma frailty model for linkage analysis with application to interval-censored migraine data. *Biostatistics* 10, 187–200.

Jonker, M., Boomsma, D. (2010) A frailty model for interval censored family survival data, applied to the age at onset of non-physical problems. *Lifetime Data Analysis* 16, 299–315.

Juel, K., Helweg-Larsen, K. (1999) The Danish registers of causes of death. *Danish Medical Bulletin* 46, 354–357.

Kalbfleisch, J., Prentice, R. (2002) *The Statistical Analysis of Failure Time Data*. Wiley, New York.

Kalwitzki, M, Weiger, R., Axmann-Krcmar, D., Rosendahl, R. (2002) Caries risk analysis: considering caries as an individual time-dependent process. *International Journal of Paediatric Dentistry* 12, 132–142.

Kaplan, E., Meier, P. (1958) Nonparametric estimation from incomplete observations. *Journal of the American Statistical Association* 53, 457–481.

Keiding, N., Andersen, P., Klein, J. (1997) The role of frailty models and accelerated failure time models in describing heterogeneity due to omitted covariates. *Statistics in Medicine* 16, 215–224.

Keiding, N. (1998) Selection effects and nonproportional hazards in survival models and models for repeated events. In: Proceedings of the 19th International Biometric Conference, Cape Town, pp. 241–250.

Keiding, N., Andersen, P. (eds.) (2006) *Survival and Event History Analysis*. Wiley, New York.

Khazaeli, A., Xiu, L., Curtsinger, J.W. (1995) Stress experiments as a means of investigating age-specific mortality in Drosophila melanogaster. *Experimental Gerontology* 30, 177–184.

Kheiri, S., Meshkani, M.R., Faghihzadeh, S. (2005) A correlated frailty model for analysing risk factors in bilateral corneal graft rejection for Keratoconus: a Bayesian approach. *Statistics in Medicine* 24, 2681–2693.

Kheiri, S., Kimber, A., Meshkani, M.R. (2007) Bayesian analysis of an inverse Gaussian correlated frailty model. *Computational Statistics and Data Analysis* 51, 5317–5326.

Kimber, A.C. (1996) A Weibull-based score test for heterogeneity. *Lifetime Data Analysis* 2, 63–71.

Kimber, A.C., Zhu, C.Q. (1999) Diagnostics for a Weibull frailty model. In: *Statistical Inference and Design of Experiments*. U.J. Dixit, M.R. Satam (eds.) Narosa Publishing House, New Delhi, pp. 36–46.

Klein, J.P., Moeschberger, M.L. (2003) *Survival Analysis - Techniques for Censored and Truncated Data*. Springer, New York.

Klein, J.P. (1992) Semiparametric estimation of random effects using the Cox model based on the EM algorithm. *Biometrics* 48, 795–806.

Klein, J.P., Moeschberger, M., Li, Y., Wang, S. (1992) Estimating random effects in the Framingham Heart Study. In: *Survival Analysis: State of the Art*. J. Klein, P. Goel (eds.), Kluwer, Dordrecht, pp. 99–120.

Klein, J.P., Pelz, C., Zhang, M.-J. (1999) Random effects for censored data by a multivariate normal regression model. *Biometrics* 55, 497–506.

Komárek, A., Lesaffre, E., Legrand, C. (2007) Baseline and treatment effect heterogeneity for survival times between centers using a random effects accelerated failure time model with flexible error distribution. *Statistics in Medicine* 26, 5457–5472.

Kondo, K. (1977) The log-normal distribution of the incubation time of exogenous diseases. *Japanese Journal of Human Genetics* 21, 217–237.

Korsgaard, I.R., Andersen, A.H. (1998) The additive genetic gamma frailty model. *Scandinavian Journal of Statistics* 25, 255–270.

Korsgaard, I.R., Madsen, P., Jensen, J. (1998) Bayesian inference in the semiparametric log normal frailty model using Gibbs sampling. *Genetics, Selection, Evolution* 30, 241–256.

Kortram, R. A., Lenstra, A. J., Ridder, G., van Rooij, A. C. M. (1995) Constructive identification of the mixed proportional hazards model. *Statistica Neerlandica* 49, 269–281.

Kosorok, M.R., Lee, B.L., Fine, J.P. (2004) Semiparametric inference for proportional hazards frailty regression models. *Annals of Statistics* 32, 1448–1491.

Koziol, J.A., Green, S.B. (1976) A Cramer–von Mises statistic for randomly censored data. *Biometrika* 63, 465–474.

Kuk, A.Y.C., Chen, C.-H. (1992) A mixture model combining logistic regression with proportional hazards regression. *Biometrika* 79, 531–541.

Kuß, O., Blankenburg, T., Haerting, J. (2008) A relative survival model for clustered responses. *Biometrical Journal* 50, 408–418.

Lam, K., Kuk, Y. (1997) A marginal approach to estimation in frailty models. *Journal of the American Statistical Association* 92, 985–990.

Lam, K.F., Lee, Y.W., Leung, T.L. (2002) Modeling multivariate survival data by a semiparametric random effects proportional odds model. *Biometrics* 58, 316–323.

Lam, K., Lee, Y. (2004) Merits of modelling multivariate survival data using random effects proportional odds model. *Biometrical Journal* 46, 331–42.

Lam, K., Fong, D., Tang, O. (2005) Estimating the proportion of cured patients in a censored sample. *Statistics in Medicine* 24, 1865–1879.

Lambert, P., Collett, D., Kimber, A., Johnson, R. (2004) Parametric accelerated failure time models with random effects and an application to kidney transplant survival. *Statistics in Medicine* 23, 3177–3192.

Lancaster, T. (1979) Econometric methods for the duration of unemployment. *Econometrica* 47, 939–956.

Lancaster, T., Nickell, S. (1980) The analysis of re-employment probabilities for the unemployed. *Journal of the Royal Statistical Society (A)* 143, 141–165

Lawless, J.F. (2002) *Statistical Models and Methods for Lifetime Data*. Wiley, New York.

Lee, S., Lee, S. (2003) Testing heterogeneity for frailty distribution in shared frailty model. *Communications in Statistics, Theory and Methods* 32, 2245–2253.

Lee, E.W., Wei, L.J., Amato, D.A. (1992) Cox-type regression analysis for large numbers of small groups of correlated failure time observations. In: *Survival Analysis: State of the Art*. J. Klein, P. Goel (eds.), Kluwer Academic Publishers, Dordrecht, pp. 237–247.

Lee, S., Wolfe, R.A. (1998) A simple test for independent censoring under the proportional hazards model. *Biometrics* 54, 1176–1182.

Legrand, C., Ducrocq, V., Janssen, P., Sylvester, R., Duchateau, L. (2005) A Bayesian approach to jointly estimate centre and treatment by centre heterogeneity in a proportional hazards model. *Statistics in Medicine* 24, 3789–3804.

Legrand, C., Duchateau, L., Sylvester, R., Janssen, P., van der Hage, J., van der Velde, C.J.H., Therasse, P. (2006) Heterogeneity in disease free survival between centers: lessions learned from an EORTC breast cancer trial. *Clinical Trials* 3, 10–18.

Legrand, C., Duchateau, L., Janssen, P., Ducrocq, V., Sylvester, R. (2008) Validation of prognostic indices using the frailty model. *Lifetime Data Analysis* 15, 59–78.

Li, H. (1999) The additive genetic gamma frailty model for linkage analysis of age-of-onset variation. *Annals of Human Genetics* 63, 455–468.

Li, H. (2002) An additive genetic gamma frailty model for linkage analysis of diseases with variable age of onset using nuclear families. *Lifetime Data Analysis* 8, 315–334.

Li, H., Zhong, X. (2002) Multivariate survival models induced by genetic frailties, with application to linkage analysis. *Biostatistics* 3, 57–75.

Li, C.-S., Taylor, J.M.G., Sy, J.P. (2001) Identifiability of cure models. *Statistics & Probability Letters* 54, 389–395.

Li, Y., Betensky, R., Louis, D., Cairncross, J. (2002) The use of frailty hazard models for unrecognized heterogeneity that interacts with treatment: considerations of efficiency and power. *Biometrics* 58, 232–236.

Liang, K.-Y., Self, S., Bandeen-Roche, K., Zeger, S. (1995) Some recent developments for regression analysis of multivariate failure time data. *Lifetime Data Analysis* 1, 403–415.

Lichtenstein, P., de Faire, U., Floderus, B., Svartengren, M., Svedberg, P., Pedersen, N.L. (2002) The Swedish Twin Registry: a unique resource for clinical, epidemiological and genetic studies. *Journal of Internal Medicine* 252, 184–205.

Lillard, L.A. (1993) Simultaneous equations for hazards: marriage duration and fertility timing. *Journal of Econometrics* 56, 189–217.

Lillard, L.A., Brian, M.J., Waite, M.J. (1995) Premarital cohabitation and subsequent marital dissolution: a matter of self-selection? *Demography* 32, 437–457.

Lillard, L.A., Panis, C. (2000) *aML User's Guide and Reference Manual*. Econ-Ware, Los Angeles, CA.

Lim, H.J., Liu, J., Melzer-Lange, M. (2007) Comparison of methods for analyzing recurrent events data: application to the emergency department visits of firearm victims. *Accident Analysis and Prevention* 39, 290–299.

Lin, D.Y. (1994) Cox regression analysis of multivariate failure time data: the marginal approach. *Statistics in Medicine* 13, 2233–2247.

Lin, D., Robins, J., Wei, L. (1996) Comparing two failure time distributions in the presence of depending censoring. *Biometrika* 83, 381–393.

Lindeboom, M., Van Den Berg, G.J. (1994) Heterogeneity in models for bivariate survival: the importance of the mixing distribution. *Journal of the Royal Statistical Society (B)* 56, 49–60.

Lindstrom, D.P. (1996) Economic opportunity in Mexico and return migration from the United States. *Demography* 33, 357–374.

Link, W.A. (1989) A model for informative censoring. *Journal of the American Statistical Association* 84, 749–752.

Littell, R.C., Milliken, G., Stroup, W., Wolfinger, R.D., Schabenberger, O. (2006) *SAS for Mixed Models* (2nd edition). SAS Publishing, Cary, NC.

Liu, L., Wolfe, R.A., Huang, X. (2004) Shared frailty models for recurrent events and a terminal event. *Biometrics* 60, 747–756.

Liu, L., Huang, X. (2008) The use of Gaussian quadrature for estimation in frailty proportional hazard models. *Statistics in Medicine* 27, 2665–83.

Liu, L., Yu, Z. (2008) A likelihood reformulation method in non-normal random effects models. *Statistics in Medicine* 27, 3105–3124.

Locatelli, I. (2003) *Frailty models for twins duration data: a Bayesian approach*. Ph.D. thesis, University Luigi Bocconi, Milano.

Locatelli, I., Lichtenstein, P., Yashin, A.I. (2004) The heritability of breast cancer: a Bayesian correlated frailty model applied to Swedish twins data. *Twin Research* 7, 182–191.

Longini, I.M., Halloran, M.E. (1996) A frailty mixture model for estimating vaccine efficacy. *Applied Statistics* 45, 165–173.

Ma, R., Krewski, D., Burnett, R.T. (2003) Random effects Cox models: a Poisson modelling approach. *Biometrika* 90, 157–169.

Macdonald, A.S. (1999) Modeling the impact of genetics on insurance. *North American Actuarial Journal* 3, 83–105.

Machin, D., Cheung, Y.B., Parmar, M. (2006) *Survival Analysis: a Practical Approach*. Wiley, Chichester.

Mahé, C., Chevret, S. (1999) Estimating regression parameters and degree of dependence for multivariate failure time data. *Biometrics* 55, 1078–84.

Makeham, W.M. (1860) On the law of mortality and the construction of annuity tables. *Journal of the Institute of Actuaries* 8, 301–310.

Maller, R.A., Zhou, X. (1996) *Survival Analysis with Long-Term Survivors*. Wiley & Sons, Chichester.

Maller, R.A., Zhou, X. (2002) Analysis of parametric models for competing risks. *Statistica Sinica* 12, 725–750.

Maller, R.A., Zhou, X. (2003) Testing for individual heterogeneity in parameter models for event-history data. *Mathematical Methods of Statistics* 12, 276–304.

Mallick, M., Ravishanker, N. (2004) Multivariate Survival Analysis with PVF Frailty Models. In: *Advances in Ranking and Selection, Multiple Comparisons, and Reliability Methodology and Applications*. N. Balakrishnan, H.N. Nagaraja, N. Kannan (eds.), Birkhäuser, pp. 369–384.

Mallick, M., Ravishanker, N. (2006) PVF frailty models with a flexible baseline hazard. *International Journal of Statistics and Systems* 1, 57–80.

Mallick, M., Ravishanker, N., Kannan, N. (2008) Bivariate positive stable frailty models. *Statistics and Probability Letters* 78, 2371–2377.

Manatunga, A.K., Oakes, D. (1999) Parametric analysis of matched pair survival data. *Lifetime Data Analysis* 5, 371–387.

Manda, S.O.M. (2001) A comparison of methods for analysing a nested frailty model to child survival in Malawi. *Australian and New Zealand Journal of Statistics* 43, 7–16.

Manda, S.O.M., Meyer, R. (2005) Bayesian inference for recurrent event data using time-dependent frailty. *Statistics in Medicine* 24, 1263–1274.

Mantel, N., Bohidar, N.R., Ciminera, J.L. (1977) Mantel–Haenszel analyses of litter-matched time-to-response data, with modifications for recovery of interlitter information. *Cancer Research* 37, 3863–3868.

Manton, K., Stallard, E. (1981) Methods for evaluating the heterogeneity of aging processes in human populations using vital statistics data: Explaining the black/white mortality crossover by a model of mortality selection. *Human Biology* 53, 47–67.

Manton, K., Stallard, E., Vaupel, J. (1981) Methods for comparing mortality experience of heterogeneous populations. *Demography* 18, 389–410.

Manton, K., Stallard, E., Vaupel, J. (1986) Alternative models for heterogeneity of mortality risks among the aged. *Journal of the American Statistical Association* 81, 635–644.

Manton, K.G., Vaupel, J.W. (1995) Survival after the age of 80 in the United States, Sweden, France, England, and Japan. *New England Journal of Medicine* 333, 1232–1235.

Marenberg, M.E., Risch, N., Berkman, L.F., Floderus, B., de Faire, U. (1994) Genetic susceptibility to death from coronary heart disease in a study of twins. *New England Journal of Medicine* 330, 1041–1046.

Marshall, A. W., Olkin, I. (1988) Families of multivariate distributions. *Journal of the American Statistical Association* 83, 834–841.

Marshall, A.W., Olkin, I. (2007) *Life Distributions.* Springer, Berlin.

Martinussen, T., Pipper, C.B. (2005) Estimation in the positive stable shared frailty proportional hazards model. *Lifetime Data Analysis* 11, 99–115.

Martinussen, T., Scheike, T. (2006) *Dynamic Regression Models for Survival Data.* Springer, Berlin.

Massonnet, G., Janssen, P., Burzykowski, T. (2008) Fitting conditional survival models to meta-analytic data by using a transformation toward mixed-effects models. *Biometrics* 64, 834–842.

Matsuyama, Y., Sakamoto, J., Ohashi, Y. (1998) A Bayesian hierarchical survival model for the institutional effects in a multi-centre cancer clinical trial. *Statistics in Medicine* 17, 1893–1908.

McCall, B.P. (1994) Testing the proportional hazards assumption in the presence of unmeasured heterogeneity. *Journal of Applied Econometrics* 9, 321–334.

McGilchrist, C.A., Aisbett, C.W. (1991) Regression with frailty in survival analysis. *Biometrics* 47, 461–466.

McGilchrist, C.A. (1993) REML estimation for survival models with frailty. *Biometrics* 49, 221–225.

McGilchrist, C., Yau, K. (1996) Survival analysis with time dependent frailty using a longitudinal model. *Australian Journal of Statistics* 38, 53–60.

McGue, M., Vaupel, J.W., Holm, N., Harvald, B. (1993) Longevity is moderately heritable in a sample of Danish twins born 1870-1880. *Journal of Gerontology: Biological Sciences B* 48, B237–B244.

Melino, A., Sueyoshi, G.T. (1990) A simple approach to the identifiability of the proportional hazards model. *Economics Letters* 33, 63–68.

Metropolis, N., Rosenbluth, A., Rosenbluth, M., Teller A., Teller, E. (1953) Equations of state calculations by fast computing machines. *Journal of Chemical Physics* 21, 1087–1091.

Miller, R.G. (1981) *Survival Analysis.* Wiley & Sons, New York.

Miller, R.G. (1983) What price Kaplan–Meier? *Biometrics* 39, 1077–1081.

Moger, T.A., Aalen, O.O., Halvorsen, T.O., Storm, H.H., Tretli, S. (2004a) Frailty modelling of testicular cancer incidence using Scandinavian data. *Biostatistics* 5, 1–14.

Moger, T.A., Aalen, O.O., Heimdal, K., Gjessing, H.K. (2004b) Analysis of testicular cancer data using a frailty model with familial dependence. *Statistics in Medicine* 23, 617–632.

Moger, T.A., Aalen, O.O. (2005) A distribution for multivariate frailty based on the compound Poisson distribution with random scale. *Lifetime Data Analysis* 11, 41–59.

Moreno, L. (1994) Frailty selection in bivariate survival models: a cautionary note. *Mathematical Population Studies* 4, 225–233.

Morgan, M.V., Adams, G.G., Campain, A.C., Wright, F.A.C. (2005) Assessing sealant retention using a Poisson frailty model. *Community Dental Health* 22, 237–245.

Morley, E., Perry, H. M., Miller, D. K. (2002) Something about frailty. *Journal of Gerontology: Medical Sciences* 57A, M698–M704.

Mudholkar, G.S., Srivastava, D.K., Kollia, G. (1996) A generalization of the Weibull distribution with application to the analysis of survival data. *Journal of the American Statistical Association* 91, 1575–1583.

Mueller, L.D., Drapeau, M.D., Adams, C.S., Hammerle, C.W., Doyal, K.M., Jazayeri, A.J., Ly, T., Beguwala, S.A., Mamidi, A.R., Rose, M.R. (2003) Statistical tests of demographic heterogeneity theories. *Experimental Gerontology* 38, 373–386.

Murphy, S.A. (1994) Consistency in a proportional hazards models incorporating a random effect. *Annals of Statistics* 22, 712–731.

Murphy, S.A. (1995) Asymptotic theory for the frailty model. *Annals of Statistics* 23, 182–198.

Murphy, S.A., Rossini, A., van der Vaart, A.W. (1997) Maximum likelihood estimation in the proportional odds model. *Journal of the American Statistical Association* 92, 968–976.

Murthy, D.N.P., Xie, M., Jiang, R. (2003) *Weibull Models.* Wiley, New York.

Naylor, J., Smith, A. (1982) Applications of a method for the efficient computation of posterior distribution. *Applied Statistics* 31, 214–225.

Neal, R. (1997) Markov chain Monte Carlo methods based on 'slicing' the density function. Technical Report 9722, Department of Statistics, University of Toronto, Canada.

Neale, M.C., Cardon, L.R. (1992) *Methodology for Genetic Studies of Twins and Families.* Kluwer, Dordrecht.

Nelsen, R.B. (2006) *An Introduction to Copulas.* Springer, New York.

Nelson, W. (1972) Theory and applications of hazard plotting for censored failure data. *Technometrics* 14, 945–965.

Nelson, K.P., Lipsitz, S.R., Fitzmaurice, G.M., Ibrahim, J., Parzen, M., Strawderman, R. (2006) Use of the probability integral transformation to fit nonlinear mixed-effects models with nonnormal random effects. *Journal of Computational and Graphical Statistics* 15, 39–57.

Nickell, S. (1979) Estimating the probability of leaving unemployment. *Econometrica* 47, 1249–1266.

Nielsen, G.G., Gill, R.D., Andersen, P.K., Sørensen, T.I.A. (1992) A counting process approach to maximum likelihood estimation in frailty models. *Scandinavian Journal of Statistics* 19, 25–43.

Noh, M., Ha, I.D., Lee, Y. (2006) Dispersion frailty models and HGLMs. *Statistics in Medicine* 25, 1341–1354.

Oakes, D. (1982) A concordance test for independence in the presence of censoring. *Biometrics* 38, 451–455.

Oakes, D. (1989) Bivariate survival models induced by frailties. *Journal of the American Statistical Association* 84, 487–493.

Oakes, D., Jeong, J.-H. (1998) Frailty models and rank tests. *Lifetime Data Analysis* 4, 209–228.

O'Quigley, J., Stare, J. (2002) Proportional hazards models with frailties and random effects. *Statistics in Medicine* 21, 3219–3233.

Orbe, J., Ferreira, E., Nùñez-Antòn, V. (2002) Comparing proportional hazards and accelerated failure time models for survival analysis. *Statistics in Medicine* 21, 3493–3510.

Panis, C., Lillard, L. (1995) Child mortality in Malaysia: explaining ethnic differences and the recent decline. *Population Studies* 49, 463–479.

Pack, S.E., Morgan, B.J.T. (1990) A mixture model for interval-censored time-to-response quantal assay data. *Biometrics* 46, 749–757.

Paik, M.C., Tsai, W.-Y., Ottman, R. (1994) Multivariate survival analysis using piecewise gamma frailty. *Biometrics* 50, 975–988.

Pan, W. (2001) Using frailties in the accelerated failure time model. *Lifetime Data Analysis* 7, 55–64.

Pankratz, V.S., de Andrade, M., Therneau, T. M. (2005) Random-effects Cox proportional hazards model: general variance components methods for time-to-event data. *Genetic Epidemiology* 28, 97–109.

Pareto, V. (1897) *Cours d'Economie Politique.* Rouge, Paris.

Parmar, M., Machin, D. (1995) *Survival Analysis: A Practical Approach.* Wiley & Sons, New York.

Parner, E. (1998) Asymptotic theory for the correlated gamma-frailty model. *Annals of Statistics* 26, 183–214.

Peng, Y., Dear, K.B.G., Denham, J.W. (1998) A generalized F mixture model for cure rate estimation. *Statistics in Medicine* 17, 813–830.

Peng, Y., Zhang, J. (2008a) Estimation method of the semiparametric mixture cure gamma frailty model. *Statistics in Medicine* 27, 5177–5194.

Peng, Y., Zhang, J. (2008b) Identifiability of a mixture cure frailty model. *Statistics and Probability Letters* 78, 2604–2608.

Petersen, J. H. (1998) An additive frailty model for correlated lifetimes. *Biometrics* 54, 646–661.

Petersen, L., Sørensen, T.I.A., Andersen, P.K. (2010) A shared frailty model for case-cohort samples: Parent and offspring relations in an adoption study. *Statistics in Medicine* 29, 924–931.

Peterson, A.V. (1977) Expressing the Kaplan–Meier estimator as a function of empirical subsurvival functions. *Journal of the American Statistical Association* 72, 854–858.

Peto, R., Lee, P.N., Paige, W.S. (1972) Statistical analysis of the bioassay of continuous carcinogens. *British Journal of Cancer* 26, 258–261.

Pickles, A., Crouchley, R., Simonoff, E., Eaves, L., Meyer, J., Rutter, M., Hewitt, J., Silberg, J. (1994) Survival models for developmental genetic data: age of onset of puberty and antisocial behavior in twins. *Genetic Epidemiology* 11, 155–170.

Pike, M.C. (1966) A method of analysis of a certain class of experiments in carcinogesis. *Biometrics* 22, 142–161.

Prentice, R.L., Williams, B.J., Peterson, A.V. (1981) On the regression analysis of multivariate failure time data. *Biometrika* 68, 373–379.

Price, D.L., Manatunga, A.K. (2001) Modelling survival data with a cured fraction using frailty models. *Statistics in Medicine* 20, 1515–1527.

Qiou, Z., Ravishanker, N., Dey, D. (1999) Multivariate survival analysis with positive stable frailties. *Biometrics* 55, 637–644.

Ridder, G. (1990) The non-parametric identification of generalized accelerated failure-time models. *Review of Economic Studies* 57, 167–182.

Ries, L.A.G., Kosary, C.L., Hankey, B.F. (eds.) (1999) *SEER Cancer Statistics Review 1973-1999*. National Cancer Institute, Bethesda, MD.

Ripatti, S., Palmgren, J. (2000) Estimation of multivariate frailty models using penalised partial likelihood. *Biometrics* 56, 1016–1022.

Ripatti, S., Larsen, K., Palmgren, J. (2002) Maximum likelihood inference for multivariate frailty models using an automated MCEM algorithm. *Lifetime Data Analysis* 8, 349–360.

Roberts, G.O. (1996) Markov chain concepts related to sampling algorithms. In: *Markov Chain Monte Carlo in Practice*. W.R. Gilks, S. Richardson, D.J. Spiegelhalter (eds.), Chapman & Hall, London.

Rocha, C.S. (1996) Survival models for heterogeneity using the non-central chi-squared distribution with zero degrees of freedom. In: *Lifetime Data: Models in Reliability and Survival Analysis*. Jewell, N. et al. (eds.) Kluwer Academic Publishers, Dordrecht, pp. 275–279.

Rockwood, K. (2005) Frailty and its definition: a worthy challenge. *Journal of the American Geriatric Society* 53, 1069–1070.

Rockwood, K., Mitnitski, A. (2007) Frailty in relation to the accumulation of deficits. *Journal of Gerontology (A)* 62, 722–727.

Rondeau, V., Commenges, D., Joly, P. (2003) Maximum penalized likelihood estimation in a gamma-frailty model. *Lifetime Data Analysis* 9, 139–53.

Rondeau, V., Gonzales, J. (2005) frailtypack: a computer program for the analysis of correlated failure time data using penalized likelihood estimation. *Computer Methods and Programs in Biomedicine* 80, 154–164.

Rondeau, V., Filleul, L., Joly, P. (2006) Nested frailty model using maximum penalized likelihood estimation. *Statistics in Medicine* 25, 4036–4052.

Rondeau, V., Mathoulin-Pelissier, S., Jacqmin-Gadda, H., Brouste, V., Soubeyran, P. (2007) Joint frailty models for recurrent events and death using maximum penalized likelihood estimation: application on cancer events. *Biostatistics* 8, 708–721.

Rondeau, V., Michiels, S., Liquet, B., Pignon, J.P. (2008) Investigating trial and treatment heterogeneity in an individual patient data meta-analysis of survival data by means of the penalized maximum likelihood approach. *Statistics in Medicine* 27, 1894–1910.

Rondeau, V., Mazroui, Y., Gonzales, J. (2010) FRAILTYPACK: An R package for the analysis of correlated survival data with frailty models using penalized likelihood estimation. *Journal of Statistical Software*, forthcoming.

Rose, M.R., Rauser, C.L., Mueller, L.D., Benford, G. (2006) A revolution for aging research. *Biogerontology* 7, 269–277.

Rosenthal, T.C., Puck, S.M. (1999) Screening for genetic risk of breast cancer. *American Family Physician* 59, 99–104.

Sahu, S.K., Dey, D.K., Aslanidou, H., Sinha, D. (1997) A Weibull regression model with gamma frailties for multivariate survival data. *Lifetime Data Analysis* 3, 123–137.

Sahu, S.K., Dey, D.K. (2004) On a Bayesian multivariate survival model with skewed frailty. In: *Skew-Elliptical Distributions and Their Applications: A Journey Beyond Normality.* M. Genton (ed.), Chapman & Hall/CRC, Boca Raton, FL, pp. 321–338.

Samuelsen, S. (2003) Exact inference in the proportional hazard model: possibilities and limitations. *Lifetime Data Analysis* 9, 239–260.

Sankaran, P.G., Gleeja, V.L. (2008) Proportional reversed hazard and frailty models. *Metrika* 68, 333–342.

Sargent, D. (1998) A general framework for random effects survival analysis in the Cox proportional hazards setting. *Biometrics* 54, 1486–1497.

Sartwell, P.E. (1966) The incubation period and the dynamics of infectious disease. *American Journal of Epidemiology* 83, 204–216.

Sastry, N. (1997) A nested frailty model for survival data, with an application to the study of child survival in northeast Brazil. *Journal of the American Statistical Association* 92, 426–435.

Schmermund, A., Stang, A., Möhlenkamp, S., Eggebrecht, H., Baumgart, D., Gilbert, V., Grönemeyer, D., Seibel, R., Erbel, R. (2004) Prognostic value of electron-beam computed tomography-derived coronary calcium scores compared with clinical parameters in patients evaluated for coronary artery disease. *Zeitschrift für Kardiologie* 93, 696–705.

Schmidt, P., Witte, A. (1989) Predicting criminal recidivism using split population survival time models. *Journal of Econometrics* 40, 141–159.

Schmoor, C., Schumacher, M. (1997) The effect of covariate omission and categorization when analyzing randomized trials with the Cox model. *Statistics in Medicine* 16, 225–237.

Schnier, C., Hielm, S., Saloniemi, H.S. (2004) Comparison of the breeding performance of cows in cold and warm loose-housing systems in Finland. *Preventive Veterinary Medicine* 62, 135–151.

Schumacher, M., Olschewski, M., Schmoor, C. (1987) The impact of heterogeneity on the comparison of survival times. *Statistics in Medicine* 6, 773–784.

Schumacher, M. (1989) Frailty-Modelle und ihre Anwendung in der Medizin. *Biometrie und Informatik in Medizin und Biologie* 20, 89–100.

Self, S.G., Liang, K.L. (1987) Asymptotic properties of maximum likelihood estimators and likelihood ratio test under nonstandard conditions. *Journal of the American Statistical Association* 82, 605–610

Semenchenko, G., Khazaeli, A., Curtsinger, J., Yashin, A. (2004a) Stress resistance declines with age: analysis of data from a survival experiment with *drosophila melanogaster*. *Biogerontology* 5, 17–30.

Semenchenko, G., Anisimov, V., Yashin, A. (2004b) Stressors and anti-stressors: how do they influence life span in *HER-2/neu* transgenic mice? *Experimental Gerontology* 39, 1499–1511.

Shih, J.H., Louis, T.A. (1995a) Inferences on the association parameter in copula models for bivariate survival data. *Biometrics* 51, 1384–1399.

Shih, J.H., Louis, T.A. (1995b) Assessing gamma frailty models for clustered failure time data. *Lifetime Data Analysis* 1, 205–220.

Shih, J.H. (1998) A goodness-of-fit test for association in a bivariate survival model. *Biometrika* 85, 189–200.

Shih, J.H., Lu, S.-E. (2009) Semiparametric estimation of a nested random effects model for the analysis of multi-level clustered failure time data. *Computational Statistics and Data Analysis* 53, 3864–3871.

Shu, Y., Klein, J.P. (1999) A SAS macro for the positive stable frailty model. *American Statistical Association Proceedings of the Statistical Computing Section* 47–52.

Silva, G.L., Amaral-Turkman, M.A. (2004) Bayesian analysis of an additive survival model with frailty. *Communications in Statistics – Theory and Methods* 33, 2517–2533.

Sinha, D., Dey, K. (1997) Semiparametric Bayesian analysis of survival data. *Journal of the American Statistical Association* 92, 1195–1212.

Sklar, A. (1959) Fonctions de répartition à n dimensions et leurs marges. *Publications de l'Institut Statistique de L'Université de Paris* 8, 229–31.

Smith, P.J. (2002) *Analysis of Failure and Survival Data.* Chapman & Hall/CRC, London.

Smith, A.F.M., Skene, A.M., Shaw, J.E.H., Naylor, J.C. (1987) Progress with numerical and graphical methods for practical Bayesian statistics. *The Statistician* 36, 75–82.

Spiegelhalter, D.J., Thomas, A., Best, N.G., Gilks, W. (1996) BUGS Examples, Volume 1, Version 0.5.

Spiegelhalter, D.J., Thomas, A., Best, N.G. (1999) WinBUGS Version 1.2. User Manual.

Spiegelhalter, D.J., Best, N.G., Carlin, B.P., van der Linde, A. (2002) Bayesian measures of model complexity and fit. *Journal of the Royal Statistical Society (B)* 64, 583–639.

Spiekerman, C.F., Lin, D.Y. (1998) Marginal regression models for multivariate failure time data. *Journal of the American Statistical Association* 93, 1164–1175.

Spilerman, S. (1972) Extensions of the mover–stayer model. *American Journal of Sociology* 78, 599–626.

Sun, J. (2006) *The Statistical Analysis of Interval-censored Failure Time Data*. Springer, New York.

Svensson, E., Moger, T.A., Tretli, S., Aalen, O.O., Grotmol, T. (2006) Frailty modelling of colorectal cancer incidence in Norway: indications that individual heterogeneity in risk is related to birth cohort. *European Journal of Epidemiology* 21, 587–593.

Sy, J.P., Taylor, J.M. (2000) Estimation in a Cox proportional hazards cure model. *Biometrics* 56, 227–236.

Tableman, M., Kim, J.S. (2004) *Survival Analysis using S: Analysis of Time-to-event Data*. Chapman & Hall/CRC, London.

Therneau, T.M., Grambsch, P.M. (2000) *Modeling Survival Data*. Springer, New York.

Therneau, T.M., Grambsch, P.M., Pankratz, V.S. (2003) Penalized survival models and frailty. *Journal of Computational and Graphical Statistics* 12, 156–175.

Tomazella, V., Louzada-Neto, F., da Silva, G.L. (2006) Bayesian modeling of recurrent events data with an additive gamma frailty distribution and a homogeneous Poisson process. *Journal of Statistical Theory and Applications* 5, 417–429.

Tomazella, V., Martins, C., Bernardo, J. (2008) Inference on the univariate frailty model: a Bayesian reference analysis approach. *Bayesian Inference and Maximum Entropy Methods in Science and Engineering* 1073, 340–347.

Trussell, J., Richards, T. (1985) Correcting for unmeasured heterogeneity in hazard models using the Heckman–Singer procedure. *Sociological Methodology* 15, 242–276.

Tsai, W., Jewell, N., Wang, M. (1987) A note on the product-limit estimator under right censoring and left truncation. *Biometrika* 74, 883–886.

Tsiatis, A. (1975) A nonidentifiability aspect of the problem of competing risks. *Proceedings of the National Academy of Sciences* 72, 20–22.

Turnbull, B.W. (1976) The empirical distribution function with arbitrarily grouped, censored and truncated data. *Journal of the Royal Statistical Society (B)* 38, 290–295.

Tweedy, M. (1984) An index which distinguishes between some important exponential families. In: *Statistics: Applications and New Directions. Proceedings of the Indian Statistical Institute Golden Jubilee International Conference*. J. Ghosh, J. Roy (eds.), Indian Statistical Institute, Calcutta, pp. 579–604.

Vaida, F., Xu, R. (2000) Proportional hazards model with random effects. *Statistics in Medicine* 19, 3309–3324.

van den Berg, G.J. (1992) Nonparametric tests for unobserved heterogeneity in duration models. Working Paper, Free University of Amsterdam, Amsterdam.

van den Berg, G.J. (2001) Duration models: specification, identification, and multiple durations. In: *Handbook of Econometrics.* (Volume V) J.J. Heckman, E. Leamer (eds.) North-Holland, Amsterdam.

van den Berg, G.J., Doblhammer-Reiter, G., Christensen, K. (2008) Being born under adverse economic conditions leads to a higher cardiovascular mortality rate later in life – evidence based on individuals born at different stages of the business cycle. Discussion paper 3635. Forschungsinstitut zur Zukunft der Arbeit.

Vaupel, J.W., Carey, J.R., Christensen, K., Johnson, T.E., Yashin, A.I., Holm, N.V., Iachine, I.A., Kannisto, V., Khazaeli, A.A., Liedo, P., Longo, V.D., Zeng, Y., Manton, K.G., Curtsinger, J.W. (1998). Biodemographic trajectories of longevity. *Science* 280, 855–860.

Vaupel, J., Manton, K., Stallard, E. (1979) The impact of heterogeneity in individual frailty on the dynamics of mortality. *Demography* 16, 439–54.

Vaupel, J.W., Yashin, A.I. (1985) Heterogeneity's ruses: some surprising effects of selection on population dynamics. *The American Statistician* 39, 176–185.

Verweij, P.J., van Houwelingen, H.C., Stijnen, T. (1998) A goodness-of-fit test for Cox's proportional hazards model based on martingale residuals. *Biometrics* 54, 1517–1526.

Viswanathan, B., Manatunga, A. (2001) Diagnostic plots for assessing the frailty distribution in multivariate survival data. *Lifetime Data Analysis* 7, 143–155.

von Bortkiewicz, L. (1898) *Das Gesetz der kleinen Zahlen.* Teubner, Leipzig.

Vu, H.T.V., Knuiman, M.W. (2002) A hybrid ML-EM algorithm for calculation of maximum likelihood estimates in semiparametric shared frailty models. *Computational Statistics and Data Analysis* 40, 173–187.

Vu, H.T.V. (2003) Parametric and semiparametric conditional shared gamma frailty models with events before study entry. *Communications in Statistics, Simulation and Computation* 32, 1223–1248.

Vu, H.T.V. (2004) Estimation in semiparametric conditional shared frailty models with events before study entry. *Computational Statistics and Data Analysis* 45, 621–637.

Wang, S.T., Klein, J.P., Moeschberger, M.L. (1995) Semi-parametric estimation of covariate effects using the positive stable frailty model. *Applied Stochastic Models and Data Analysis* 11, 121–133.

Warwick, J., Tabar, L., Vitak, B., Duffy, S.W. (2004) Time-dependent effects on survival in breast carcinoma. *Cancer* 100, 1331–1336.

Wassell, J.T., Moeschberger, M.L. (1993) A bivariate survival model with modified gamma frailty for assessing the impact of interventions. *Statistics in Medicine* 12, 241–248.

Wei, L., Glidden, D. (1997) An overview of statistical methods for multiple failure time data in clinical trials. *Statistics in Medicine* 16, 831–839.

Wei, L.J., Lin, D.Y., Weissfeld, L. (1989) Regression analysis of multivariate incomplete failure time data by modeling marginal distributions. *Journal of the American Statistical Association* 84, 1065–1073.

Weibull, W. (1939) A statistical theory of the strength of materials. Ingenior Ventenskaps Akademien Handlinger 151. Generalstabens Litografiska Anstalts Förlag, Stockholm.

Whittemore, A., Altshuler, B. (1976) Lung cancer incidence in cigarette smokers: further analysis of Doll and Hill's data for British physicians. *Biometrika* 32, 805–816.

Wienke, A. (1998) An asymptotically optimal adaptive selection procedure in a proportional hazards model with conditionally independent censoring. *Biometrical Journal* 40, 963–978.

Wienke, A., Christensen, K., Holm, N., Yashin, A. (2000) Heritability of death from respiratory diseases: an analysis of Danish twin survival data using a correlated frailty model. In: *Medical Infobahn for Europe.* A. Hasman et al. (eds.), IOS Press, Amsterdam, pp. 407–411.

Wienke, A., Holm, N., Skytthe, A., Yashin, A.I. (2001) The heritability of mortality due to heart diseases: a correlated frailty model applied to Danish twins. *Twin Research* 4, 266–274.

Wienke, A., Christensen, K., Skytthe, A., Yashin, A.I. (2002) Genetic analysis of cause of death in a mixture model with bivariate lifetime data. *Statistical Modelling* 2, 89–102.

Wienke, A., Lichtenstein, P., Yashin, A.I. (2003a) A bivariate frailty model with a cure fraction for modeling familial correlations in diseases. *Biometrics* 59, 1178–1183.

Wienke, A., Holm, N., Christensen, K., Skytthe, A., Vaupel, J., Yashin, A.I. (2003b) The heritability of cause-specific mortality: a correlated gamma-frailty model applied to mortality due to respiratory diseases in Danish twins born 1870 – 1930. *Statistics in Medicine* 22, 3873–3887.

Wienke, A. (2004) Die Vererbbarkeit der Todesursache: ein correlated-frailty Modell angewendet auf Dänische Zwillinge, geboren 1870 – 1930. In: *Lebenserwartung und Mortalität.* R. Scholz, J. Flöthmann (eds.), Materialien zur Bevölkerungswissenschaft 111, Wiesbaden, pp. 81–98.

Wienke, A., Herskind, A., Christensen, K., Skytthe, A., Yashin, A. (2005a) The heritability of CHD mortality in Danish twins after controlling for smoking and BMI. *Twin Research and Human Genetics* 8, 53–59.

Wienke, A., Arbeev, K., Locatelli, I., Yashin, A.I. (2005b) A comparison of different correlated frailty models and estimation strategies. *Mathematical Biosciences* 198, 1–13.

Wienke, A., Locatelli, I., Yashin, I. (2006a) The modelling of a cure fraction in bivariate time-to-event data. *Austrian Journal of Statistics* 35, 67–76.

Wienke, A., Lichtenstein, P., Czene, K., Yashin, A.I. (2006b) The role of correlated frailty models in studies of human health, ageing and longevity. In: *Applications to Cancer and AIDS Studies, Genome Sequence Analysis, and Survival Analysis.* N. Balakrishnan, J. Auget, M. Mesbah, G. Molenberghs (eds.), Birkhäuser, Boston, pp. 151–166.

Wienke, A., Ripatti, S., Palmgren, J., Yashin, A.I. (2010) A bivariate survival model with compound Poisson frailty. *Statistics in Medicine* 29, 275–83.

Wintrebert, C.M.A., Putter, H., Zwinderman, A.H., van Houwelingen, J.C. (2004)Centre-effect on survival after bone marrow transplantation: application of time-dependent frailty models. *Biometrical Journal* 46, 512–25.

Wintrebert, C.M.A. (2007) Statistical modelling of repeated and multivariate survival data. PhD thesis, Leiden University Medical Center, Leiden.

Wong, M.C.M., Lam, K.F., Lo, E.C.M. (2006) Multilevel modelling of clustered grouped survival data using Cox regression model: an application to ART dental restorations. *Statistics in Medicine* 25, 447–457.

Wu, D., Rea, S.L., Yashin, A.I., Johnson, T.E. (2006) Visualizing hidden heterogeneity in isogenic populations of C. elegans. *Experimental Gerontology* 41, 261–270.

Xu, R. (2004) Proportional hazards mixed models: a review with application to twin models. *Advances in Methodology and Statistics* 1, 205–212.

Xu, L., Zhang, J. (2010) An EM-like algorithm for the semiparametric accelerated failure time gamma frailty model. *Computational Statistics and Data Analysis* 54, 1467–1474.

Xue, X., Brookmeyer, R. (1996) Bivariate frailty model for the analysis of multivariate survival time. *Lifetime Data Analysis* 2, 277–290.

Xue, X., Ding, Y. (1999) Assessing heterogeneity and correlation of paired failure times with the bivariate frailty model. *Statistics in Medicine* 18, 907–918.

Yamaguchi, T., Ohashi, Y. (1999) Investigating centre effects in a multicentre clinical trial of superficial bladder cancer. *Statistics in Medicine* 18, 1961–1971

Yamaguchi, T., Ohashi, Y., Matsuyama, Y. (2002) Proportional hazard models with random effects to examine centre effects in multicentre cancer clinical trials. *Statistical Methods in Medical Research* 11, 221–236.

Yashin, A.I., Begun, A., Iachine, I.A. (1999a) Genetic factors in susceptibility to death: a comparative analysis of bivariate survival models. *Journal of Epidemiology and Biostatistics* 4, 53–60.

Yashin, A.I., Herskind, A.-M., Begun, A.Z., Iachine, I.A. (1999b) Survival models for genetic analysis with random effects depending on observed covariates. Unpublished draft.

Yashin, A.I., Iachine, I.A. (1995a) Genetic analysis of durations: Correlated frailty model applied to survival of Danish twins. *Genetic Epidemiology* 12, 529–538.

Yashin, A.I., Iachine, I.A. (1995b) Survival of related individuals: an extension of some fundamental results of heterogeneity analysis. *Mathematical Population Studies* 5, 321–39.

Yashin, A.I., Iachine, I.A. (1996) Random effect models of bivariate survival: quadratic hazard as a new alternative. In: *Transactions of Symposium i Anvendt Statistik*. G. Kristensen (ed.), Institute of Economy, Odense University, pp. 87–101.

Yashin, A.I., Iachine, I.A. (1997) How frailty models can be used for evaluating longevity limits: taking advantage of an interdisciplinary approach. *Demography* 34, 31–48.

Yashin, A.I., Iachine, I. (1999a) Dependent hazards in multivariate survival problems. *Journal of Multivariate Analysis* 71, 241–261.

Yashin, A.I., Iachine, I. (1999b) What difference does the dependence between durations make? Insights for population studies of aging. *Lifetime Data Analysis* 5, 5–22.

Yashin, A.I., Manton, K.G. (1997) Effects of unobserved and partially observed covariate processes on system failure: a review of models and estimation strategies. *Statistical Science* 12, 20–34.

Yashin, A.I., Manton, K.G., Iachine, I.A. (1996) Genetic and environmental factors in duration studies: multivariate frailty models and estimation strategies. *Journal of Epidemiology and Biostatistics* 1, 115–120.

Yashin, A.I., Vaupel, J.W., Iachine, I.A. (1993) Correlated individual frailty: an advantageous approach to survival analysis of bivariate data. Working Paper: Population Studies of Aging 7, Odense University.

Yashin, A.I., Vaupel, J.W., Iachine, I.A. (1995) Correlated individual frailty: an advantageous approach to survival analysis of bivariate data. *Mathematical Population Studies* 5, 145–159.

Yau, K., McGilchrist, C. (1997) Use of generalised linear mixed models for the analysis of clustered survival data. *Biometrical Journal* 39, 3–11.

Yau, K.K.W., McGilchrist, C.A. (1998) ML and REML estimation in survival analysis with time dependent correlated frailty. *Statistics in Medicine* 17, 1201–1213.

Yau, K.K.W. (2001) Multilevel models for survival analysis with random effects. *Biometrics* 57, 96–102.

Yin, G., Ibrahim, J.G. (2005) A class of Bayesian shared gamma frailty models with multivariate failure time data. *Biometrics* 61, 208–216.

Yu, B., Peng, Y. (2008) Mixture cure models for multivariate survival data. *Computational Statistics and Data Analysis* 52, 1524–1532.

Zahl, P.-H. (1994) Correlated frailty models - modelling of unobserved correlated risks of death. *Norwegian Journal of Epidemiology* 4, 90–94.

Zahl, P. (1997) Frailty modelling for the excess hazard. *Statistics in Medicine* 16, 1573–1585.

Zdravkovic, S., Wienke, A., Pedersen, N.L., Marenberg, M.E., Yashin, A.I., de Faire, U. (2002) Heritability of death from coronary heart disease: a 36 years follow-up of 20,966 Swedish twins. *Journal of Internal Medicine* 252, 247–254.

Zdravkovic, S., Wienke, A., Pedersen, N.L., Marenberg, M.E., Yashin, A.I., de Faire, U. (2004) Genetic influences on CHD-death and the impact of known risk factors: comparison of two frailty models. *Behavior Genetics* 34, 585–591.

Zhang, J., Peng, Y. (2007) An alternative estimation method for the accelerated failure time frailty model. *Computational Statistics and Data Analysis* 51, 4413–4423.

Zheng, M., Klein, J.P. (1995) Estimates of marginal survival for dependent competing risks based on assumed copula. *Biometrika* 82, 127–138.

Zhong, X., Li, H. (2004) Score tests of genetic association in the presence of linkage based on the additive genetic gamma frailty model. *Biostatistics* 5, 307–327.

Index

accelerated failure time, 45, 50, 51, 58, 145

additive frailty model, 58

Archimedian copula, 138, 166, 209, 213

asymptotic distribution, 230

at risk, 39, 41, 42, 46, 56, 60, 63, 67, 74, 123, 125, 229

binary frailty, 67, 68, 123, 231, 239

bivariate distribution, 215, 218

bivariate survival function, 152, 159, 166, 195, 198, 210, 211, 215, 216, 243

breast cancer, 3, 12, 13, 95, 124, 125, 177, 183, 184, 187, 188, 195, 196, 239, 248

censoring, 9, 11–13, 15, 19, 20, 23, 24, 29, 41, 46, 47, 52, 123, 124, 127, 129, 130, 132, 164, 169, 179, 197, 205, 207, 231, 232, 234, 239, 240, 244, 261

Central Limit Theorem, 34

competing risks, 46, 152, 169, 179, 204, 206, 207, 223, 238

compound Poisson distribution, 107, 111, 114

compound Poisson frailty, 115, 123, 125, 185, 187, 188, 194

concordance analysis, 169, 261

conditional independence, 134, 164, 167, 202

conditional likelihood, 2, 79, 81, 140, 164, 199

conditional survival function, 163, 164, 210

confounding, 106, 180

copula, 2, 166, 192, 195, 204, 209, 211–215, 217–222, 252

copula representation, 166, 192

coronary heart disease, 9, 10, 172, 179

correlated compound Poisson frailty, 162, 187, 188, 194, 217, 245, 247, 248

correlated frailty, 160, 162–164, 170, 181, 184, 187, 193, 194, 198, 199, 201–203, 207, 237, 240, 261, 263

correlated gamma frailty, 144, 162, 166–169, 171–174, 176, 178, 185, 187, 188, 194, 195, 198, 204, 207, 209, 212, 213, 215, 217, 219, 220, 232, 234, 238, 245–247, 253

correlated log-normal frailty, 162, 173, 177, 179, 181–183

cross-ratio function, 220–222

crossing-over, xii, 76, 77, 95, 131

cure model, 67, 123, 125, 185, 188, 195, 196

current status data, 3, 14, 24, 90, 145–147, 173, 174, 176

Danish Twin Registry, 3, 8, 10, 179

Danish twins, 3, 8, 10, 110, 139, 167, 168, 172, 177, 213, 214, 224, 263

dependent censoring, 23, 52, 205

EBCT, 3, 4, 39, 41, 81, 86

EM algorithm, 1, 58, 62, 84, 86–89, 143, 161, 173, 181, 190, 198, 201, 214, 225–227, 241, 242

Erlangian distribution, 36